A Clinician's Guide to Chronic Diseases

A Clinician's Guide to Chronic Diseases

Editor: Simon Bishop

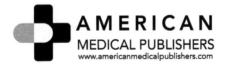

AMERICAN
MEDICAL PUBLISHERS
www.americanmedicalpublishers.com

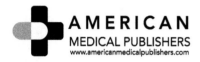

Cataloging-in-Publication Data

A clinician's guide to chronic diseases / edited by Simon Bishop.
   p. cm.
Includes bibliographical references and index.
ISBN 978-1-63927-844-2
1. Chronic diseases. 2. Chronic diseases--Diagnosis. 3. Chronic diseases--Treatment.
I. Bishop, Simon.
RA644.5 .C55 2023
362.16--dc23

American Medical Publishers,
41 Flatbush Avenue,
1st Floor, New York,
NY 11217, USA

ISBN 978-1-63927-844-2 (Hardback)

Contents

Preface

The purpose of the book is to provide a glimpse into the dynamics and to present opinions and studies of some of the scientists engaged in the development of new ideas in the field from very different standpoints. This book will prove useful to students and researchers owing to its high content quality.

Chronic diseases refer to those conditions that often last for three months or more, and have the potential to get worse with time. These diseases are more common in older people, and can typically be managed but not cured. Diabetes, cancer, stroke, arthritis and heart diseases are the most common types of chronic diseases. These diseases have symptoms specific to the disease, but can also cause subtle symptoms like mood disorders, pain and exhaustion. Several chronic diseases are caused by a combination of risk factors, such as physical inactivity, tobacco use, excessive alcohol consumption and poor nutrition. Chronic diseases can be treated in a variety of ways including psychological therapy, surgery, radiotherapy and physical therapy. However, the use of medication is the most prevalent therapeutic method. This book explores all the important aspects of chronic diseases in the modern day. It provides significant information for clinicians to help develop a good understanding of these diseases.

At the end, I would like to appreciate all the efforts made by the authors in completing their chapters professionally. I express my deepest gratitude to all of them for contributing to this book by sharing their valuable works. A special thanks to my family and friends for their constant support in this journey.

Editor

Self-Care Experiences of Adults with Chronic Disease in Indonesia

Nurul Akidah Lukman (ID), **Annette Leibing, and Lisa Merry**

Faculty of Nursing, University of Montreal, Canada H3T 1A8

Correspondence should be addressed to Nurul Akidah Lukman; nurul.akidah.lukman@umontreal.ca

Academic Editor: Ivor J. Katz

We conducted a literature review to document what is known regarding the self-care experiences and various influencing factors among adults living with chronic disease in Indonesia, from the perspective of those living with the illness. We searched CINAHL and Google Scholar to identify peer-reviewed research focused on men and/or women living with a chronic disease (the most prevalent) in urban or rural settings in Indonesia. Using a "Self-Care of Chronic Illness" framework as a guide, information on self-care experiences and how various factors influence these experiences, was extracted and synthesized. Nine studies were included (3 quantitative; 6 qualitative). Self-care involves maintaining well-being through different strategies (e.g., foot hygiene, seeking information/care, praying, diet, resting, and simplifying life), following prescribed treatments, and using traditional remedies. Religion sometimes serves as a means for taking care of one's health (e.g., prayer), or as a source of motivation to self-care, while in other instances, it results in a fatalistic attitude. Which treatments (conventional versus traditional) are sought, it is affected by an understanding of the disease and treatments, which is shaped by beliefs, values, emotions, health literacy, and SES. The literature shows that family, especially women, has a key role in providing support. Community organizations also play an important supportive role, particularly for patients in rural areas. Significant barriers to healthcare include costs and care not being well-adapted to the psychosocial needs and contexts of patients. The literature highlights a disconnection between the self-care experiences and how healthcare and support are delivered. To better support self-care, healthcare professionals should use a personalized approach; however, more research is needed to gain a better understanding of what patients want and expect regarding how religion, beliefs, life circumstances, and the use of alternative therapies should be addressed within the patient-professional dynamic.

1. Introduction

Rising morbidity rates and a high prevalence of death due to chronic disease, including cardiovascular disorders (35%), respiratory illnesses (6%), and diabetes (6%), are of growing concern in Indonesia [1]. For those living with a chronic disease, it has a significant impact on functioning, quality of life, and well-being, while for society, it has implications for productivity and healthcare costs. Although prevention and health promotion initiatives are needed to curb the rising rates of chronic disease, there is also a need to improve healthcare and services in order to better support those already affected by an illness [2].

Self-care is an essential aspect of chronic disease management [3]. It involves the actions and behaviors implemented by an individual towards monitoring and managing their chronic illness and maintaining health [4]. Self-care experiences are complex as individuals may have different perspectives on their illness, and their priorities, expectations for support, and how they go about carrying-out their self-care may vary. These experiences are also shaped by several factors, including cultural beliefs and values, biomedical knowledge/health literacy, confidence and skill, support from others, and access to care [4]. Indonesia's population is ethnically diverse; there are over 300 ethnic groups, each with their own culture and convictions [5, 6], and these influence health

TABLE 1: CINAHL search strategy.

#	Query	Results
S19	S17 AND S18 AND S16	13
S18	S4 OR S6 OR S7 OR S8 OR S9 OR S10 OR S11 OR S12 OR S13 OR S14 OR S15	704,073
S17	S1 OR S2 OR S3 OR S5	87,054
S16	(MH "Indonesia")	2,978
S15	(MH "Dialysis+")	21,117
S14	(MH "Hemodialysis+")	14,629
S13	(MH "Osteoarthritis+")	25,399
S12	(MH "Kidney Failure, Chronic+") OR (MH "Liver Failure+") OR (MH "Kidney Diseases+")	79,339
S11	(MH "Kidney Failure, Chronic+") OR (MH "Renal Insufficiency, Chronic+") OR (MH "Chronic Disease+") OR (MH "Kidney Diseases+") OR (MH "Noncommunicable Diseases") OR (MH "Kidney, Cystic+")	131,481
S10	(MH "Heart Failure+") OR (MH "Myocardial Ischemia+")	122,998
S9	(MH "Cardiovascular Diseases+")	521,800
S8	(MH "Diabetes Mellitus, Type 2")	54,568
S7	(MH "Hypertension+")	70,017
S6	(MH "Hypertension") OR (MH "Pulmonary Arterial Hypertension") OR (MH "Hypertension, White Coat") OR (MH "Hypertension, Renovascular") OR (MH "Hypertension, Pulmonary") OR (MH "Hypertension, Isolated Systolic") OR (MH "Intra- Abdominal Hypertension") OR (MH "Persistent Fetal Circulation Syndrome") OR (MH "Intracranial Hypertension") OR (MH "Hypertension, Portal") OR (MH "Hypertension, Renal")	65,422
S5	(MH "Long Term Care")	24,508
S4	(MH "Chronic Disease+") OR (MH "Kidney Failure, Chronic+")	77,143
S3	(MH "Self-Efficacy")	19,148
S2	(MH "Self-Management") OR (MH "Self Care+")	45,532
S1	(MH "Self Care+")	45,532

TABLE 2: Inclusion and exclusion criteria.

Inclusion criteria	Exclusion criteria
(1) Studied the self-care experiences of adults (men and/or women) with chronic illness living in Indonesia	(1) Studied self-care experiences from the perspective of a healthcare professional
(2) Focused on the most prevalent chronic diseases among Indonesian adults (i.e., hypertension, cardiovascular diseases, chronic kidney diseases, type 2 diabetes mellitus, arthritis, and chronic obstructive pulmonary disease)	(2) Studied the self-care experiences of individuals living with chronic diseases across a number of countries (e.g., low-middle-income countries and south-east Asian countries) without any specific mention of Indonesia
(3) Peer-reviewed empirical research (qualitative, quantitative, or mixed methods' studies)	(3) Focused on pregnant women living with a chronic illness
	(4) Focused on individuals living with cancer
(4) Published in English or *Bahasa*	(5) Commentaries, theoretical/discussion papers, books, book reviews, editorials, abstracts, conference abstracts/proceedings, and newspaper/magazine articles

beliefs and practices [6], including the use of complementary/alternative medicine [7–10]. Indonesians are also known for their religiosity, and for many, faith and spirituality have an important role in how they make sense of and face an illness [10–12]. Education levels also vary among Indonesians [13], and this affects health literacy, which in turn also has an effect on health behaviors and treatment choices [7–12, 14–16]. Culturally, Indonesians tend to be collective and family-oriented [15, 17] and have more traditional views on gender roles, which shape expectations regarding support and assistance for when one is sick or suffering [7, 9, 14, 15]. Additionally, access to healthcare and support services may differ depending on where one lives and on their socioeconomic status (SES) [7–10, 12, 16]. To adequately care for and promote self-care, it is therefore imperative for policymakers and healthcare providers in Indonesia to understand the self-care experiences of those living with a chronic illness and how various factors may influence these experiences.

The aim of this review was to document what is known regarding the self-care experiences and various influencing factors among adults living with chronic illness in Indonesia, from the perspective of those living with the illness.

2. Materials and Methods

We used an integrative approach and aimed to include a mix of empirical research in the review [18]. We used the "Middle Range Theory of Self-care of Chronic Illness" by Riegel et al. [4] as a framework. In this theory, self-care is defined as the actions and behaviors implemented by an individual towards monitoring and managing their chronic illness and maintaining health [4]. *Self-care maintenance* refers to the behaviors performed by patients to sustain general well-being and to preserve health physically, emotionally, socially, and spiritually [4]. For those with chronic illness, this often includes lifestyle practices such as preparing healthy food, coping with stress, exercising, and maintaining social activities [4]. *Self-care monitoring* refers to the routines and actions that chronic illness patients use to assess the illness (e.g., checking blood glucose levels in patients with diabetes and weight checks in patients with heart failure) so that interventions may then be implemented towards controlling symptoms and/or improving outcomes [4]. *Self-care management* is the active implementation of the treatments and taking medications to manage the disease and prevent health deterioration [4]. Although the specifics of monitoring, maintenance, and management vary, all of these components are part of the self-care experience irrespective of the illness.

According to theory by Riegel et al., a number of factors influence self-care experiences including one's skill level and motivation, functional and cognitive (biomedical knowledge and health literacy) abilities, cultural beliefs and values, lifestyle habits, support from others, and access to care. Some of these are particularly relevant to adults' self-care experiences in Indonesia, including culture and values, biomedical knowledge/health literacy, support from others, and access to care. *Culture and values*, including *religious beliefs*, affect attitudes and perceptions of health and disease, including their causes, and how one should respond to and treat the illness. *Culture* also influences lifestyle choices, which can be essential in maintaining health when living with a chronic disease [4]. *Biomedical knowledge* and *literacy* levels are influenced by education (formal and informal) and will affect how an illness, symptoms, and treatments are understood, while *support from family, friends, community,* and *healthcare professionals (HCPs)* can be a key in helping patients enact self-care, for example, decision-making regarding treatment choices, providing emotional and practical support [4]. Finally, *access to healthcare services* is a significant factor in self-care as it influences which treatments, including medicines and lifestyle recommendations, are followed [4]. Each of these factors (support, access to care, biomedical knowledge/health literacy, and beliefs), as well as the others mentioned in the theory (e.g., motivation and skill), are overlapping and have an influence on one another.

2.1. Search Strategy. We searched the CINAHL database. Subject headings and keywords used related to self-care (e.g., self-care, self-management, self-efficacy, and long-term care), chronic disease (e.g., chronic disease, chronic illness, long-term disease, hypertension, high blood pressure, diabetes mellitus type 2, type 2 diabetes mellitus, cardiovascular disease, heart failure, chronic kidney disease, end-stage renal disease, osteoarthritis, arthritis, hemodialysis, and dialysis), and Indonesia (Indonesia, Indonesian, and Indonesian patients). No language or year limitations were applied. The search was conducted during the month of May 2019. The detailed search strategy is presented in Table 1.

Additional studies were also identified by perusing the reference lists of included literature and searching for "related articles" via Google Scholar.

2.2. Inclusion and Exclusion Criteria. The inclusion and exclusion criteria are summarized in Table 2. To be included, studies must have described or examined the self-care experiences of adults (men and/or women) living with a chronic illness in Indonesia, including rural and urban areas. Studies that examined self-care experiences of people with chronic illness across several countries (e.g., low-middle-income countries and south-east Asian countries) without any specific mention regarding Indonesia were excluded (i.e., results for Indonesians had to be reported separately). The literature was also restricted to studies that focused on the most prevalent chronic diseases in Indonesia (i.e., hypertension, cardiovascular diseases, chronic kidney diseases, type 2 diabetes mellitus, arthritis, and chronic obstructive pulmonary disease) [1]. Studies that focused on people with cancer were excluded since cancer presents unique challenges and because it is also considered an acute illness that involves intensive treatments and hospitalization. We also excluded pregnant women living with a chronic illness, since pregnancy is a distinct life event and a time when women are experiencing a range of physical, emotional, and social changes that also require care and support. Since the objective was to understand self-care experiences from the point of view of those living with the illness, we excluded studies that examined self-care from the perspective of healthcare professionals. We only considered peer-reviewed research, including quantitative, qualitative, and mixed methods' studies published in English and *Bahasa*.

All citations were downloaded and managed using Endnote X9 software. NAL was responsible for screening and selecting the literature. This process consisted of three steps: (1) a review of titles in order to eliminate duplicates and records that clearly did not meet the inclusion/exclusion criteria, (2) a review of abstracts to identify potentially relevant papers, and (3) a review of full-texts to confirm eligibility.

2.3. Data Extraction, Collation, and Reporting. For all articles meeting the inclusion criteria, we extracted the following data: (1) paper characteristics (i.e., authors and publication year) and (2) study information, including the objective, research design, population (e.g., age group, education level, and socioeconomic status) and chronic illnesses (e.g.,

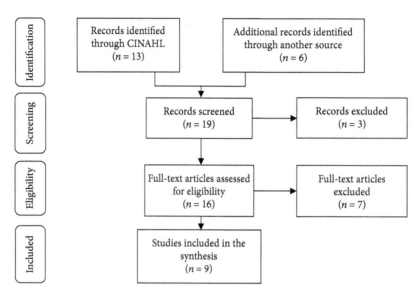

FIGURE 1: Identification and selection of the literature.

hypertension) studied, research location (city/region, urban vs. rural), data collection methods, and key findings/themes. We also extracted information about self-care experiences and how the various factors influenced these experiences. We used the Riegel et al. [4] framework as a guide for this process. NAL read each article in full and extracted the information into tables in a word document. LM and AL supervised and supported NAL through ongoing discussions; LM also reviewed three papers to confirm the quality and completeness of the data extracted. The paper characteristics and study information were summarized into tables. The information on self-care experiences and the influencing factors were synthesized into a narrative text and organized under the following headings: religion; biomedical knowledge and health literacy; cultural expectations; support from family, peer, HCPs, and community; and barriers to care. All authors contributed to the synthesis and writing of the results.

3. Results

Figure 1 presents the results from the literature search. Nineteen records were identified (13 through the database searches, 1 through the review of reference lists, and 5 through Google Scholar); three were excluded because they were conference abstracts/proceedings. Sixteen full-text papers were then assessed for eligibility and seven articles were subsequently eliminated because they did not meet the inclusion criteria (i.e., participants did not have a chronic illness, had cancer or were pregnant, or the study focused on the perspectives of healthcare professionals). Nine papers (English publications), including six qualitative and three quantitative studies, were selected for the integrative synthesis. A summary of the included literature is presented in Table 3.

Table 4 summarizes the characteristics of the included papers. All nine were published within the last 10 years, and most were published in 2018 and 2019. Studies were con-

ducted in a mix of urban and rural settings, and the participants were mostly female ($n = 7$), elderly ($n = 5$), low educated ($n = 5$), and living with diabetes ($n = 4$) or hypertension ($n = 3$). Regarding the factors influencing self-care, all of the studies considered access to care and biomedical knowledge, health literacy, and/or culture ($n = 9$), while peer support was only mentioned in two papers.

3.1. Chronic Illness Self-Care Experiences and Influencing Factors

3.1.1. Religion. Research on the self-care experiences of Indonesians living with chronic illness shows that religion and faith can have a significant influence on experiences, both positively and negatively [10–12].

The positive effects of religion are evident across Indonesians with different illnesses and living in various regions and settings. For example, in the study with Muslim Indonesians living with end-stage renal disease (ESRD) undergoing hemodialysis in urban regions of Pekanbaru, a male participant mentioned that prayer gave him spirit and serenity and helped him sleep [10]. Going to the mosque or listening to the radio online to hear Islamic preaching also motivated some participants to seek medical treatment and to "not give up" on their illness [10]. Similarly, in the study of Muslim patients with type 2 diabetes mellitus (T2DM) living in urban regions in Yogyakarta, examining the relation between prayer and foot care behavior, results showed a significant association between praying and adopting good foot care behavior; the more patients prayed, the more likely they were to adopt good foot care [11]. The study explained that praying was an occasion, up to five times a day, for patients to wash their feet and therefore it helped them to maintain good hygiene and prevent foot ulcers [11]. The study also explained that patients were more likely to engage in good foot care behaviors because they perceived the illness as God's way of reminding them to take care of their health [11]. It therefore encouraged them to take responsibility for

TABLE 3: Summary of included literature.

Study	Study objective	Location and setting	Sample	Research design	Methods	Key findings/themes
Amelia et al. [14]. "Analysis of Factors Affecting the Self-Care Behaviours of Diabetes Mellitus Type 2 Patients in Binjai, North Sumatera-Indonesia"	To determine the most dominant factor affecting the self-care behavior of patients with type 2 diabetes mellitus	Binjai, North Sumatera-Indonesia. Urban	115 respondents—male and female, middle-aged adults and elderly, less educated, high and low socioeconomic status (SES)	Descriptive quantitative and explanatory research	Questionnaires	Self-care behaviors of type 2 diabetes mellitus in Binjai were significantly influenced by motivation, self-efficacy, communication, knowledge, and attitude. Motivation was the most dominant factor.
Bayhakki et al. [10]. "Self-Caring in Islamic Culture of Muslim Persons with End-Stage Renal Disease and Hemodialysis: An Ethnographic Study"	To explore self-caring among Islamic persons living with end-stage renal disease undergoing hemodialysis	Pekanbaru, Indonesia. Urban	12 participants—male and female, middle-aged adults and elderly, less educated, high and low SES	Ethnography	Interview, observation, medical records	Identified themes: (1) Meaning of self-caring (2) Actions in self-caring (3) Islamic influences to self-care living (4) Cultural influences to self-care living
Dewi et al. [8]. "Maintaining Balance and Harmony': Javanese Perceptions of Health and Cardiovascular Disease"	To understand patients' perceptions of health and cardiovascular disease	Yogyakarta, Indonesia. Urban	78 informants—male and female, high and low SES	Qualitative description	Focus group discussion, individual interview	Identified themes: (1) The cause of heart disease (2) Men have no time for health (3) Women are caretakers for health (4) Different information seeking pattern (high vs. low SES) (5) The role of community
Indrayana et al. [11]. "Illness Perception as a Predictor of Foot Care Behavior among People with Type 2 Diabetes Mellitus in Indonesia"	To characterize the relationships among demographic factors, foot care knowledge, illness perception, including local beliefs and foot care practices among people with type 2 diabetes mellitus	Yogyakarta, Indonesia. Urban	200 patients—male and female, middle-aged adults and elderly, less educated, high and low SES	Cross-sectional study	Foot care knowledge questionnaire, the brief illness perception questionnaire, the diabetes foot self-care behavior questionnaire, and local beliefs about diabetes mellitus were measured using a developed questionnaire	(1) Knowledge regarding foot care was strongly correlated with foot care behaviors (2) Perception about illness, including the consequences, the timeline, the treatment control, the identity, the concern, and the coherence, was correlated with foot care behaviors (3) The "food-related and spiritual beliefs" factor was related to foot care behaviors

TABLE 3: Continued.

Study	Study objective	Location and setting	Sample	Research design	Methods	Key findings/themes
						(4) The participants who agreed more that "diabetes is only related to food problems; diabetes is a temptation from God; refusing foods and drinks served by another person is impolite" were more likely to have better foot care behaviors
Kristianingrum et al. [15]. "Perceived Family Support among Older Persons in Diabetes Mellitus Self-Management"	To explore perceived family support by older persons in diabetes mellitus self-management	East Java, Indonesia. Urban and rural	9 older people—male and female, educated and less educated	Descriptive phenomenology	Semistructured interview, field notes	Family support included daily activity assistance, help with accessing health services, food preparation, financial support, psychological support, advice, and solutions regarding self-management.
Ligita et al. [7]. "How People Living with Diabetes in Indonesia Learn about Their Disease: A Grounded Theory Study"	To generate a theory explaining the process by which people with diabetes learn about their disease in Indonesia	Pontianak, the capital city of West Kalimantan Province, Indonesia. Urban	28 participants—from inpatient and outpatient settings	Grounded theory	Face to face and telephone interviews	The core category and social process of the theory was *Learning, choosing, and acting: self-management of diabetes in Indonesia*; this process includes five major distinctive categories: seeking and receiving diabetes-related information, processing received information, responding to recommendations, appraising the results, and sharing with others. People with diabetes acted after they had received recommendations that they considered to be trustworthy. Resource issues (affordability and accessibility of therapies) and physiological and psychological reasons influenced peoples' choice of recommendations.

TABLE 3: Continued.

Study	Study objective	Location and setting	Sample	Research design	Methods	Key findings/themes
Mizutani et al. [12]. "Model Development of Healthy-Lifestyle Behaviours for Rural Muslim Indonesians with Hypertension: A Qualitative Study"	To explore the perceptions of middle-aged husbands and wives, whose lives were affected directly or indirectly by hypertension, on their healthy-lifestyle behaviors and related reasons for practicing the behaviors	West Java District, Indonesia. Rural	12 married couples	Qualitative description and case study	Semistructured interview	(1) Behaving healthy by eating well, doing physical activity, resting, not smoking, managing stress, seeking health information, seeking healthcare, providing care for family and community, and fulfilling their obligations to God (2) Reasons for practicing healthy-lifestyle behaviors were beliefs, competence, religious support, prior experience, social support, and health system support (3) Reasons for not practicing healthy-lifestyle behaviors were personal, social, and environmental barriers
Rahmawati and Bajorek [9]. "Understanding Untreated Hypertension from Patients' Point of View: A Qualitative Study in Rural Yogyakarta Province, Indonesia"	To explore perspectives about hypertension from patients who do not take antihypertensive medications	Yogyakarta, Indonesia. Rural	30 participants—middle-aged and older adults	Qualitative description	Face to face semistructured interviews	Identified themes: (1) Alternative medicines for managing high blood pressure (2) Accessing healthcare services (3) The need for antihypertensive medications (4) Existing support and patients' expectations Reluctance to take antihypertensive medications was influenced by patients' beliefs in personal health threats and the effectiveness of antihypertensive medications, high self-efficacy for taking alternative medicines, the lack of recommendations regarding hypertension

TABLE 3: Continued.

Study	Study objective	Location and setting	Sample	Research design	Methods	Key findings/themes
						treatment, and barriers to accessing supplies of medicines.
Rahmawati and Bajorek [16]. "Access to Medicines for Hypertension: A Survey in Rural Yogyakarta Province, Indonesia"	To explore how and where people in rural villages in Indonesia obtain their supplies of antihypertensive medications	Yogyakarta, Indonesia. Rural	384 participants—male and female, middle-aged and older adults, high and low SES	Descriptive quantitative	Researcher-administered questionnaire	Among 384 participants, 203 people reported had taken medication for the latest 30 days before the data collection. 97 of 203 participants (50%) obtained hypertensive medications from public health services, while 61 participants (30%) get the medications from private healthcare providers (e.g., private hospital, community pharmacy, private nurse, private doctor, and private nurse), and 45 participants (22%) reported obtaining the medications from varied sources (e.g., pharmacy, community health centre)

TABLE 4: Descriptive summary of literature.

Descriptor	Studies $N = 9$
Year of publication	
2010	1
2016	1
2017	1
2018	3
2019	3
Location	
Urban	4
Rural	4
Urban and rural	1
Gender	
Females only	6
Males and females	1
Not specified	2
Education	
Educated	1
Less educated	5
Not specified	3
Population studied	
Middle-aged adults	2
Elderly	4
Middle-aged adults and elderly	1
Not specified	2
Socioeconomic status	
Low income	3
Middle income	1
Low and middle income	1
Not specified	4
Medical diagnosis	
Hypertension	3
Diabetes	4
Cardiovascular disease	1
End-stage renal disease	1
Factors influencing self-care	
Religion	3
Biomedical knowledge and health literacy	9
Cultural expectation	8
Family support	4
Peer support	2
Support from healthcare providers	4
Community support	3
Barriers to care	6

their health and to follow recommended foot care in order to avoid foot ulcers and other complications [11].

In other instances, Indonesians believe that self-care is important but, ultimately, that they have little control over their situation and that it is God who is the one to decide their fate. This fatalistic approach was shown in a study with middle-aged, Muslim women participants living in a rural area, and who had hypertension; these women believed that if they fulfilled their obligations to God, for example, by praying and fasting, that then health would be delivered by God [12]. Their faith was strong, and they believed that everything, including disease and health, was determined by God [12].

3.1.2. Biomedical Knowledge and Health Literacy. Research on the self-care experiences in Indonesia reflects the educational and cultural diversity of the country's population and shows variations in how illnesses and treatments are perceived and understood, and how self-care is practiced [7–12, 14–16].

For some Indonesians, self-efficacy (i.e., confidence and belief in one's ability to achieve a goal), which is associated with high-level education, is an essential and positive contributor to their self-care behavior [9, 12, 14]. In other words, for some patients, a better medical understanding of the disease results in more active and engaged self-care. In two studies, self-efficacy was shown to be positively associated with diet management, taking medications, seeking treatment, and engaging in other prescribed health and care-related activities [9, 14]. Similarly, in another study, one male participant knew that resting would make him feel better and reduce his stress [12]. In the same study, another male participant addressed his stress by going for walks or accompanying his wife shopping. And still in the same study, another participant discussed the importance of controlling his diet and was motivated and integrated this change into his lifestyle. In each of these cases, the patients had biomedical knowledge/health literacy and confidence which helped them enact changes towards improving their health.

In contrast, a patients' lack of health literacy (i.e., capacity to access, understand, and use health information towards making appropriate health decisions) can lead to not taking care of oneself [7, 9]. For example, some patients living with hypertension in rural regions in Yogyakarta did not recognize that a systolic pressure of 150 mmHg wasn't healthy, and since they did not feel any symptoms, they did not seek any medical treatment [9]. Similarly, in another study, some patients believed that their diabetes was "not too bad" if they had boils on their leg [7]. They thought this was only a small wound and not as severe as the foot ulcers of other patients they knew and therefore believed it was not necessary to seek care [7]. Overall, a lack of understanding of the illness and its symptoms prohibited the patients from taking action.

Knowledge about treatments and their effects is also varied and may be shaped by health literacy as well as beliefs and values [7, 9, 12]. For example, in one study, some Indonesians with type 2 diabetes mellitus believed that medications contained chemical materials and that they were dangerous for their body, and therefore, they decided to stop consuming the medication one week after they were prescribed [7]. However, in another study, patients who were aware of their health problems, had an understanding of their medical care, and had had positive experiences in improving their health reported buying medicines, taking prescribed treatments, and seeking medical attention [12]. Similarly, some participants in another study knew that hypertensive medication would bring a positive effect on their body if they took it regularly and therefore they made many efforts to maintain and follow their treatment as indicated.

Understanding the advantages of self-care also seems to be a motivating factor for some Indonesian patients to act towards managing their illness and improving their health [10, 11]. In one study, for example, the participants saw their hemodialysis as an essential therapy to follow for them to feel well and to improve their quality of life [10]. They also recognized that controlling fluid intake, reducing the toxins in their body through diet, resting, and using massage, helped them to manage and control their symptoms including weakness and pain [10]. The positive outcomes therefore stimulated them to further engage in these behaviors [10]. Similarly, in another study with patients living with type 2 diabetes mellitus, when patients believed foot care was a useful treatment, they would perform the foot care behavior [11]. The study explained that patients who believed that their treatment was effective were more motivated to perform better foot care.

In a similar vein, fear of negative outcomes or previous bad outcomes can also stimulate patients to act and better monitor and manage their illness [9, 11, 12]. In one study, some patients with hypertension practiced a healthy lifestyle (e.g., checked their blood pressure regularly, controlled their diet, and exercised) due to their previous experience of having a stroke (a complication of hypertension) [12]. Conversely, the potential adverse consequences and severity of the illness can demotivate patients. For example, when patients in the study by Indrayana et al. felt that their T2DM prognosis was poor, they were less likely to have proper foot care behavior [11]. The study explained that perceiving serious consequences of their illness causes stress and decreases patients' intention and drive to perform foot care. In another study, demotivation in self-care was also noted; however, this was due to the feeling that the medications were not effective [9]. The older patients in the study had tried many treatments and had made many efforts to treat their hypertension, but in the end, felt there was little effect or progress [9]. They therefore preferred to remain untreated as long as they could continue to work and "not feel too dizzy" [9]. This decision was also motivated by the fact that these patients felt that given their older age, they just needed to simplify their life and accept and live with their illness and its outcomes, whatever they may be [9].

Knowledge and where information is sought are influenced by various factors including gender, SES, and personal characteristics. In the study by Dewi et al., in high SES households, both men and women tended to seek health information from various sources, including mass media, magazines, television, and websites, while in low SES homes, women were mostly responsible for the task of finding information and their sources were not as broad [8]. Low SES women did not do research online or by reading, but rather, they tended to seek information from peers or relatives who were living with a similar condition [8]. In the study by Ligita et al., participants reported that they examined and decided what information to use based on their prior knowledge, own experiences, and personal judgment [7]. They also asked for the opinions of others in whom they had confidence (e.g., HCPs, peers, and family) before finally choosing to trust or distrust information [7]. In the same study, some participants also did research before deciding on whether or not to use a treatment (e.g., they searched for information online as they wanted to inform themselves about the function and the side effects of traditional treatments recommended by a friend before choosing to use it or not).

Finally, irrespective of having biomedical knowledge and/or a desire to participate in certain self-care activities (e.g., an active lifestyle), life circumstances can be an important determining factor in actual behavior. For example, men with CVD in the study by Dewi et al. felt that they did not have enough time to exercise [8]. Similarly, in the study by Mizutani et al., some participants living with hypertension hesitated to do exercise because the location of the sports centre was far from their living area [12]. In the same study, other participants wanted to improve their chronic condition by exercising, but they felt that exercising in hot weather would actually worsen their condition [12]. In both studies, participants also believed that their job and farming activities (e.g., planting the fruit, digging, and walking around), respectively, were sufficient as a form of exercise since it was physically demanding [12].

3.1.3. Cultural Expectations. Many beliefs around chronic illness and responses are influenced by culture [8, 11]. The eating behaviors of Indonesians, for example, are often determined by cultural and religious traditions, and these can influence self-care in complex ways. For example, in the study by Indrayana et al., "accepting food and drinks served by another person" was significantly associated with positive foot care behavior [11]. The study explained that participants might have believed that they were not allowed socially or culturally to refuse food served by another person and therefore they compensated by performing better foot care behaviors [11]. Similarly, people with chronic illness may also seek to compensate for the negative effects of smoking [8]. Smoking is a common habit and widely socially accepted in Indonesia, especially among men, and as such is very difficult to quit, even in the face of illness [8]. Compensation is therefore a strategy that may be used to maintain health, rather than to quit the habit [8]. For example, high SES males in the study by Dewi et al. perceived smoking as unhealthy but felt it was needed to help them cope with their job [8]. Therefore, to compensate, they believed that they needed to exercise [8].

Gender roles, which are culturally determined, can also affect how a chronic disease is perceived and self-care is practiced [8]. For example, male patients with cardiovascular disease (CVD) in the study by Dewi et al. believed that they were responsible for earning money to support the family and therefore they needed to prioritize their job and felt that they did not have time to attend to their health [8]. High SES male patients, however, reported that they believed that engaging in a healthy lifestyle could improve their outcomes, but did not have time for these activities and therefore managed and monitored their CVD only by necessary medical examinations and care [8]. Conversely, male patients of low SES believed that their heart disease was their destiny and that they had no control in changing the outcome of their condition [8]. They felt that any activities aimed at prevention would be useless [8].

Culture and beliefs also shape the choice on which treatments and care are used [7, 8]. For example, in Ligita et al., some patients with T2DM living in Pontianak (the capital of the Indonesian province of West Kalimantan) preferred to use unconventional therapies, as they believed that taking medications and drinking less water, as were recommended by healthcare professionals (HCPs), would exacerbate their illness [7]. Instead of prescribed medications or treatments, these patients therefore used traditional medicines and other treatments, for example, a magnet device around their waist [7], which is believed by some people to heal diabetic neuropathy by increasing the blood flow on their lower extremities and reducing their blood glucose levels [19]. Similarly, in the study by Dewi et al., Javanese patients living in Yogyakarta perceived that "too much exposure to wind" was what contributed to them developing cardiovascular disease (CVD); they also referred to CVD as "angin duduk" (sitting wind sickness) [8]. They also believed that their "angin duduk" could only be cured by rubbing the back with traditional oil and then scratching it with the coin [8].

For some, herbal medicine is used as the core treatment for their illness and medical treatment is considered the last resort [7, 9]. In these cases, the use of alternative medicines lowers patients' intentions and motivation to seek medical treatment and leads them to visit doctors only when their condition is severe [7, 9]. For example, in the study by Rahmawati and Bajorek, some patients preferred to treat their hypertension by consuming certain foods including cucumbers, melons, watermelon juice, grated carrots, and said that they only visited medical services when they felt natural approaches had no effect [9]. Similarly, in a study of patients with T2DM, just following their diagnosis, some sought out traditional medicines and decided to use these instead of medically recommended treatments to manage their glucose levels and treat their blurred vision [7].

In some instances, traditional medicine and healers are believed to be complementary to medical treatment [7, 10]. For example, in the study by Bayhakki et al., some patients with end-stage renal disease (ESRD), while undergoing hemodialysis, also used a traditional treatment called *bedah ayam* (also known as "chicken surgery"; i.e., an alternative treatment that involves a healer slaughtering a chicken and performing rituals with the dead chicken in order to remove the illness from a patient's body) [10]. In the same study, some participants used massage and consumed tamarind extract to relieve pain as it contains antioxidants and has anti-inflammatory effects [20]. Similarly, in the study by Ligita et al., some patients with T2DM also used herbal medication as a complementary treatment to their insulin injections [7].

Some Indonesians decide not to use traditional therapies at all and prefer to only follow medically prescribed treatments [7]. This decision appears to be influenced by a combination of factors, including fear of traditional medicines,

support to use prescribed medicine, and beliefs that conventional therapies are more effective [7]. For example, in one study, a female participant did not trust alternative therapies that were suggested by her friend because she feared overdosing since she did not know what amount of the medication would be appropriate for her [7]. Moreover, it was important for her that there be medical evidence showing the effectiveness of the treatment in order for her to feel comfortable taking it [7].

Lastly, for some, traditional approaches may be used initially to manage and treat illness and to maintain health, but then due to adverse effects, are stopped [7–10]. This was evident in the study by Dewi et al., where some patients with CVD who had used traditional methods including rubbing their back with oil and scratching it with a coin reported it had had no effect for them or for other patients with CVD that they knew who had used it [8]. Those with ESRD, in the study by Bayhakki et al., who had used the *bedah ayam*, massage, and tamarind extract, also reverted to only using hemodialysis due to feeling no effect from alternative approaches [10]. In the study by Rahmawati and Bajorek where patients living with hypertension consumed fruit as a primary treatment and natural method for staying healthy, this too was stopped because it had no effect on their blood pressure [9]. Finally, in another study, some participants with T2DM also stopped using herbal medicines because it caused them to be hypoglycaemic [7].

3.1.4. Family Support. Family support includes giving motivation, financial help, and daily life assistance and may be provided by different family members [7, 9, 14, 15]. For example, in the study by Kristianingrum et al., some female participants with T2DM received support from their daughters to iron and wash their clothes, to remind them to consume food, and to take medicine [15]. The women were also accompanied to visit medical services, given money to buy the medications, and encouraged not to do housework and to rest by their sons [15]. Similarly, some older patients in the study by Rahmawati and Bajorek also relied on their children to buy medications and to prepare healthy meals for them [9]. Studies also show that siblings and spouses provide assistance to their ill family members [7, 15]. For example, in two studies, siblings helped by giving reminders to monitor blood sugar levels, by accompanying their brothers/sisters to visit medical services, and by providing support to follow recommended diets [7, 15]. Lastly, some women in the study by Kristianingrum et al. were helped by their husbands to prepare meals and to take a bath [15].

Family can also be a source of intrinsic motivation for self-care by providing a sense of purpose [10]. In one study, some participants reported that they underwent hemodialysis because they wanted to be well and survive their illness so that they could be around to see their children's success [10]. They also felt that their families needed them, and this therefore inspired them to stay healthy [10].

Family support in some instances is gendered. For some Indonesian men, they consider that their family members, especially women, are responsible for assisting with their self-care [8, 10, 12, 15]. For example, in the study by

Bayhakki et al., some men with ESRD asked their wives to drive, prepare meals, and help them go to the restroom [10]. Similarly, in the study by Kristianingrum et al. with Indonesians with T2DM living in urban and rural regions in East Java, male participants also relied on women to help them for a bath, to cook for them, and to remind them to control their stress and eat healthy food [15]. Also, in another study, some of the male participants relied on their wives to remind them not to work so hard [12]. In Dewi et al., women also reported that they felt it was their responsibility to care for their sick family members [8].

Support from family can have both positive and negative effects on self-care [7, 11]. In the study by Amelia et al., motivation from the family, including encouragement and support to eat healthy food and nutrient intake, was positively associated with patients' self-care behavior [11]. Positive feedback helped patients maintain a healthy diet and to control their blood glucose levels [11]. Also, in the same study, money provided from family to cover regular medical examinations was also associated with patients seeking and accessing medical care [11]. Conversely, in another study, a participant reported that they had stopped using insulin to treat their diabetes, after being advised by their older sister that they would become dependent on the medication [7]. Out of respect for the sister and the belief that they had been given good advice, the participant had followed his sister's recommendation [7].

Lastly, some patients, especially older adults, hesitate to ask for help/support from their family, unless they are in an urgent situation [9]. For example, in the study by Rahmawati and Bajorek, some older participants did not want to bother their children when they felt a headache or dizzy [9]. They preferred to self-care independently without any help [9]. They would, however, ask their children to help to accompany them to visit the "village nurse" when they felt very ill [9].

3.1.5. Peer Support. Fellow patient support also seems to be a key source of support for some Indonesians living with chronic illness in Indonesia [7, 12]. For example, in one study, some patients mentioned that sharing experiences with other patients living with similar conditions including information about symptoms and treatment was helpful for them in dealing with their illness [7]. Similarly, in another study, some of the male patients stopped smoking on the advice of friends who also had the same disease and who had been advised by their doctors to stop smoking in order to lower their blood pressure [12].

3.1.6. Support from Healthcare Professionals. Healthcare professionals (HCPs) seem to mainly provide informational support. For example, in the study by Amelia et al., which analyzed factors affecting self-care behavior of patients with T2DM, it was found that information provided about the development, prevention, and treatment of illness by physicians was significantly associated with positive self-care behavior, including controlling blood sugar levels and engaging in other activities to generally maintain health [14]. Similarly, in the study by Ligita et al., some participants reported

that HCPs provided them information regarding the treatment and the effects of taking medication regularly versus irregularly, and they used this knowledge to prevent complications of their diabetes [7]. In two other studies conducted in rural areas in Indonesia, patients with hypertension reported obtaining information about reducing salty food and sweets [9, 12]; while in the study by Rahmawati and Bajorek, some patients received information about physical activity from the village midwife, as ways to help manage their diseases.

Informational support from HCPs is not always helpful. This is largely due to information not being well-communicated and/or poorly understood by the patient. This was evident in the study by Ligita et al., where there was a communication breakdown between the HCPs and the patient, and so the patient came to his own conclusions about how best to manage his diabetes. His understanding was that as long as he took the medications, he could eat whatever he wanted [7].

3.1.7. Community Support. Support from the community has also been shown to be essential in the self-care experiences of Indonesians [8, 10, 12]. This includes support from neighbors, the religious community, and community organizations [8, 10, 12]. The latter also includes care and support from lay healthcare workers.

In the study by Bayhakki et al., some Muslims with ESRD mentioned that they were visited by members of their mosque and this enhanced their spirit and motivated them to take better care of themselves [10]. Neighbors and *Kader* (i.e., a health volunteer worker in the community who visits patients and provides care at home) can also be helpful in patients' self-care [12]. In the study by Mizutani et al., some women patients reported being helped by their neighbors, such as escorting them to medical appointments, and were also reminded or accompanied by the *Kader* to visit community support services [12]. In some cases, *Kader* also provides direct care (e.g., blood pressure check and giving health information) [12].

In the study by Dewi et al., participants received support from the *Pemberdayaan Kesejahteraan Keluarga (PKK)*—an influential women's group that encourages community participation towards improving family welfare—and *Pos Bina Terpadu Penyakit Tidak Menular (Posbindu PTM)*—a women's group that supports the health of people living with noncommunicable diseases (NCD). These are two well-known organizations in Indonesia that are located in the community and provide a range of support care, including medical examinations (e.g., blood pressure and cholesterol level measurement/checks), and health education to patients—these services are predominantly delivered by lay healthcare workers (i.e., individuals with little training and formal healthcare education) [8, 12]. These organizations are therefore key community supports for many Indonesians with chronic illness as they are helpful to patients by providing direct support to aid them in monitoring and managing their illnesses [8].

Both gender and SES are essential factors in community support. In the study by Dewi et al., it was women of low

SES who were responsible for supporting health at the community level through community organizations, such as the *PKK* and *Posbindu PTM*. These organizations were also mainly relied upon by men participants of low SES [8]. For high SES participants, they did not depend as much on the support of PKK and Posbindu PTM and preferred to visit professional medical services instead [8].

3.1.8. Barriers to Care. Barriers to seeking and using care and treatments include cost, fear, or discomfort associated with treatments, location of services, negative experiences, and length/severity of the illness. Cost was an issue in the study by Ligita et al., where participants with T2DM hesitated to take medication because they were too expensive [7]. Fear was also an issue in this study where some patients were afraid to do self-injections (of insulin), while some were also worried about the side effects of these injections, including fainting, which could prohibit them from performing their daily activities. Similarly, in the study by Rahmawati and Bajorek, some patients with hypertension also hesitated to seek care because they could not cover the expense [9]. In the same study, some patients also stopped using medications because the smell of the medication made them nauseous or they were tired of taking the medications.

Time and convenience are issues that are usually associated with a patient's employment situation and their sense of responsibility to provide for the family. As already mentioned above, in the study by Mizutani et al. and Dewi et al. with Indonesians living with hypertension and CVD, respectively, male participants positioned themselves as breadwinners who needed to earn money, and therefore, they felt that they did not have time to pursue their health [8, 12]. Their priority was to work and support the family [8, 12].

Challenges associated with the location of healthcare services are mainly when patients live in rural areas. In two studies, several participants hesitated to seek care because the location of healthcare services was far from where they lived and the route to get there was rough terrain and they did not have appropriate vehicles to take these roads [9, 12]. In the study by Rahmawati and Bajorek, for some, especially elderly, walking was also difficult and added to the challenge of getting to health services [9]. For the patients in these studies, it was felt that seeking care in such conditions would actually exacerbate their illness [9, 12].

Generally, patients living in rural areas seem to prefer to access care that is close by and accessible by walking, whether it is community or larger healthcare services [16]. However, services in rural centres often rely on HCPs coming from urban settings, who are sometimes late, and this can be a barrier to care [9]. As shown in Rahmawati and Bajorek, this can create more frustration and results in patients feeling disappointed and losing trust in the care-providers and services and therefore further lead to patients not seeking services [9].

Conversely, positive experiences and outcomes when care is sought can stimulate further use of services. For example, in the study by Mizutani et al., several patients with hypertension reported that they regularly checked their condition in *Posbindu PTM* because they felt that the information (e.g., diet recommendations) that was given was very useful for them [12].

Length of time living with an illness is another determining factor on where health services are accessed. In the survey by Rahmawati and Bajorek, participants who were recently diagnosed with hypertension would obtain their care and medication at the community organizations and hospitals nearby (e.g., *Puskesmas*, *Posbindu PTM*, and public hospital) [16]. However, patients who had been living with the disease longer were more likely to obtain their medications in larger hospitals or private pharmacies (e.g., private doctor, private nurse, or private midwife) [16]. The study explained that people with a recent diagnosis perceived that their illness was not severe and therefore did not require more "complex" care or medication, while those who had been living with the disease for a while felt that their condition required more advanced care that could only be provided in private or larger healthcare facilities [16].

Along the same lines, the advanced condition of patients is also sometimes a determining factor on when medical care is sought. This was evident in the study by Bayhakki et al., where participants with ESRD only sought medical treatment if they were no longer able to care for themselves or when the condition was very severe [10]. Similarly, in the study by Rahmawati and Bajorek, some older patients with hypertension reported that they would never visit medical services as long as they felt that they could manage their condition themselves (e.g., take a rest and take available medication) and the symptoms were not bothering their work and/or daily life activities [9]. They felt healthcare services would only be necessary if they felt very ill [9].

Lastly, the expensive cost of medical visits, having a low socioeconomic status, the location of health services, and fear of being given poor prognoses from the HCPs can also contribute to patients' self-medicating rather than using prescription drugs. This was evident in three studies among older Indonesians with hypertension living in rural areas where several participants tended to buy over the counter medications (without prescription) in *Warung* [9, 12, 16], a small family-owned business (e.g., restaurant, café, minimarket) in Indonesia [21], or in pharmacies, to treat their blood pressure [9, 12, 16]. In Rahmawati and Bajorek, patients preferred to take prescribed medication as a treatment to lower their blood pressure only when the location of the health services was not far from their living area [16].

4. Discussion

The literature reviewed provides several insights on self-care among Indonesians living with chronic illness in Indonesia including (1) the importance of religion and faith in how one lives with their illness; (2) the variation in responses to an illness that are influenced by a person's background and life experiences; (3) the role of family and community, especially women for self-care support; and (4) the range of barriers that people face in accessing care and services.

The findings of the review highlight how in Indonesia religion may serve as a means for taking care of one's health (e.g., through prayer), or as a source of motivation to partake in self-care. Practicing the Muslim faith provides not only psychological well-being but also physical wellness [10]. This includes, for example, hearing Islamic preaching which can increase one's patience in order to better face illness and be an empowering force to self-care [10], as well as adopting good foot care behavior (i.e., washing the feet), as this is part of the prayer ritual [11]. The role of religion in self-care has also been shown in research conducted in other non-Western countries. For example, a study done in Ghana with people living with end-stage kidney disease, faith was shown to be a driving motivator and method for staying well [22]. Care providers' can thus promote faith and religious practices as a means to support their patients' self-care [10, 22, 23].

In other instances, religion however seems to result in a fatalistic attitude and approach to health. These such attitude and approach to living with an illness have also been observed in other research, where similar to our findings, patients believed that their illness was God's plan and that it was up to God to decide their fate [22]. They also had a strong belief that God would keep them well as long as they fulfilled their obligations to God. "Fulfilling obligations" and being rewarded by God may be interpreted in various ways within and across religious affiliations and thus may have different implications for self-care [23]. For some, they may interpret it to mean that they should solely rely on a reward from God for good health, and not engage in any active disease management or monitoring, whereas others may interpret it to mean that they should actively treat their illness and partake in activities to stay well as part of God's work in addition to their other religious obligations. Care providers should therefore be cognizant of how religion may operate and influence self-care and provide an opportunity to discuss with their patients so that they may understand their patients' beliefs and views and adjust their care accordingly [10, 22, 23].

Our findings also show that Indonesians' responses to living with a chronic illness, including which sort of treatments (conventional versus traditional) are sought, are very much influenced by one's knowledge and understanding of the disease and treatments. In turn, knowledge and understanding are shaped by culture, beliefs, emotions, life experiences, and circumstances and by the level of education/SES and health literacy. Varied responses and behaviors to living with an illness have also been shown in other research conducted in low- and middle-income countries. These studies also found that patients have different views and practices related to diet, exercise, foot care, and which medical and nonmedical treatment they seek as part of their disease management and health promotion activities [22, 24–27]. These results therefore suggest that to best promote self-care, care providers should consider the cultural and social diversity of their patients and adapt their care accordingly. In Indonesia, however, the predominant healthcare model is that HCPs are the experts and that patients should comply with their medical instructions. Currently, there is little collaboration with patients or adaptation to care based on patients' needs or preferences [8]. The results of the review also showed that HCPs mainly provide support in the form of prescribing

medications and making recommendations on lifestyle behaviors. Therefore, there seems to be a disconnection between the realities of patients, their self-care experiences, and how healthcare is delivered.

Regarding support, the literature reviewed showed that family, especially women, has a key role in supporting sick family members including direct assistance with self-care as well as emotional encouragement. This is consistent with what is known regarding the role women tend to play in family life in Indonesia. In addition, in Indonesian culture, caring for family members is perceived as an obligation and a form of adhering to religion [15]. Similar to our findings, other research has shown that family is often closely involved and may provide a range of support and care to their sick loved ones, especially in low-resource countries/areas [22, 26, 27]. This research also highlights that family support can be positive as well present challenges, for example, causing tension between the ill family member and their family caregivers regarding how to stay healthy and manage the illness [22, 26, 27]. Given the extensive involvement of family, in particular, female family members, family should not only be included in the care process of the ill family member but also support should be made available to them in order to ensure that they do not experience caregiver burnout. This is especially so in the context where women may not communicate their challenges as they are culturally expected to care for their ill family and where women's roles in Indonesia are expanding and more and more women are entering the workforce (i.e., take more roles outside the home) in order to help the family economically, which is increasing their overall workload [28].

In Indonesia, women also seem to play a pivotal role in supporting self-care via their involvement in community organizations (i.e., *PKK* and *Posbindu PTM)*. The literature suggests that community organizations are essential resources for ill patients, particularly for low-SES and those living in rural areas where medical services are less available. As the burden of chronic disease increases, these community services will need to be strengthened, not only to safeguard against these resources being depleted (and women taking on further responsibilities) but also to ensure that health inequities between low and high-SES patients are not exacerbated. Currently, there are fewer HCPs working in rural areas compared to urban centres. Moreover, given the geographical distance of the rural service centres from the cities, laywomen as well as *Kader* provide services with little supervision or input from professionals [29]. Consequently, care tends to be suboptimal and largely focused on just providing medication; little attention is given to prevention and health promotion [29]. Therefore, more education, training, and supervision of laywomen and *Kader* are needed to improve the quality of service delivered in smaller, rural communities [29]. Supervision may be enhanced by improving (virtual) collaborations between community services and medical education institutions [29]. Increasing healthcare human resources, especially the number of nurses, and implementing strategies to improve the distribution of HCPs across the country (e.g., salary incentives, paid housing, and professional development opportunities) are also required [30].

Lastly, the research shows that some Indonesians face barriers in trying to use health information and services, including the cost, time and inconvenience, the location of services, and emotions and fears around care. Cost and location of services are known access barriers and are not unique to Indonesia [22, 24, 26, 27]. However, given the significant social and economic inequities that exist in Indonesia, the negative effects of these barriers are amplified, especially in remote areas where they are more common. Since 2014, in an effort to try and overcome cost issues, the government introduced *BPJS* (*Badan Penyelenggara Jaminan Sosial*), a free universal health coverage. However, only patients living in urban areas benefited since rural areas lacked the infrastructure and care personnel to deliver services. This further reinforces the need to implement strategies towards making healthcare more widely available across the country. Moreover, since health-seeking behavior and use of services are shaped by emotions and fears, which are influenced by personal beliefs, education levels, previous experiences with the healthcare system, and how advanced their illness is, this further emphasizes that lay care-providers and HCPs should be giving psychosocial support and doing more to personalize care to promote the use of services. The healthcare system, including community services, also need to be better adapted to the life circumstances of patients. The literature however reveals little about what patients expect and would like exactly from healthcare professionals, including how religion, beliefs, life circumstances, and the use of alternative therapies should be addressed and managed within this patient-professional dynamic. Future research in this area is warranted.

4.1. Implications for Care and Policy. Given the need for more personalized care, implementation of a person-centred care (PCC), an established healthcare approach used in many high-income countries (e.g., UK, USA, and Australia), may have relevance in Indonesia [6]. In PCC, healthcare providers deliver care that considers a patient's values and characteristics and centres on the patient's personal experience. Self-efficacy is also a central concept to this approach whereby interventions aim to enhance a patient's level of knowledge, competence, and confidence towards further empowering them to make decisions and to actively participate in being healthy [6]. A PCC approach also involves inviting and including relatives in the care process, which aligns with Indonesian's collective and family-oriented culture. PCC has been shown to improve patient capability to self-care and also their satisfaction in services [6].

There are a number of factors to consider, however, if changes in the approach to healthcare delivery or PCC are to be implemented in Indonesia. Firstly, the decentralization of healthcare has resulted in public health institutions and hospitals becoming more profit-oriented rather than focused on the quality of care. Decentralization was meant for local governments to have more power to adapt and implement healthcare to best suit their populations' needs; however, this has not happened [6]. Instead, there has been poor planning and implementation, and HCPs have been limited in what they can do, and thus, access and quality of care have reduced

[6]. Secondly, while a personalized care approach has been introduced through nursing education, nurses unfortunately lack authority and therefore have little influence on how care is delivered [6]. Kader and community personnel have even less clout. In Indonesia, physicians have a more prestigious status and are considered the experts for clinical management [6]. Consequently, nurses have less independence in delivering healthcare and cannot adapt their care to patients' needs [6]. In rural areas, as described previously, the Kader and community personnel are simply not equipped to provide personalized care. In order to implement changes in the healthcare system and to improve access and quality to care, political will, financial investment, and policy changes at all levels of government, national and local, would be needed. The government also needs to do more to elevate the professional status of nurses and to reinforce their identity as health professionals so that patients and society will gain trust in them and they will then be able to function more independently, especially in rural areas where fewer services are available [6]. To this end, nurses need more standardized training and education to improve their knowledge, skills, and capacity in delivering interventions. To further promote personalized care (or PCC) across the healthcare system, it also needs to be further integrated into medical school so that physicians are also more likely to adopt and endorse this approach.

4.2. Limitations and Strengths. This review has a number of limitations. Firstly, the search only used one database and only included peer-reviewed publications; grey literature, especially in Bahasa, may have provided useful information that was not captured in journal articles. Secondly, the review focused on the most prevalent chronic illnesses in Indonesia and included only the perspectives of patients; experiences with less common illnesses and the views of HCPs and family caregivers' may have offered different information. Thirdly, male and younger participants were less represented in the studies, providing less insight about the experiences of these groups. Fourthly, while some studies considered gender, age, SES, and severity/length of time living with the illness as influencing factors, generally, there was a limited examination of these in the studies.

This review, however, does have strengths. Although the number of papers included was small, our approach was inclusive, and the literature covered a broad range of chronic illness self-care experiences across different ethnic and social populations in Indonesia. We also examined each paper in-depth and used the "Middle Range Theory of Self-Care of Chronic Illness" as a guide, in order to produce an extensive, detailed portrayal of self-care experiences and the various influencing factors [4].

4.3. Future Research. Future research should explore what patients expect and would like from healthcare professionals regarding how religion, cultural beliefs, life circumstances, and the use of alternative therapies should be addressed in care. Since men and younger people are underrepresented in the review, further understanding of the self-care experiences of these groups is also needed. Furthermore, analysis of how self-care experiences may differ and change over the illness trajectory is also warranted.

5. Conclusions

The research shows that Indonesians living with chronic illness experience self-care in a variety of ways and that there is a disconnection between these experiences and how healthcare and support are delivered. The review suggests that to better support self-care, healthcare professionals should use a more personalized approach. More research, however, is needed to gain a better understanding of what patients' want and expect from healthcare professionals to better monitor and manage their illness and to stay healthy.

Acknowledgments

NAL received bursaries from Lembaga Pengelola Dana Pendidikan (LPDP) (Indonesia Endowment Fund for Education), the University Institute with Regard to Cultural Communities (SHERPA), Montreal, Canada, and Faculty of Nursing, University of Montreal. LM was supported by a research scholar junior 1 award from the Fonds de Recherche du Québec - Santé (FRQS). The article processing charges were paid from LM's general research funds.

References

[1] World Health Organization, Indonesia, 2016https://www.who.int/nmh/countries/idn_en.pdf.

[2] D. Kusuma, N. Kusumawardani, A. Ahsan, S. K. Sebayang, V. Amir, and N. Ng, "On the verge of a chronic disease epidemic: comprehensive policies and actions are needed in Indonesia," *International Health*, vol. 11, no. 6, pp. 422–424, 2019.

[3] P. A. Grady and L. L. Gough, "Self-management: a comprehensive approach to management of chronic conditions," *American Journal of Public Health*, vol. 104, no. 8, pp. e25–e31, 2014.

[4] B. Riegel, T. Jaarsma, and A. Stromberg, "A middle-range theory of self-care of chronic illness," *Advances in Nursing Science*, vol. 35, no. 3, pp. 194–204, 2012.

[5] J. Hays, "Facts and details : religion in Indonesia," 2008, http://factsanddetails.com/indonesia/History_and_Religion/sub6_1f/entry-3975.html.

[6] W. N. Dewi, D. Evans, H. Bradley, and S. Ullrich, "Person-centred care in the Indonesian health-care system," *International Journal of Nursing Practice*, vol. 20, no. 6, pp. 616–622, 2014.

[7] T. Ligita, K. Wicking, K. Francis, N. Harvey, and I. Nurjannah, "How people living with diabetes in Indonesia learn about their disease: a grounded theory study," *PLoS One*, vol. 14, no. 2, article e0212019, 2019.

[8] F. S. T. Dewi, L. Weinehall, and A. Ohman, "'Maintaining balance and harmony': Javanese perceptions of health and cardiovascular disease," *Global Health Action*, vol. 3, no. 1, article 4660, 2010.

[9] R. Rahmawati and B. Bajorek, "Understanding untreated hypertension from patients' point of view: a qualitative study in rural Yogyakarta province, Indonesia," *Chronic Illness*, vol. 14, no. 3, pp. 228–240, 2017.

[10] Bayhakki, U. Hatthakit, and P. Thaniwatthananon, "Self-caring in Islamic culture of Muslim persons with ESRD and hemodialysis: an ethnographic study," *Enfermería Clínica*, vol. 29, pp. 38–41, 2019.

[11] S. Indrayana, S.-E. Guo, C.-L. Lin, and S.-Y. Fang, "Illness perception as a predictor of foot care behavior among people with type 2 diabetes mellitus in Indonesia," *Journal of Transcultural Nursing*, vol. 30, no. 1, pp. 17–25, 2018.

[12] M. Mizutani, J. Tashiro, Maftuhah, H. Sugiarto, L. Yulaikhah, and R. Carbun, "Model development of healthy-lifestyle behaviors for rural Muslim Indonesians with hypertension: a qualitative study," *Nursing & Health Sciences*, vol. 18, no. 1, pp. 15–22, 2016.

[13] Badan Pusat Statistik, "Laporan Bulanan Data Sosial Ekonomi Agustus 2019 (Monthly report of socio-economy status in Indonesia)," 2019, https://www.bps.go.id/publication/2019/08/06/420f612f722ac869e32051b3/laporan-bulanan-data-sosial-ekonomi-agustus-2019.html.

[14] R. Amelia, A. Lelo, D. Lindarto, and E. Mutiara, "Analysis of factors affecting the self-care behaviors of diabetes mellitus type 2 patients in Binjai, North Sumatera-Indonesia," *Asian Journal of Microbiology Biotechnology & Environmental Science*, vol. 20, no. 2, pp. 361–367, 2018.

[15] N. D. Kristianingrum, W. Wiarsih, and A. Y. Nursasi, "Perceived family support among older persons in diabetes mellitus self-management," *BMC Geriatrics*, vol. 18, Supplement 1, p. 304, 2018.

[16] R. Rahmawati and B. Bajorek, "Access to medicines for hypertension: a survey in rural Yogyakarta province, Indonesia," *Rural and Remote Health*, vol. 18, article 4393, 2018.

[17] Cultural Atlas, "Indonesian culture : family," 2019, https://culturalatlas.sbs.com.au/indonesian-culture/indonesian-culture-family.

[18] M. Dixon-Woods, S. Agarwal, D. Jones, B. Young, and A. Sutton, "Synthesising qualitative and quantitative evidence: a review of possible methods," *Journal of Health Services Research and Policy*, vol. 10, no. 1, pp. 45–53, 2005.

[19] M. R. Vann, "How to avoid online diabetes treatment scams that may be harmful," 2017, https://www.everydayhealth.com/type-2-diabetes/living-with/avoiding-diabetes-scams/.

[20] K.-A. Jennings, "What is tamarind? A tropical fruit with health benefits," 2016, https://www.healthline.com/nutrition/tamarind.

[21] Wowshack, "Why the warung is a special part of Indonesian society," 2017, https://www.wowshack.com/warung-special-part-indonesian-society/.

[22] E. A. Boateng, L. East, and C. Evans, "Decision-making experiences of patients with end-stage kidney disease (ESKD) regarding treatment in Ghana: a qualitative study," *BMC Nephrology*, vol. 19, no. 1, p. 371, 2018.

[23] I. Permana, P. Ormandy, and A. Ahmed, "Maintaining harmony: how religion and culture are interwoven in managing daily diabetes self-care," *Journal of Religion and Health*, vol. 58, no. 4, pp. 1415–1428, 2019.

[24] C. Guell and N. Unwin, "Barriers to diabetic foot care in a developing country with a high incidence of diabetes related amputations: an exploratory qualitative interview

study," *BMC Health Services Research*, vol. 15, no. 1, p. 377, 2015.

[25] Z. M. Hassan, "Mobile phone text messaging to improve knowledge and practice of diabetic foot care in a developing country: feasibility and outcomes," *International Journal of Nursing Practice*, vol. 23, article e12546, 2017.

[26] E. Mendenhall and S. A. Norris, "Diabetes care among urban women in Soweto, South Africa: a qualitative study," *BMC Public Health*, vol. 15, no. 1, article 1300, 2015.

[27] N. Abrahams, L. Gilson, N. S. Levitt, and J. A. Dave, "Factors that influence patient empowerment in inpatient chronic care: early thoughts on a diabetes care intervention in South Africa," *BMC Endocrine Disorders*, vol. 19, no. 1, p. 133, 2019.

[28] L. Parker and M. Ford, *Women and Work in Indonesia*, Routledge, 2008.

[29] Y. Christiani, J. E. Byles, M. Tavener, and P. Dugdale, "Exploring the implementation of poslansia, Indonesia's community-based health programme for older people," *Australasian Journal on Ageing*, vol. 35, no. 3, pp. E11–E16, 2016.

[30] G. Walt, *WHO's world health report 2003*, British Medical Journal Publishing Group, 2004.

Association of ABO and Rh Blood Group Phenotypes with Type 2 Diabetes Mellitus at Felege Hiwot Comprehensive Referral Hospital Bahir Dar, Northwest Ethiopia

Biruk Legese,[1] **Molla Abebe ⓘ,**[2] **and Alebachew Fasil ⓘ**[2]

[1]*Infectious Disease Screening Division, Amhara National Regional State Health Bureau, Bahir Dar Blood Bank Laboratory, Bahir Dar, Ethiopia*
[2]*Department of Clinical Chemistry, School of Biomedical and Laboratory Sciences, College of Medicine and Health Sciences, University of Gondar, Gondar, Ethiopia*

Correspondence should be addressed to Alebachew Fasil; alebachewfasil333@gmail.com

Academic Editor: Jochen G. Schneider

Background. ABO and Rh blood group antigens are thought to be among genetic determinants of type 2 diabetes mellitus. Identification of blood group phenotypes are more associated with type 2 diabetes mellitus. It will be helpful for individuals who are susceptible blood groups to take care of themselves by avoiding other predisposing factors and taking preventive measures. *Methods.* Hospital-based comparative cross-sectional study was carried out from February to April 2019 at Felege Hiwot Comprehensive Referral Hospital. Sociodemographic and clinical data were collected with a semistructured pretested questionnaire. ABO and Rh Blood group were determined by slide and test tube methods. Biochemical parameters were determined with Mindray BS-200E fully automated clinical chemistry analyzer. Data were analyzed by IBM SPSS version 20 statistical software. Chi-square test and logistic regression analysis were employed for data analysis. A P value of < 0.05 was considered statistically significant. *Results.* From a total of 424 participants included for this study, blood group O was found higher in frequency with 74 (34.9%) and 97 (45.75%) for cases and healthy controls, respectively. ABO blood groups showed significant association with T2DM, a chi-square value of 12.163 and P value of 0.007. However, the Rh blood group was not associated with T2DM. Binary logistic regression analysis revealed that blood group B had a higher risk (OR: 2.12, 95% CI: 1.33-3.32) and blood group O had decreased risk (OR: 0.636, 95% CI: 0.43-0.94) of T2DM as compared to other blood groups. *Conclusion.* ABO blood group antigens showed significant association with type 2 diabetes mellitus. Blood group B was associated with an increased risk and O blood group with decreased risk of type 2 diabetes mellitus.

1. Introduction

Diabetes mellitus (DM) is a metabolic disorder of multiple etiologies characterized by chronic hyperglycemia with disturbances of carbohydrate, fat, and protein metabolisms resulting from defects in insulin secretion, insulin action, or both [1, 2]. Several pathological processes are involved in the development of DM that range from autoimmune destruction of the β cells of the pancreas with consequent insulin deficiency to abnormalities that result in resistance to insulin action [3].

Blood group antigens are thought to be among hereditary determinants and play a vital role to understand genetics and disease susceptibility [4]. Since the discovery of blood groups in 1900, there have been interests to discover a possible association between ABO and Rh blood groups and different diseases [5]. Along with their expression on red blood cells, ABO antigens are also expressed on the surface of many human cells and tissues, including the epithelium, sensory neurons, platelets, and the vascular endothelium [6]. Thus, the clinical significance of the ABO and Rh blood group system extends beyond transfusion medicine, and several studies have suggested an important involvement of the ABO and Rh blood group antigens in the development of different diseases [7, 8]. The data obtained from different studies showed that the ABO and Rh blood group antigens are associated with gastric cancer, salivary gland tumors, duodenal ulcer, colorectal cancer, thyroid disorders, ovarian tumors, coronary heart disease, and DM especially T2DM [9–13].

The pathophysiologic mechanisms for the association between ABO blood group phenotypes with T2DM and associated factors are not well understood. However, there are some possible assumptions: the first is that the ABO blood group is linked to specific molecules related to T2DM. Genome-wide association studies documenting that variants at ABO gene loci, especially A and B antigens, are associated with increased levels of plasma lipid and inflammatory markers such as soluble intercellular adhesion molecule 1 (ICAM-1), E-selectin, P-selectin, and tumor necrosis factor-2 (TNF-2), are well known risk factors of DM. These molecules are well-known mediators of inflammation that affects insulin and its receptors and contributed to the development of DM [14, 15].

The ABO gene on chromosome 9q34 encodes glycosyl transferases that catalyze the transfer of nucleotide donor sugars to the H antigen to form the A and B antigens. The transferase enzymes and nucleotide donor sugars also induce the production of inflammatory mediators like interleukin 6 and TNF-α in the endothelium [16].

Inflammatory cytokines secreted by endothelium exert an endocrine effect conferring insulin resistance in the liver, skeletal muscle, and vascular endothelial tissue, ultimately leading to the clinical expression of T2DM. These inflammatory markers also lead to an acute phase response with increased hepatic production of C-reactive protein (CRP), a sensitive marker of low-grade systemic inflammation which directly promotes insulin resistance [17].

ABO blood types may also be associated with gut bacteria composition, which may be linked to T2DM. In T2DM, gut dysbiosis contributes to the onset and maintenance of insulin resistance. Different strategies that reduce dysbiosis can improve glycemic control. Evidence in animals and humans reveals the differences between the gut microbial composition in healthy individuals and those with T2DM. Changes in the intestinal ecosystem could cause inflammation, alter intestinal permeability, and modulate metabolism of bile acids, short-chain fatty acids, and metabolites that act synergistically on metabolic regulation systems contributing to insulin resistance [18].

Diabetes mellitus is the most common metabolic disorder affecting people worldwide both in developing and developed countries. People living with DM were estimated to be 451 million in the world by 2017. These figures were expected to increase to 693 million in 2045 [19]. Asia is a major area of the rapidly emerging T2DM global epidemic, with China and India being the top two epicenters [20]. In the African region, the average prevalence was 4.9% in 2013, having Reunion (15.4%), Seychelles (12.1%), and Gabon (10.7%) as the top three countries with higher prevalence [21]. In Ethiopia in 2016, the prevalence of DM was found to be 6.5% [22]. ABO and Rh blood groups are among the genetic factors that

contribute to the occurrence of T2DM [23]. The major human blood group systems are ABO and Rh. The frequency distribution of these blood groups varies markedly in different races and ethnic and socioeconomic groups.

Several researches have been conducted to show the association between the ABO and Rh blood groups with T2DM but the results were not consistent and such a study is yet to be conducted in Ethiopia. Therefore, this study is aimed at ascertaining the association of the ABO and Rh blood groups with T2DM among adults with T2DM at Felege Hiwot Comprehensive Referral Hospital, Bahir Dar, Northwest Ethiopia,

2. Methods and Materials

2.1. Study Area. The study was conducted at FHCRH Diabetic Clinic. The hospital is located in the capital city of Amhara regional state, Bahir Dar, Northwest Ethiopia, about 565 kilometers far away from the capital city of Ethiopia, Addis Ababa. The hospital is one of the biggest hospitals in the Amhara region that provide health services and serves as the referral center for other district hospitals in the region. The hospital is providing services for more than 7 million people.

2.2. Study Design and Period. A hospital-based comparative cross-sectional study was conducted from February to April 2019 to assess the association of the ABO and Rh blood groups with DM and associated factors among adults with T2DM attending clinic at FHCRH, Bahir Dar, Ethiopia.

2.3. Population

2.3.1. Source Population. All patients served at FHCRH were the source population for cases, and apparently, healthy volunteer blood donors at Bahir Dar Blood bank (BBBS) were the source population for controls.

2.3.2. Study Population. All T2DM patients who had follow-up at FHCRH DM Clinic during the study period that met the eligibility criteria, volunteers, and apparently healthy blood donors who donated blood during the study period at Bahir Dar Blood Bank were included as the study population. During data collection, identification of T2DM from T1DM was done by analyzing the patient's chart.

2.4. Sample Size and Sampling Technique. The sample size was determined by using the double population proportion general formula ($N = 2 \times (p)(1 - p)(z\beta + (z \propto)/2)2/(p1 - p2)2$), where N was sample size, p estimates of the double population proportion, $p1$ proportion ofthe B blood group among healthy controls, $p2$ was the proportion of the B blood group among T2DM patients, Z_β was power, and $Z_{\alpha/2}$ was the level of significance.

Proportions of the B blood group among DM patients ($p2 = 33.06\%$) and apparently healthy controls ($p1 = 18.62$ %) from a study done in Malaysia [24], 95% confidence level, 0.05 level of significance, power = 90, and the ratio of controls to cases = 1 were considered and entered into Epi Info version7 software. The total sample size was 424, 212 for each group. Study participants were selected by systematic random sampling technique.

2.5. Data Collection Methods. Sociodemographic and clinical data were collected with the semistructured pretested questionnaire by trained nurses. Height and weight of study participants were measured with stadiometer and digital weight scale (Zhongshan Frecom Electronic Company Limited, China), respectively. Blood pressure of the study participants was measured by trained nurses with manual aneroid sphygmomanometer manufactured by Shanghai Caremate Medical Co., Ltd., Shanghai, China.

The ABO blood group of study participants was determined by the slide method using known anti-A and anti-B sera (Spinreact, Spain). The Rh blood group of participants was determined with the slide method and those tested Rh negative were tested again by the test tube method with anti-D and anti-human globulin sera (Spinreact, Spain). Triglyceride (TRG), low-density lipoprotein (LDL), high-density lipoprotein (HDL), total cholesterol (TC), and fasting blood glucose levels of DM patients were determined with Mindray BS-200E (Mindray Medical International Ltd., China). The manufacturer's instruction for each parameter was followed. Glucose, TRG, and TC were determined using glucose oxidase, glycerokinase peroxidase, and cholesterol oxidase peroxidase methods, respectively.

2.6. Data Management and Quality Control. The questionnaire was pretested on participants equivalent to 5% of the sample size of the study at the University of Gondar Comprehensive Referral Hospital for its accuracy, consistency, and to estimate the time needed to complete the questionnaire prior to actual data collection. A one-day training was given for data collectors on the objective of the study, consenting, techniques of interview, laboratory test procedures, and their quality control. Data collectors were monitored throughout the whole data collection period. Sociodemographic and clinical data were collected by trained nurses under the supervision of the principal investigator, and the quality of measuring devices was checked daily. In order to assure the quality of the laboratory result, standard operating procedures in preanalytical, analytical, and postanalytical stages were followed. The quality of results was assured by running quality control samples (Humatrol P and Humatrol N) daily. Known A and B cell suspension used to check the quality of anti-A and anti-B sera. The quality control sample results for biochemical profiles were monitored using a Levey-Jennings (LJ) chart.

2.7. Data Analysis and Interpretation. The data were checked for completeness, cleaned, arranged, and categorized manually. Then, it was entered and analyzed by SPSS version 20 (IBM, USA). Descriptive statistics were performed for sociodemographic and clinical data, and odds ratio and chi-square values were derived to show the correlation between the ABO blood groups and DM and DM-associated factors. The bivariable logistic and multivariable regression analyses were employed. Variables having a P value ≤ 0.2 were incorpo-

rated into multivariable logistic regression analysis, and a P value < 0.05 was considered statistically significant.

2.8. Ethical Considerations. Ethical clearance was obtained from the Research and Ethical Review Committee of the School of Biomedical and Laboratory Sciences, College of Medicine and Health Sciences, University of Gondar. Seal of approval was obtained from FHCRH and BBBS. A full explanation about the purpose of the study was made to the authorized bodies of FHCRH. A permission letter was taken from the medical director of the hospital and head of the DM clinic. To ensure confidentiality of the data, study participants were identified using codes and unauthorized persons had no access to the collected data. Data was collected after full written consent was obtained from each participant. The study was beneficial to study participants as it helped them to know their blood groups and lipid profile level. Abnormal lipid profile results were reported to physicians and nurses at the DM clinic.

3. Results

3.1. Sociodemographic Characteristics. Males (216) comprised 50.9% of the study participants. The median age of the study participants was 37.4 years (range: 18-89 years). Most of T2DM study participants were married157 (74.1%), self-employed 56 (26.4%), and unable to read and write 100 (47.2%).

3.2. Clinical Data of Study Participants. Sixty-five (30.7%) of T2DM cases had a family history of DM. Out of 212 T2DM cases, 4.2%, 26.9%, 62.7%, 63.7%, and 55.7% were cigarette smokers, alcohol drinkers, eat fruits and vegetables sometimes, and did not perform physical exercise, and have normal BMI, respectively. One hundred and sixty-five (77.8%) of T2DM patients had poor glycemic control. Among T2DM patients 51.4%, 62.7%, 78.3%, and 51.4% showed normal TRG, LDL, HDL, and TC, respectively (Table 1).

Among DM patients, blood group O 74 (34.9%) was the most frequent followed by B 70 (33.0%), A 59 (27.8%), and AB 9 (4.2%), and 191 (90.1%) were Rh 'D' positive (Figure 1). Among healthy controls blood group O 97 (45.8%) was most frequent followed by A 68 (32.1%), B 40 (18.9%), and AB 7 (3.3%), and 195 (92%) were Rh 'D' positive (Figure 2).

3.3. Association of ABO and Rh Blood Group Phenotypes with T2DM. ABO blood groups were significantly associated with T2DM with a chi-square value of 12.163 and P value of 0.007, but Rh blood group was not associated with T2DM (Table 2).

Binary logistic regression analysis indicated that blood group B individuals were 2.12 times more risk to develop T2DM as compared to other ABO blood groups (OR: 2.12; 95% CI: 1.33-3.32). On the other hand, blood group O was protective against T2DM as compared to other blood groups (OR: 0.636; 95% CI: 0.43-0.94). The Rh blood group was not significantly different between the two groups (Table 3).

3.4. Factors Associated with ABO and Rh Blood Group Phenotypes. Family history of DM, physical exercise, DBP,

TABLE 1: Clinical data of DM patients attending at FHCRH, Bahir Dar, Northwest Ethiopia, 2019 ($n = 212$).

Variables		Frequency	Percentage
Family history of DM	Yes	65	30.7
	No	147	69.3
Cigarette smoking habit	Yes	9	4.2
	No	203	95.8
Alcohol drinking habit	Nondrinker	155	73.1
	Light	15	7.1
	Moderate	31	14.6
	Heavy	11	5.2
Eat fruits and vegetables	Do not eat at all	62	29.2
	Some times	133	62.7
	Every day	17	8.0
Physical exercise	Inactive	135	63.7
	Medium	69	32.5
	Highly active	8	3.8
SBP	≤135	125	59.0
	>135	87	41.0
DBP	≤85	146	68.9
	>85	66	31.1
BMI	Underweight	10	4.7
	Normal weight	118	55.7
	Overweight	74	34.9
	Obese	10	4.7
Glycemic control	Good (FBS ≤ 152)	47	22.2
	Poor (FBS > 152)	165	77.8
TRG	≤150 mg/dL	109	51.4
	>150 mg/dL	103	48.6
LDL	≤100 mg/dL	133	62.7
	>100 mg/dL	79	37.3
HDL	≥40 mg/dL	166	78.3
	<40 mg/dL	46	21.7
TC	≤200 mg/dL	109	51.4
	>200 mg/dL	103	48.6

Note: BMI: body mass index; DM: diabetes mellitus; DBP: diastolic blood pressure; HDL: high-density lipoprotein; LDL: low-density lipoprotein; SBP: systolic blood pressure; TRG: triglycerides.

BMI, TRG, and HDL cholesterol were not statistically associated with ABO blood group phenotypes. However, SBP (AOR = 2.353, $P = 0.019$) was associated with blood group A; individuals with blood group A were 2.353 times more at risk to be hypertensive as compared to other blood groups. Increased alcohol drinking habit (AOR = 3.362, $P < 0.0001$) and decreased total cholesterol (AOR = 0.496, $P = 0.029$) were associated with blood group B compared with the other blood groups (Table 4).

4. Discussion

Many studies have been conducted in order to investigate the possible relationship between the ABO and Rh blood group phenotypes with T2DM and its associated factors. The results have been proved to be inconsistent and differed from one study to another [24–27]. The results of the present study supported the assumption that ABO blood group phenotypes are associated with the risk of developing T2DM. Our finding was similar with studies done in Saudi Arabia [28] and Malaysia [24, 29]. Contrary to the current findings, studies conducted in India [30], Iran [27], and Algeria [26] reported nonstatistically significant association between DM and any of ABO blood group phenotypes. The possible reason for this contradiction might be sample size, age and gender distribution, and a difference in racial and environmental factors which may affect the distribution of ABO blood group phenotypes and disease occurrence [23].

Findings of the current study revealed that study participants with blood group B were more affected by T2DM as compared with healthy controls. The rationales behind this observed association might be the existence of higher levels

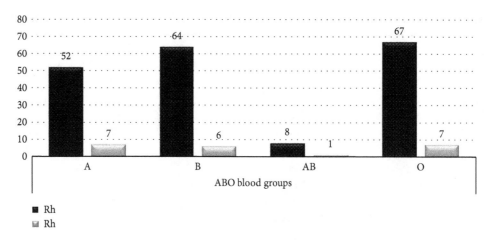

FIGURE 1: Frequency of the ABO and Rh blood group phenotypes among T2DM patients.

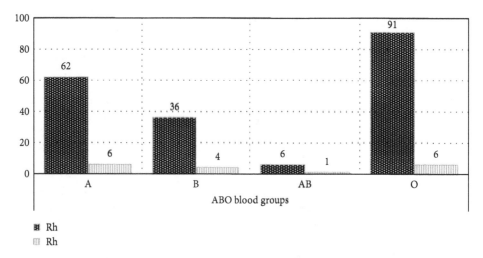

FIGURE 2: Frequency of the ABO and Rh blood group phenotypes among healthy controls.

TABLE 2: The association of ABO blood group phenotypes with T2DM at FHCRH, Bahir Dar, northwest Ethiopia, 2019 ($n = 424$).

Blood groups	T2DM patients	Controls	X^2	P value
A	59 (46.5%)	68 (53.5%)		
B	70 (63.6%)	40 (36.4%)	12.163	0.007
AB	9 (56.2%)	7 (43.8%)		
O	74 (43.3%)	97 (56.7%)		
Rh 'D'+	191 (49.5%)	195 (50.5%)	0.463	0.496
Rh 'D'-	21 (55.3%)	17 (44.7%)		

of inflammatory mediators like factor VIII-VWF complex, ICAM-1, and TNF-2 in blood group B individuals. It is well stated that systemic inflammation is the main cause of insulin resistance and ultimately plays a role in the development of T2DM [31, 32]. Similar results were reported by studies in Qatar [25], Saudi Arabia [28], India [30, 33, 34], Malaysia [24], and France [23]. However, a study conducted in Pakistan [5] indicated that blood groups B and A were less likely to develop p to T2DM as compared to other blood groups. The possible justifications for the observed difference may

be geographical and racial differences which may affect the genetic expression of disease and the frequency of ABO blood group antigens [33].

Blood group 'O' individuals were less likely to develop T2DM compared to other ABO blood types. In line with this study, studies in Qatar [25], Saudi Arabia [28], Malaysia [29], and India [35] reported a similar result. A study in Iran [36] also showed a decreased risk of O blood group to develop DM, but the association was not statistically significant. The reason for this protective effect of the O blood group might be the low level of inflammatory mediators like factor VIII-VWF complex, intercellular adhesion molecule-1 (ICAM-1), and TNF-2 [31, 32]. Inconsistent to the current result, a study in India [37] reported that blood group O had increased risk of developing DM as compared to other blood groups. The reasons for the observed difference might be the geographical, environmental, and genetic differences in which these studies were conducted.

In the current study, even though the frequency of the A blood group was slightly higher among controls ($n = 68$) than DM patients ($n = 59$), it did not show statistically significant association with T2DM. Concordant results to the current

TABLE 3: Association of the ABO and Rh blood group phenotypes with T2DM at FHCRH, Bahir Dar, Northwest Ethiopia, 2019 ($n = 424$).

Study group	Non-A	A	COR (95% CI)	P value
Control	144 (67.9%)	68 (32.1%)	1	
DM	153 (72.2%)	59(27.8%	0.817 (0.538-1.24)	0.34
	Non-B	B		
Control	172 (81.1%)	40 (18.9%)	1	
DM	142 (67.0%)	70 (33.0%)	2.12 (1.33-3.32)	0.001
	Non-O	O		
Control	115 (54.2%)	97 (45.8%)	1	
DM	138 (65.1%)	74 (34.9%)	0.636 (0.43-0.94)	0.023
	Non-AB	AB		
Control	205 (96.7%)	7 (3.3%)	1	
DM	203 (95.8%)	9 (4.2%)	1.298 (0.474-3.55)	0.611
	Rh+	Rh-		
Control	195 (50.5%)	17 (44.7%)	1	
DM	191 (49.5%)	21 (55.3%)	1.261 (0.645-2.464)	.497
	Non-B+	B+		
Control	176 (83%)	36 (17%)	1	
DM	149 (70.3%)	63 (29.7%)	2.067 (1.300-3.288)	0.002
	Non-O+	O+		
Control	121 (57.1%)	91 (42.9%)	1	
DM	145 (63.4%)	67 (36.6%)	0.614 (0.413-0.914)	0.016

Note: COR: crude odds ratio; DM: diabetes mellitus.

finding were reported in Qatar [25] and Malaysia [38]. However, studies in Pakistan [5], Malaysia [35], and Egypt [39] revealed that blood group A was significantly associated with T2DM.

From this study, blood group AB was not associated with T2DM. However, a study done in Egypt [39] showed that blood group AB was protective against T2DM, and another study in India [37] showed that the AB blood group was higher among T2DM patients as compared to healthy controls. The reasons for this variation might be the geographical, genetic, and environmental difference in the study area.

The result of the present study showed that the Rh factor was not associated with T2DM. Similar results were reported by studies in India [37] and Algeria [26]. However, a study conducted in Pakistan [5] indicated that Rh-negative blood groups and T2DM had a significant association. On the other side, research done in Iran [40] showed that Rh-positive blood groups are positively associated with T2DM.

In our study, O+ and B+ blood groups were significantly associated with the risk of T2DM. In support of the present study, a study in France [23] reported that blood group B+ showed a higher risk for DM; another study from Nigeria [41] conducted on both types of diabetes types reported that O+ blood group was significantly lower in diabetics patients than in the control population.

In the current study, ABO blood groups showed an association with DM-associated factors. Blood group A was significantly and positively associated with hypertension (increased systolic blood pressure) as compared to other blood groups. Studies conducted in Bosnia and Herzegovina [42] and India [43] among African-origin populations also

reported similar findings to the current finding. Discordant to our results, a study conducted in Egypt [39] revealed that blood group B had a significantly higher risk for hypertension. Studies conducted in Iran [40] and India [44] also attested different results compared to the current study, in which individuals with blood group B had significantly increased risk of developing hypertension.

The result of our study revealed that blood group B was associated with a decreased level of total cholesterol as compared to other blood groups. Contrary to the current results, a study in Egypt demonstrated that individuals with blood group B showed a significant elevation in total cholesterol and triglyceride levels [39]. Another research in Nigeria also revealed that blood group A individuals had increased levels of LDL cholesterol as compared to other blood groups [45]. The current study also showed an association between alcohol drinking habits with ABO blood groups. In this case, blood group B was associated with alcohol drinking habit in DM patients. In line with our result, a study in Nigeria [46] revealed that alcohol drinking habit was associated with ABO blood groups.

The mechanisms for the observed association between ABO blood group phenotypes with T2DM are still unknown. There are some possible suggested assumptions. The first suggestion was that the human ABO antigen locus might influence inflammatory mediators, such as factor VIII-von Willebrand factor (VWF) complex, which is present in higher levels in non-O individuals [31]. In addition, ABO blood group antigens have been linked with plasma-soluble ICAM-1 and TNF-R levels. These both markers have been associated with an increased type 2 diabetes risk thus

TABLE 4: Association of ABO blood group phenotypes with biochemical and anthropometric measurements at FHCRH, Bahir Dar, northwest Ethiopia 2019 (n =212).

Variables		Non-A	A	COR (95% CI)	AOR (95% CI)	P value
SBP	Normal	99 (79.2%)	26 (20.8%)		1	
	Hypertensive	54 (62.1%)	33 (37.9%)	2.327 (1.26-4.29)	2.353 (1.15-4.815)	0.019*
LDL	Normal	91 (68.4%)	42 (31.6%)		1	
	Abnormal	62 (78.5%)	17 (21.5%)	0.594 (0.31-1.137)	0.493 (0.244-0.995)	0.048*
HLD	Normal	122(73.5%)	44 (26.5%)		1	
	Abnormal	31 (67.4%)	15 (32.6%)	1.32 (0.662-2.72)	1.64 (0.774-3.477)	0.197
TC	Normal	83 (76.1%)	26 (23.9%)		1	
	Abnormal	70 (68.0%)	33 (32.0%)	1.5 (0.822-2.75)	1.885 (0.96-3.69)	0.065
		Non-B	B			
SBP	Normal	80 (64.0%)	45 (36.0%)		1	
	Hypertensive	62 (71.3%)	25 (28.7%)	0.72 (0.397-1.294)	0.704 (0.353-1.406)	0.320
DBP	Normal	94 (64.4%)	52 (35.6%)		1	
	Hypertensive	48 (72.7%)	18 (27.3%)	0.678(0.358-1.284)	0.771 (0.377-1.575)	0.475
TC	Normal	65 (59.6%)	44 (40.4%)		1	
	Abnormal	77 (74.8%)	26 (25.2%)	0.499 0,277-0.897)	0.496 (0.265-0.931)	0.029*
Alcohol	No	115 (74.2%)	40 (25.8%)		1	
	Yes	27 (47.4%)	30 (52.6%)	3.19(1.694-6.012)	3.316 (1.728-6.362)	<0.001*

Note: * Statistically significant association. Abbreviations: Non-A: blood groups other than A; Non-B: blood groups other than B; SBP: systolic blood pressure; DBP: diastolic blood pressure; LDL: low-density lipoprotein; HDL: high-density lipoprotein; TC: total cholesterol.

providing a potential explanation for the observed relationships [32].

5. Limitations of the Study

The limitation of this study was the inability to determine the association of ethnic backgrounds with blood groups for the study participants with T2DM.

6. Conclusions

From the findings of this study, ABO blood group phenotypes are significantly associated with T2DM. In this study, B blood group was found to be positively associated with T2DM, while O blood group has negative association with T2DM. However, blood groups A, AB, and Rh were not associated with T2DM. This study also sought to determine the relationship between ABO and Rh blood group phenotypes with DM-associated factors, and it was realized that blood group A is associated with an increased systolic BP, and blood group B is significantly associated with decreased levels of total cholesterol.

Acknowledgments

First of all, we are glad to acknowledge data collectors, Felege Hiwot Comprehensive Referral Hospital and Bahir Dar blood bank staff, for their cooperation during data collection. Our gratitude also goes to the study participants for their willingness to be part of this study.

References

[1] W. Kerner and J. Brückel, "Definition, classification and diagnosis of diabetes mellitus," Experimental and Clinical Endocrinology & Diabetes, vol. 122, no. 7, pp. 384–386, 2014.

[2] G. Roglic, "WHO Global report on diabetes: a summary," International Journal of Noncommunicable Diseases, vol. 1, no. 1, p. 3, 2016.

[3] American Diabetes Association, "Diagnosis and classification of diabetes mellitus," Diabetes care, vol. 36, Supplement 1, pp. S67–S74, 2012.

[4] D. Dodiya, A. Patel, and J. Jadeja, "A ssociation of ABO blood group with diabetes mellitus," International Journal of Basic and Applied Physiology, vol. 5, no. 1, pp. 63–66, 2016.

[5] A. G. Waseem, M. Iqbal, O. Khan, and M. Tahir, "Association of diabetes mellitus with ABO and Rh blood groups," The Annals of Pakistan Institute of Medical Sciences, vol. 8, no. 2, pp. 134–136, 2012.

[6] M. Franchini and G. Lippi, "The intriguing relationship between the ABO blood group, cardiovascular disease, and cancer," BMC Medicine, vol. 13, no. 1, p. 7, 2015.

[7] G. M. Liumbruno and M. Franchini, "Beyond immunohaematology: the role of the ABO blood group in human diseases," Blood Transfusion, vol. 11, no. 4, pp. 491–499, 2013.

[8] M. Franchini, E. J. Favaloro, G. Targher, and G. Lippi, "ABO blood group, hypercoagulability, and cardiovascular and cancer risk," *Critical Reviews in Clinical Laboratory Sciences*, vol. 49, no. 4, pp. 137–149, 2012.

[9] H. Wazirali, R. A. Ashfaque, and J. W. Herzig, "Abo blood group frequency in Ischemic heart disease patients in Pakistani population," *Pakistan Journal of Medical Sciences*, vol. 30, no. 3, pp. 1–3, 1969.

[10] G. Edgren, H. Hjalgrim, K. Rostgaard et al., "Risk of gastric cancer and peptic ulcers in relation to ABO blood type: a cohort study," *American Journal of Epidemiology*, vol. 172, no. 11, pp. 1280–1285, 2010.

[11] L. Klechova and T. Gosheva-Antonova, "ABO and Rh blood group factors in thyroid gland diseases," *Vutreshni bolesti*, vol. 19, no. 4, pp. 75–79, 1980.

[12] B.-L. Zhang, N. He, Y.-B. Huang, F.-J. Song, and K.-X. Chen, "ABO blood groups and risk of cancer: a systematic review and meta-analysis," *Asian Pacific Journal of Cancer Prevention*, vol. 15, no. 11, pp. 4643–4650, 2014.

[13] C. Montavon Sartorius, A. Schoetzau, H. Kettelhack et al., "ABO blood groups as a prognostic factor for recurrence in ovarian and vulvar cancer," *PLoS One*, vol. 13, no. 3, article e0195213, 2018.

[14] J. A. Jankowski, *Inflammation and Gastrointestinal Cancers: Springer Science & Business Media*, Springer, Berlin, Heidelberg, 2011.

[15] A. Bahar, L. Asadian, S. Abediankenai, S. S. Namazi, and Z. Kashi, "Coronary heart disease and ABO blood group in diabetic women: a case-control study," *Scientific Reports*, vol. 9, no. 1, pp. 1–6, 2019.

[16] M. A. Gates, M. Xu, W. Y. Chen, P. Kraft, S. E. Hankinson, and B. M. Wolpin, "ABO blood group and breast cancer incidence and survival," *International journal of cancer*, vol. 130, no. 9, pp. 2129–2137, 2012.

[17] J.-P. Bastard, M. Maachi, C. Lagathu et al., "Recent advances in the relationship between obesity, inflammation, and insulin resistance," *European cytokine network*, vol. 17, no. 1, pp. 4–12, 2006.

[18] F. Aykas, D. Avci, F. Arik et al., "There is a relation between blood subgroups and insulin resistance," *Acta Medica Mediterranea*, vol. 33, no. 6, pp. 987–990, 2017.

[19] N. H. Cho, J. E. Shaw, S. Karuranga et al., "IDF Diabetes Atlas: global estimates of diabetes prevalence for 2017 and projections for 2045," *Diabetes research and clinical practice*, vol. 138, pp. 271–281, 2018.

[20] Y. Zheng, S. H. Ley, and F. B. Hu, "Global aetiology and epidemiology of type 2 diabetes mellitus and its complications," *Nature Reviews Endocrinology*, vol. 14, no. 2, pp. 88–98, 2018.

[21] L. Guariguata, D. R. Whiting, I. Hambleton, J. Beagley, U. Linnenkamp, and J. E. Shaw, "Global estimates of diabetes prevalence for 2013 and projections for 2035," *Diabetes research and clinical practice*, vol. 103, no. 2, pp. 137–149, 2014.

[22] S. B. Aynalem and A. J. Zeleke, "Prevalence of diabetes mellitus and its risk factors among individuals aged 15 years and above in Mizan-Aman town, Southwest Ethiopia, 2016: a cross sectional study," *International journal of endocrinology*, vol. 1, no. 1, pp. 1–7, 2018.

[23] G. Fagherazzi, G. Gusto, F. Clavel-Chapelon, B. Balkau, and F. Bonnet, "ABO and Rhesus blood groups and risk of type 2 diabetes: evidence from the large E3N cohort study," *Diabetologia*, vol. 58, no. 3, pp. 519–522, 2015.

[24] K. Sukalingam and K. Ganesan, "Rh blood groups associated with risk to obesity and diabetes mellitus: a report on Punjabi population in Selangor, Malaysia," *International Journal of Integrative Medical Sciences*, vol. 2, no. 4, pp. 105–109, 2015.

[25] A. Bener and M. Yousafzai, "The distribution of the ABO blood groups among the diabetes mellitus patients," *Nigerian journal of clinical practice*, vol. 17, no. 5, pp. 565–568, 2014.

[26] S. M. Dali, M. A. Aour, F. Belmokhtar, R. Belmokhtar, and F. Boazza, "The relationship between ABO/Rh blood groups and type 2 diabetes mellitus in Maghnia, western Algeria," *South African Family Practice*, vol. 53, no. 6, pp. 568–572, 2014.

[27] F. Moinzadeh, G. M. Najafabady, and A. Toghiani, "Type 2 diabetes mellitus and ABO/Rh blood groups," *Journal of research in medical sciences: the official journal of Isfahan University of Medical Sciences*, vol. 19, no. 4, p. 382, 2014.

[28] S. Meo, F. Rouq, F. Suraya, and S. Zaidi, "Association of ABO and Rh blood groups with type 2 diabetes mellitus," *European Review for Medical and Pharmacological Sciences*, vol. 20, no. 2, pp. 237–242, 2016.

[29] B. Mandal, R. S. A. Basu, A. Sinha, A. Maiti, and K. Bhattacharjee, "Association of ABO blood groups with type-2 diabetes mellitus and its complications," *Journal of Diabetes, Metabolic Disorders & Control*, vol. 5, no. 1, pp. 1–7, 2018.

[30] S. Sharma, J. Kumar, R. Choudhary, and N. Soni, "Study of association between ABO blood groups and diabetes mellitus," *Scholars Journal of Applied Medical Sciences*, vol. 2, no. 1A, pp. 34–37, 2014.

[31] B. Umadevi, M. Roopakala, W. D. C. Silvia, and P. K. Kumar, "Role of von Willebrand factor in type 2 diabetes mellitus patients," *Journal of evolution of medical and dental sciencees*, vol. 5, no. 81, pp. 6075–6079, 2016.

[32] M. Barbalic, J. Dupuis, A. Dehghan et al., "Large-scale genomic studies reveal central role of ABO in sP-selectin and sICAM-1 levels," *Human molecular genetics*, vol. 19, no. 9, pp. 1863–1872, 2010.

[33] D. Dodiya, A. Patel, and J. Jadeja, "Association of ABO blood groups with diabetes mellitus," *International Journal of Basic and Applied Physiology*, vol. 5, no. 1, 2016.

[34] T. Chandra and A. Gupta, "Association and distribution of hypertension, obesity and ABO blood groups in blood donors," *Iranian journal of pediatric hematology and oncology*, vol. 2, no. 4, pp. 140–145, 2012.

[35] M. Kamil, H. Ali Nagi Al-Jamal, and N. Mohd Yusoff, "Association of ABO blood groups with diabetes mellitus," *Libyan Journal of Medicine*, vol. 5, no. 1, p. 4847, 2010.

[36] R. Azizi, S. Manoochehry, S. K. Razavi-Ratki, S. M. S. Hosseini, M. Vakili, and N. Namiranian, "Distribution of ABO and Rh blood groups among diabetes type 2 patients in Yazd Diabetes Research Center (2015-2016)," *Iranian Journal of Diabetes & Obesity (IJDO)*, vol. 8, no. 4, pp. 191–195, 2016.

[37] T. Aggarwal, D. Singh, B. Sharma, S. S. Siddiqui, and S. Agarwal, "Association of ABO and Rh blood groups with type 2 diabetes mellitus in Muzaffarnagar city," *National Journal of Physiology, Pharmacy and Pharmacology*, vol. 8, no. 2, pp. 167–170, 2018.

[38] K. Ganesan and S. B. Gani, "Relationship between ABO, Rh blood groups and diabetes mellitus, obesity in Namakkal town, Tamilnadu," *International Journal of Advances in Pharmacy, Biology and Chemistry*, vol. 3, no. 4, pp. 995–998, 2014.

[39] M.-I. K. El-Sayed and H.-K. Amin, "ABO blood groups in correlation with hyperlipidemia, diabetes mellitus type II, and essential hypertension," *Asian Journal of Pharmaceutical and Clinical Research*, vol. 8, no. 5, pp. 261–268, 2015.

[40] H. S. Al-Ali, "Association of ABO and Rh blood groups with diabetes mellitus and hypertension in Basrah City," *basrah journal of science*, vol. 26, no. 1B english, pp. 29–37, 2008.

[41] U. Okon, A. Antai, E. Osim, and S. Ita, "The relative incidence of diabetes mellitus in ABO/Rh blood groups in South-Eastern Nigeria," *Nigerian journal of physiological sciences*, vol. 23, no. 1-2, 2008.

[42] A. Hercegovac, E. Hajdarević, S. Hodžić, E. Halilović, A. Avdić, and M. Habibović, "Blood group, hypertension, and obesity in the studentpopulation in northeast Bosnia and Herzegovina," *CMBEBIH 2017*, vol. 62, pp. 774–777, 2017.

[43] B. Nemesure, S. Wu, A. Hennis, M. C. Leske, and Group BES, "Hypertension, type 2 diabetes, and blood groups in a population of African ancestry," *Ethnicity and Disease*, vol. 16, no. 4, pp. 822–829, 2006.

[44] H. Sadiq, R. Anjum, S. Shaikh, S. Mushtaq, M. Negi, and P. Kasana, "A study on the correlation of ABO blood group system and hypertension," *International Journal of Applied Dental Sciences*, vol. 3, no. 4, pp. 38–41, 2017.

[45] K. Iheanacho, S. Offiah, M. Udo, M. C. Ugonabu, I. V. Onukaogu, and L. Chigbu, "Evaluation of lipid profile of different ABO blood groups," *International Journal of Research Studies in Medical and Health Sciences*, vol. 3, no. 1, p. 13, 2018, 4.

[46] U. Egesie, N. Mbaka, O. Egesie, and K. Ibrahim, "The effect of alcoholism on secretor status of blood groups A and B individuals in Jos–Nigeria," *Journal of medicine in the tropics*, vol. 7, no. 2, pp. 8–12, 2005.

3

Assessment of Prevalence, Associations, Knowledge and Practices about Diabetic Foot Disease in a Tertiary Care Hospital in Colombo, Sri Lanka

V. T. S. Kaluarachchi ®,[1] D. U. S. Bulugahapitiya,[1] M. H. Arambewela,[2] M. D. Jayasooriya,[1] C. H. De Silva,[1] P. H. Premanayaka,[1] and A. Dayananda[1]

[1]Diabetes and Endocrinology Unit, Colombo South Teaching Hospital, Kalubowila, Colombo, Sri Lanka
[2]Department of Physiology, Faculty of Medical Sciences, University of Sri Jayewardenepura, Diabetes and Endocrinology Unit, Colombo South Teaching Hospital, Kalubowila, Colombo, Sri Lanka

Correspondence should be addressed to V. T. S. Kaluarachchi; kvidumini@yahoo.com

Academic Editor: Katarzyna Zorena

Background. One in five adults in Sri Lanka has either diabetes or prediabetes, and one-third of those with diabetes are undiagnosed. Diabetic foot is a debilitating condition affecting up to 50% of patients with both type 1 and type 2 diabetes. The risk of nontraumatic lower limb amputations is 15 times higher in diabetic patients when compared with nondiabetics. Patient education about correct foot care practices is the cornerstone of prevention of diabetic foot disease. *Objective.* To assess the prevalence of diabetic foot disease, knowledge, and practices about diabetic foot care among diabetic patients. *Methods.* 334 patients attending the diabetic clinic in Colombo South Teaching Hospital were recruited according to the inclusion and exclusion criteria. Data were collected using 3 questionnaires, and they were filled using the foot examination findings, patients' medical records, and direct interviewing of the patients. *Results.* The mean age of the patients included in the study was 58.23 ± 10.65 years while the median duration of diabetes was 10.54 ± 7.32 years. 34.1% patients had peripheral neuropathy, and 29.5% had peripheral vascular disease. Diabetic foot disease according to the WHO definition was present only in 23 (6.9%) patients. There was a significant association between peripheral neuropathy and current or past foot ulcer which took more than 2 weeks to heal ($p < 0.05$). Knowledge about foot care was less among the studied population, and it was associated with poor foot care practices. Presence of diabetic foot and current or past foot ulcer which took more than 2 weeks to heal were significantly associated with the foot care knowledge and practices ($p < 0.05$) *Conclusion.* Improvement of patients' knowledge about foot care and their practices have a significant impact on the reduction of diabetic foot disease.

1. Introduction

Being a noncommunicable disease, diabetes accounts for a significant proportion of morbidity and mortality worldwide. Diabetes mellitus is a group of physiological dysfunctions characterized by hyperglycemia resulting directly from insulin resistance or inadequate insulin secretion leading to macrovascular and microvascular complications with time. Estimated community prevalence of diabetes in Sri Lankan urban population was 27.6% according to the recent study done in Sri Lanka, and this is an exponential rise over the last

3 decades [1]. This is higher than the urban prevalence of 18% shown by Katulanda et al. 12 years ago [2].

The International Working Group on the Diabetic Foot (IWGDF) has defined the diabetic foot as infection, ulceration, or destruction of tissues of the foot of a person with currently or previously diagnosed diabetes mellitus, usually accompanied by neuropathy and/or peripheral arterial disease (PAD in the lower extremity [3]. Diabetic foot is a debilitating complication of diabetes due to its effects on peripheral nerves and peripheral vessels, affecting up to 50% of patients with both type 1 and 2 diabetes. Peripheral nerve disease leads to loss of sensation predisposing to injuries while peripheral vascular disease affects the blood supply leading to poor healing. This complication significantly affects the quality of life of the patient. Furthermore, it represents at least 12–15% of the overall cost associated with diabetes and in developing countries, this is up to 40% [4].

When considering the Sri Lankan setup, the main cause of lower extremity amputations in Sri Lanka is diabetic foot ulcer according to Ubayawansa et al. [5]. They have found that diabetes was contributing to more than 50% of amputations directly or indirectly.

Many risk factors were identified as risk factors for diabetic foot such as long duration of diabetes, poor diabetic control, foot deformities, and presence of other diabetic complications [6]. According to a research done in Sri Lanka in 1996, one-third of all non-insulin-dependent diabetes patients attending the clinic had a risk of foot ulceration. 30.6% of patients had neuropathy according to the criteria used. 10.2% had a foot ulcer, a history of foot ulceration, or a lower extremity amputation due to neuropathic ulceration. 4.8% had a history of lower extremity amputation [7].

A descriptive cross-sectional study which has been done using individuals who were having diagnosed diabetic foot ulcers selected from the National Hospital of Sri Lanka in 2011 showed among those patients with foot ulcers, nonhealing ulcers were present among 82.7%, and amputations amounted to 38.2%. Also, they have found that there was a significant association between the foot care knowledge and practices ($p < 0.001$) [8].

According to a cross-sectional study done on diabetic foot: proportion, knowledge, and foot self-care practices among diabetic patients in Dar es Salaam, Tanzania, of 404 patients included in this study, 15% had foot ulcers, 44% had peripheral neuropathy, and 15% had peripheral vascular disease. In multivariate analysis, peripheral neuropathy ($p < 0.001$) and insulin treatment (OR 2.04, 95% CI) were significantly associated with presence of foot ulcer. Patients with moderate peripheral neuropathy were eight times more likely to have diabetic foot ulcer, and those with severe neuropathy were 24 times more likely to develop ulcers. Patients on insulin treatment were twice more likely to have diabetic foot ulcer than those on oral or nonpharmacological management. Foot self-care was significantly higher in patients who had received advice on foot care and in those whose feet had been examined by a doctor at least once [9].

About 85% of the diabetic-related amputations are due to foot ulcers, and this accounts for more than 50% of nontraumatic lower limb amputations [10]. This is at least 15 times greater in those with diabetes than nondiabetics. The American Diabetes Association has estimated that one in five people with diabetes who seek hospital care does so for foot problems [11].

Early proper management of diabetic foot can reduce the severity of complications such as preventable amputations and possible mortality improving overall quality of life. Based on studies, good blood sugar control, wound debridement, proper dressings, and off-loading shoes should always be a part of diabetic foot ulcer management. Furthermore, surgery to heal chronic ulcers and prevent recurrence should

be considered an essential component of management. Appropriate patient education encourages good foot care practices and thereby prevents the occurrence of diabetic foot diseases and its complications [12].

The main objective of this descriptive cross-sectional study was to assess proportion, existing knowledge, and practices on diabetic foot among patients attending the diabetic clinic at Colombo South Teaching Hospital which is situated in an urban setting in Sri Lanka. The specific objectives were to assess the proportion of diabetic foot and risk stratification of diabetic patients for diabetic foot diseases, to assess the knowledge and practices on diabetic foot diseases among diabetic patients, and to assess the disease variables and sociodemographic factors associated with diabetic foot disease.

2. Methodology and Study Instruments

This is a descriptive cross-sectional study conducted in a diabetic clinic at an urban tertiary care hospital (Colombo South Teaching Hospital) which caters to around 300 patients with diabetes on a daily basis. The referrals to the diabetic clinic are done by the other subspecialties in the hospital itself, patients attending to the outpatients departments, and direct referrals from the primary and secondary care. Even though the patient group attending the diabetic clinic is a representative sample of a Sri Lankan urban population, the sample that attended the foot clinic cannot be considered a representative sample of the Sri Lankan population. In the selected sample, the majority were females ($n = 245$) and most of the patients were above 50 years of age. This may be due to the timing of the clinic which was during the working hours of the day. This may be the reason for getting less males and less people in the 18–50-year age group.

334 patients with diabetes who are above 18 years of age were included into the study by simple random sampling. Exclusion criteria were age of 18 years or less than 18 years, mental subnormality, and inability to comply with medical instructions.

Questionnaires (Appendix 1 in Supplementary Materials (available here)) were developed to get the details about sociodemographic details and disease variables according to the previous studies done on diabetes [8]. Questionnaire to assess knowledge and practices about foot care was adopted from the foot care questionnaire used in the Diabetes Care Program of Nova Scotia [13]. Pretesting of the questionnaire was done before starting the study.

Medical officers in the diabetic clinic of Colombo South Teaching Hospital and a trained research assistant obtained the informed written consent from the patients after checking patient suitability depending on inclusion and exclusion criteria (Appendix 2 in Supplementary Materials).

Questionnaire 3 was translated into 2 other languages which are commonly used in Sri Lanka (Sinhala, Tamil). These were prepared to collect data on sociodemographic factors, disease variables, risk stratification of diabetic foot, and knowledge and practices with regard to diabetic foot. Questionnaires 1 and 2 were interviewer administered which were filled by specially trained medical officers whereas questionnaire 3 was a self-administered questionnaire.

Questionnaire 3 was filled by an interviewer if patient has difficulties in filling the form. Questionnaire 2 was administered to collect data on disease variables, medical history, investigations, complications, and diabetic foot with risk stratification. Medical history and investigation findings were taken from the patients' medical records.

Diabetic foot risk assessments were done by trained medical officers by a proper examination of the feet according to risk assessment in the Diabetic Foot Care Program of Nova Scotia. Ankle brachial pressure index (ABPI), monofilament test, and vibration sensation test using a biothesiometer were done using standard techniques.

The monofilament test was done on three sites, and the response recorded. If two out of three responses were incorrect, it was taken as peripheral neuropathy. Vibration sensation of the foot was assessed using a biothesiometer, and anything above 25 Hz was taken as peripheral neuropathy. Ankle brachial pressure index was taken as an objective measure of peripheral vascular disease, using the standard blood pressure cuff and Doppler device to detect pulse. Systolic blood pressure was measured in both arms, and the higher value was used as the denominator of the ABI. Systolic blood pressure is then measured in the dorsalis pedis and posterior tibial arteries by placing the cuff just above the ankle. The higher value is the numerator of the ABI in each limb. A value less than 0.9 was taken as the presence of peripheral vascular disease [14].

At the end of questionnaire 2, patients were categorised into one of the three categories (low, moderate, or high risk for diabetic foot disease). This risk stratification system was developed from the Diabetes Care Program of Nova Scotia [13].

Questionnaire 3 is a self-administered questionnaire which was prepared in all three languages to improve patients' understanding. The objective of this questionnaire was to assess patient's knowledge and practices on foot care, footwear, safety, and prevention of complications with regard to diabetic foot. This questionnaire was a modification of the foot care questionnaire used in the Diabetes Care Program of Nova Scotia. The patients who were having difficulty in answering the questionnaire alone were assisted by an interviewer.

Before the commencement of proper data collection, a pilot study was done using 30 patients to check the reliability of the questionnaires and to check whether the questions were understood by the patients.

2.1. Statistical Analysis. SPSS software program (Statistical Package for the Social Sciences) version 20 was used to analyse the data after collection and tabulation. Quantitative data were expressed as mean and SD (standard deviation) while the qualitative data were expressed as numbers and percentages. Chi-squared test was used with 5% level of significance to assess the differences in frequencies of the qualitative variables.

3. Results

The mean age of the patients included in the study was 58.23 ± 10.65 years while the median duration of diabetes

TABLE 1: Sociodemographic characteristics of the patients.

Patient characteristics	Frequency	Percentage (%)
Gender		
(i) Female	245	73.4
(ii) Male	89	26.6
Age groups		
(i) 21-30	4	1.2
(ii) 31-40	12	3.6
(iii) 41-50	51	15.3
(iv) 51-60	125	37.4
(v) 61-70	98	29.3
(vi) 71-80	42	12.6
(vii) 81-90	2	0.6
Foot care practice		
Frequency of self-examination of feet		
(i) Everyday	157	47.0
(ii) 2-6 times a week	49	14.7
(iii) Once a week or less	41	12.3
(iv) When there is a problem in feet	48	14.4
(v) Not examining	29	8.7
Washing feet everyday		
(i) Yes	325	97.3
(ii) No	6	1.8
Dry between toes		
(i) Yes	290	86.8
(ii) No	40	12.0
Use of moisturizer for feet		
(i) Yes	163	48.8
(ii) No	166	49.7
Cutting of toenails		
(i) Self	292	87.4
(ii) Family member	40	12.0
Use suitable shoes	112	36.8

was 10.54 ± 7.32 years. When the age is categorised into 10-year intervals, majority of the patients were in the 51-60-year age group (37%). Another 29% belonged to the 61-70-year age group.

Among these patients, 245 patients (73.4%) were females and 89 patients (26.6%) were males (Table 1). The mean BMI of the population was $25.38 \pm 4.06 \, \text{kg/m}^2$. The mean fasting blood sugar among the group was $135.6 \pm 45.5 \, \text{mg/dl}$.

Majority of patients have been educated up to the ordinary level (32%) while there were few illiterate people (2.4%). 4.5% of patients have an educational level of degree and above. Fundoscopy findings were available for 66% of the studied population ($n = 222$). 50% of them did not have diabetic retinopathy, and among the patients with diabetic retinopathy, most had nonproliferative diabetic retinopathy (12%). 77.5% of the patients were on oral hypoglycemics, and 4.8% of the patients were using insulin. 17.7% of the patients were using both insulin and oral hypoglycemics. Most of the patients stated that they take their medications regularly (91%).

When considering the macrovascular complications of diabetes mellitus in the studied population ($n = 333$), 14.1% of patients had a history of ischemic heart disease while 85% of them have not had a history of ischemic heart disease. Among 331 patients, 5 patients (1.5%) have given a history of TIA or stroke.

114 patients (34.1%) were having peripheral neuropathy while 97 patients out of 334 (29.5%) were having peripheral vascular disease. However, the diabetic foot disease according to the IWGFDF definition was present only in 50 (15%) patients (Table 2). 78 patients have experienced a foot ulcer which took more than 2 weeks to heal while 254 out of 332 patients have not had experienced a foot ulcer that took more than 2 weeks to heal.

According to the examination findings, 65.3% of patient were in the moderate-risk category while 6% were at high risk and 28.7% were at low risk (Table 3). 6.9% of patients were having diabetic foot disease according to the definition.

When considering the knowledge of the patients on foot care, 58.45% of patients had not read any handouts on foot care while 38.6% of them have never attended a class on diabetic foot care. 61.4% of patients had not read handouts about suitable footwear.

9.4% of patients were using special diabetic footwear while majority (90.6%) were not using special footwear. 46.6% of patients were self-examining their feet daily while 10.5% of them never self-examine their feet. However, 97.3% of patients wash their feet daily and 86.8 patients keep their inter toe areas dry after washing. 48.8% of patients use moisturizer to the feet. 87.4% of patients cut their toenails by themselves while 12% of patients get their family member's help to cut their toenails.

There is a significant association ($p < 0.05$) between the knowledge about foot care and the foot care practices. Also, there is a significant association between current or past foot ulcer which took more than 2 weeks to heal and the knowledge about foot care ($p < 0.05$).

4. Discussion

This descriptive cross-sectional study was conducted to assess the knowledge, attitude, and practices of foot care among the diabetic patients attending a diabetic clinic at a tertiary care hospital.

Most of the study population was females, and it was 73.45% (Table 1). The mean age of the patients included in the study was 58.23 ± 10.65 years. A descriptive cross-sectional study which has been done among individuals who were diagnosed with diabetic foot ulcers selected from the National Hospital of Sri Lanka in 2011 showed that the mean age of having diabetic foot ulcers was 58.4 years (SD ± 8.6) which is similar to our finding. When the age is categorised into 10-year intervals, majority of the patients were in the 51-60-year age group (37%) (Table 1). The mean BMI of the patients was $25.38 \pm 4.06\,kg/m^2$ which is in the overweight range of the BMI categorisation for an Asian population. The mean duration of diabetes was 10.5 years. The mean fasting blood glucose level is 135.5 mol/l which showed a poor diabetes control among the population.

TABLE 2: Frequency of diabetic foot complications.

Foot complications		Frequency	Percentage (%)
Current or past foot ulcer which took more than 2 weeks to heal	Yes	78	23.5
	No	254	76.5
Diabetic foot disease	Yes	50	15
	No	284	85

TABLE 3: Risk category of diabetic foot disease.

Risk category	Frequency	Percentage (%)
Low risk	96	28.7
Moderate risk	218	65.3
High risk	20	6

Among the study population of 333 patients, 52 (15.2%) patients had an abnormal monofilament test and 108 patients had abnormal vibration sense. Either of these was considered peripheral neuropathy. Depending on these findings, 114 (34.1%) of patients had peripheral neuropathy which is a major risk factor for foot ulceration. A study has published similar results where 44% of patients have had peripheral neuropathy and 15% of patients have had peripheral vascular disease. In their study population, presence of foot ulceration was 15% and they have found a significant association between foot ulceration and presence of peripheral neuropathy and insulin treatment [1].

Our study population was selected from the routine diabetic clinic. This may be the reason for the very low prevalence of diabetic foot disease in the study population. Most of the studies which analysed diabetic foot disease have chosen the study population from the patients already having foot problems [2]. However, our study was mainly designed to assess the proportion and knowledge, attitudes, and practices about foot care; the appropriate population would be the patients attending the general diabetic clinic.

The proportion of patients having diabetic foot according to the IWGDF definition in our study is 50 patients out of 334 (15%) patients. This prevalence is slightly higher than the pooled worldwide prevalence of diabetic foot disease found in a systematic review and meta-analysis done by Zhang et al. [12]. The prevalence of diabetic foot found in this meta-analysis was 6.3%. The definition used in this meta-analysis to define diabetic foot was similar to the WHO definition which we used for our study. A similar prevalence has been stated by Boulton, who reported that the worldwide prevalence of diabetic foot ranges from 1.4% to 5.9%, in his grand overview about diabetic foot [15]. Our prevalence is almost similar when compared to the study done by Chiwanga et al. in the Dar es Salaam, Tanzania [9], who reported the prevalence of diabetic foot ulcer as 15%. However, they have mentioned in their article that the higher prevalence is because they hired most of their patients from diabetic foot clinics. In another study done in Sudan about the prevalence of diabetic foot ulceration and the prevalence of diabetic foot ulcer and associated risk factors, they have found a higher prevalence of diabetic foot ulcer in that study group which was 18.1% [16]. When considering, Sri Lanka, there is only one study done in a diabetic clinic in the National Hospital in Sri Lanka about the prevalence of neuropathic foot ulceration; they have found that the prevalence of neuropathic foot ulceration or amputation due to neuropathic foot ulceration was 10.2% which is slightly less than our finding [7]. The major risk factor for the development of foot ulcers is the presence of peripheral neuropathy according to previous studies. The presence of both peripheral neuropathy and peripheral vascular disease is not essential to develop diabetic foot ulcers. In our study, the number of patients who had current or past foot ulcers which took more than 2 weeks to heal, which is very much suggestive of diabetic foot ulcer, was 78 (23.4%) which is higher than the prevalence of foot ulcer described in Chiwanga et al.'s study in Dar es Salaam, Tanzania [9].

When considering the peripheral vascular disease and peripheral neuropathy separately, the prevalence of peripheral neuropathy was found to be 34.1% and peripheral vascular disease was present in 29.9% of the study population.

Chiwanga et al. [9] have shown a significant association between diabetic foot ulcers and peripheral neuropathy. In our study, we found the similar results. There was a significant association between the peripheral neuropathy and current or past foot ulcers which took more than 2 weeks to heal ($p < 0.05$).

Risk stratification for diabetic foot disease was done according to the criteria used by the Nova Scotia foot risk assessment guide [13]. More than 50% of patients (61.1%) were in the moderate-risk category, and 5.7% of patients were in the high-risk category (Table 2). This is an important guide for the management of diabetic patients. Predicting the risk for foot ulceration early can prevent the limb-threatening complications of diabetic foot disease. This is important because 85% of the amputations in diabetic patients were preceded by a foot ulcer which later gets complicated with infection and gangrene [17]. Therefore, limb amputations and foot ulcerations are significantly interrelated in diabetes and the rate of amputations are 15 times higher among diabetes patients when compared to nondiabetic adults [18].

We assessed the patients' knowledge and practices using a self-administered questionnaire given to the patients in their own language. According to the findings of the questionnaire, 58.4% of patients never had an opportunity to read a handout about diabetic foot care. 38% of the patients have had read a handout about foot care. Our results are slightly higher than the percentage of patients who read handouts about diabetic foot care found in a study done in Makkha, Saudi Arabia, by Goweda et al. which was about 34% [18]. This implies the importance of educating the patients by giving handouts for the patients who are able to read. Most of our study population had a reasonable literacy indicated by the educational level questioned in the interviewer-administered questionnaire. Only 2.4% have never attended a school, and most of them were educated up to the O/L.

61.4% of patients have attended a class about foot care, and this is higher than the percentage found in the study done by Goweda et al. [18]. Regular classes about foot care

are a very effective way of educating the diabetic patients about foot care because the patients get a chance to clarify their doubts and the education can be delivered in a customised manner to cater the individual patient's needs. Further, all the newly diagnosed diabetic patients should be educated about foot care on the very first clinic visit and they should be examined for the presence of signs of diabetic foot disease in the very first clinic visit by an experienced person about diabetic foot disease because they may have had diabetes for a long time before they were diagnosed. Moreover, this gives the opportunity to risk stratify them and direct them to appropriate foot care facilities such as correct footwear and foot orthoses. This has a lot of long-term benefits such as reduction of the rate of amputations and long-term disability, reduction of the health care cost for surgeries and different expensive treatment modalities, and improvement of the quality of life of the diabetic patients. According to the literature, every 30s, there is a lower limb amputation due to diabetes [17].

33.1% of patients have read the handouts about diabetic footwear, and this is higher than the percentage found by a study done in Makkha, Saudi Arabia, by Goweda et al. [18]. In our study, only 9.4% of patients were using special footwear for diabetes. 36.8% of patients were using acceptable kinds of footwear such as adjustable shoes, shoes with wide toe space, sandals, athletic shoes, and custom-made shoes. A similar finding was observed in the study done by Goweda et al. in Makkha, Saudi Arabia. 63.2% of patients were using pointed shoes, flip-flops, or high-heeled shoes which are recognised as an improper footwear. Even though we did not find a significant statistical association between the use of appropriate footwear and the diabetic foot disease, only 8 out of 48 patients with diabetic foot disease were using a special diabetic footwear. Further, 65 out of 76 patients with current or past foot ulcer which took more than 2 weeks to heel were not using a special diabetic footwear. An appropriate footwear includes the custom-made footwear according to the patient's foot architecture (for the patients who have existing foot problems such as Charcot foot), off-loading footwear, comfortable and appropriate footwear with wide toe space, and adjustable and well-fitting footwear. An appropriate footwear should be adjustable according to the patient's pressure points in the foot, and it should be made of good-quality material appropriate to the climate of the country. Patients should also be educated about using appropriate footwear according to their activities, and they should be provided with the advices such as suitable socks, how to check the shoe before wearing it, how to identify the faults in the footwear, and what are the precautions to be taken when they are wearing the footwear for a long duration. The major barrier towards the appropriate footwear is the high cost. Custom-made shoes and good-quality shoes are expensive, and they are not freely available in the government hospitals. Even if a patient can afford a pair of good-quality footwear, they do not have the knowledge about choosing it correctly according to their needs. Some patients are reluctant to wear their expensive footwear in adverse weather conditions because they are worrying about the damage to their footwear by the weather. They also cannot afford more than one footwear because of the cost, and they tend to wear the same footwear for all the activities. Sometimes, these footwear are bulky and unsightly which prevent the patient from wearing these frequently. These problems should be addressed adequately to motivate the diabetic patients to wear the appropriate shoes. Sometimes, because of the cultural beliefs and the occupations, patients used to be barefooted. This increases the foot problems related to diabetes, and these were observed in the study conducted by Goweda et al. at Makkha, Saudi Arabia, and Taksande et al. in central rural India [18, 19].

Knowledge about diabetic foot disease was assessed by the self-administered questionnaire. The mean score was 11.28 out of 20 which is slightly higher than 50%. Most of the patients have scored above 10.

When analysing the foot care practices (Table 1), 46.6% of patients were self-examining their feet daily and this is a higher percentage when compared to the study done by Goweda et al. at Makkha, Saudi Arabia. Goweda et al. have found this percentage as 37.7%. 97.3% of patients wash their feet daily, and this is a similar finding to the aforementioned study. However, a study done in Chandigarh, India, has found that only 63.3% of diabetic patients take care of their feet by washing their feet daily [20]. In countries like Saudi Arabia, they wash their feet regularly as a religious ritual which may have accounted for this higher percentage. Our study was conducted in a tertiary care hospital which mainly serves the urban population where the awareness about cleanliness and the sanitation are much better when compared to the above study which was conducted in a rural area in India. 86.8% of patients keep their intertoe areas dry after washing which is a much higher percentage when compared to previous studies [18]. 48.8% of patients use moisturizer to the feet, and 87.4% of patients self-cut their toenails which are much more similar findings to the previous studies [18].

In this current study, there is a significant association ($p < 0.05$) between the knowledge about foot care and the foot care practices. Even though there is no statistically significant association between the presence of diabetic foot and the knowledge about foot care, most of the patients with diabetic foot disease ($n = 37$) have not had any form of knowledge about foot care (reading handouts, attending classes). The similar findings were found in previous studies according to the literature [18]. These findings confirm the importance of educating the patients about diabetic foot disease and correct foot care facilities. Proper education can prevent this limb-threatening complication which has a major impact on health care costs.

5. Conclusion

Our study concludes that there is a large group of patients who have a significant risk to develop diabetic foot disease even though the prevalence of diabetic foot disease is 15%. Also, there is a significant lack of knowledge and a high rate of improper foot care practices in this study population. Furthermore, our study shows a significant association between knowledge about foot care and foot care practices and the knowledge about foot care and the development of diabetic

foot complications. This confirms the importance of education about foot care as an effective method of primary prevention of diabetic foot complications. Proper education about diabetic foot care reduces the development of diabetic foot disease which has a major impact on the quality of life of a diabetic patient.

6. Recommendations

The main recommendation from this study is to improve the patients' knowledge about proper foot care practices. Classes, handouts, posters, and the use of mass media are some effective methods of education. Another recommendation is to increase patients' awareness about correct footwear and increase the availability of custom-made shoes at least for high-risk patients. All the diabetic patients should be examined by a qualified person to detect the features of foot disease, and all should get risk stratified. The patients should be educated according to their risk, and the follow-up plan should be individualised according to the individual patients' risk. Improvement of pediatric services in the diabetic clinics is an essential step to reduce the devastating diabetic foot complications which have a significant impact on health care costs.

References

[1] N. P. Somasundaram, I. Ranathunga, K. Gunawardana, and D. S. Ediriweera, "High prevalence of diabetes mellitus in Sri Lankan urban population – data from Colombo urban study," *Sri Lanka Journal of Diabetes Endocrinology and Metabolism*, vol. 9, no. 2, p. 8, 2019.

[2] P. Katulanda, G. R. Constantine, J. G. Mahesh et al., "Prevalence and projections of diabetes and pre-diabetes in adults in Sri Lanka-Sri Lanka Diabetes, Cardiovascular Study (SLDCS)," *Diabetic Medicine*, vol. 25, no. 9, pp. 1062–1069, 2008.

[3] J. J. Netten, S. A. Bus, J. Apelqvist et al., "Definitions and criteria for diabetic foot disease," *Diabetes/Metabolism Research and Reviews*, vol. 36, no. S1, 2020.

[4] D. Mauricio, E. Jude, A. Piaggesi, and R. Frykberg, "Diabetic foot: current status and future prospects," *Journal of Diabetes Research*, vol. 2016, Article ID 5691305, 2 pages, 2016.

[5] D. H. B. Ubayawansa, W. Y. M. Abeysekera, and M. M. A. J. Kumara, "Major lower limb amputations: experience of a tertiary care hospital in Sri Lanka," *Journal of the College of Physicians and Surgeons Pakistan*, vol. 26, pp. 620–622, 2016.

[6] A. M. Al-Wahbi, "The diabetic foot. In the Arab world," *Saudi Medical Journal*, vol. 27, pp. 147–153, 2006.

[7] D. J. Fernando, "The prevalence of neuropathic foot ulceration in Sri Lankan diabetic patients," *The Ceylon Medical Journal*, vol. 41, no. 3, pp. 96–98, 1996.

[8] C. V. M. Jinadasa and M. Jeewantha, "SP5-14 a study to determine the knowledge and practice of foot care in patients with chronic diabetic ulcers," *Journal of Epidemiology & Community Health*, vol. 65, Suppl 1, p. A449, 2011.

[9] F. S. Chiwanga and M. A. Njelekela, "Diabetic foot: prevalence, knowledge, and foot self-care practices among diabetic

patients in Dar es Salaam, Tanzania - a cross-sectional study," *Journal of Foot and Ankle Research*, vol. 8, no. 1, 2015.

[10] C. N. Dang and A. J. M. Boulton, "Changing perspectives in diabetic foot ulcer management," *The International Journal of Lower Extremity Wounds*, vol. 2, no. 1, pp. 4–12, 2003.

[11] American Diabetes Association, "Economic costs of diabetes in the U.S. in 2012," *Diabetes Care*, vol. 36, no. 4, pp. 1033–1046, 2013.

[12] P. Zhang, J. Lu, Y. Jing, S. Tang, D. Zhu, and Y. Bi, "Global epidemiology of diabetic foot ulceration: a systematic review and meta-analysis†," *Annals of Medicine*, vol. 49, no. 2, pp. 106–116, 2017.

[13] B. Harpell and L. Harrigan, "The diabetic foot: patient and provider tools," *Canadian Journal of Diabetes*, vol. 33, no. 3, p. 217, 2009.

[14] American Diabetes Association, "Peripheral arterial disease in people with diabetes," *Diabetes Care*, vol. 26, no. 12, pp. 3333–3341, 2003.

[15] A. J. M. Boulton, "The diabetic foot: grand overview, epidemiology and pathogenesis," *Diabetes/Metabolism Research and Reviews*, vol. 24, no. S1, pp. S3–S6, 2008.

[16] A. O. Almobarak, H. Awadalla, M. Osman, and M. H. Ahmed, "Prevalence of diabetic foot ulceration and associated risk factors: an old and still major public health problem in Khartoum, Sudan?," *Annals of Translational Medicine*, vol. 5, no. 17, p. 340, 2017.

[17] J. Apelqvist, "Diagnostics and treatment of the diabetic foot," *Endocrine*, vol. 41, no. 3, pp. 384–397, 2012.

[18] R. Goweda, "Assessment of knowledge and practices of diabetic patients regarding diabetic foot care, in Makkah, Saudi Arabia," *Journal of Family Medicine and Health Care*, vol. 3, no. 1, p. 17, 2017.

[19] B. Taksande, M. Thote, and U. Jajoo, "Knowledge, attitude, and practice of foot care in patients with diabetes at central rural India," *Journal of Family Medicine and Primary Care*, vol. 6, no. 2, p. 284, 2017.

[20] K. Kaur, K. Kaur, M. M. Singh, and I. Walia, "Knowledge and self-care practices of diabetics in a resettlement colony of Chandigarh," *Indian Journal of Medical Sciences*, vol. 52, no. 8, pp. 341–347, 1998.

4

Global Burden of Anxiety and Depression among Cystic Fibrosis Patient

Mistire Teshome Guta ⓘ,[1] Tiwabwork Tekalign,[1] Nefsu Awoke ⓘ,[1] Robera Olana Fite ⓘ,[2] Getahun Dendir ⓘ,[3] and Tsegaye Lolaso Lenjebo ⓘ[4]

[1]School of Nursing, College of Health Science and Medicine, Wolaita Sodo University, Wolaita Sodo, Ethiopia
[2]HaSET Program/Ethiopian Public Health Institute, Adis Abeba, Ethiopia
[3]School of Anesthesia, College of Health Science and Medicine, Wolaita Sodo University, Wolaita Sodo, Ethiopia
[4]School of Public Health, College of Health Science and Medicine, Wolaita Sodo University, Ethiopia

Correspondence should be addressed to Mistire Teshome Guta; mister.guta952@gmail.com

Academic Editor: Kosagi S. Jagannatha Rao

Aims. This systemic review and meta-analysis were aimed at determining the level of anxiety and depression among cystic fibrosis patients in the world. *Methods.* We conducted a systematic search of published studies from PubMed, EMBASE, MEDLINE, Cochrane, Scopus, Web of Science, CINAHL, and manually on Google Scholar. This meta-analysis follows the Preferred Reporting Items for Systematic Reviews and Meta-Analyses (PRISMA) guidelines. The quality of studies was assessed by the modified Newcastle-Ottawa Scale (NOS). Meta-analysis was carried out using a random-effects method using the STATA™ Version 14 software. Trim and fill analysis was done to correct the presence of significant publication bias. *Result.* From 419,820 obtained studies, 26 studies from 2 different parts of the world including 9766. The overall global pooled prevalence of anxiety and depression after correction for publication bias by trim and fill analysis was found to be 24.91(95% CI: 20.8-28.9) for anxiety. The subgroup analyses revealed with the lowest prevalence, 23.59%, (95% CI: 8.08, 39.09)) in North America and the highest, 26.77%, (95% CI: 22.5, 31.04) seen in Europe for anxiety and with the highest prevalence, 18.67%, (95% CI: 9.82, 27.5) in North America and the lowest, 13.27%, (95% CI: -10.05, 16.5) seen in Europe for depression. *Conclusion.* The global prevalence of anxiety and depression among cystic fibrosis patients is common. Therefore, close monitoring of the patient, regularly screening for anxiety and depression, and appropriate prevention techniques is recommended.

1. Background

Depression is a mental disorder characterized by feelings of depressed mood, loss of interest or pleasure in activities, and loss of energy that lasts for 2 weeks or more [1]. Depression disorder presents with depressed mood, loss of interest or pleasure, decreased energy, feelings of guilt or low self-worth, disturbed sleep or appetite, poor concentration, the problem of thinking and making decisions, and, in severe stages, recurring thoughts of death or suicide [2], whereas anxiety is a vague, subjective, nonspecific feeling of uneasiness, apprehension, tension, (excessive nervousness) fears, and a sense of impending doom, irrational avoidance of objects or situation, and anxiety attack [3]. Anxiety and

depression are the most frequently occurring mental disorders in the general population [4]. Moreover, depression often comes with symptoms of anxiety. These problems can become chronic or recurrent and lead to substantial impairments in an individual's ability to take care of his or her everyday responsibilities [5].

According to the WHO report in 2017, 300 million people around the world have depression and also, the burden of depression and other mental health conditions is on the rise globally [6]. Similarly in another study, globally more than 264 million people affected with depression [7]. The high prevalence suggests that immediate preventive measures should be implemented, such as the setting up of psychopedagogic support services for those in need

[8]. Moreover, depression is a significant determinant of quality of life and survival, accounting for approximately 50% of psychiatric consultations and 12% of all hospital admissions [9]. Cystic fibrosis (CF) is a common genetic, life-shortening chronic illness, leading to frequent infections and progressive failure of most organ systems (e.g., lungs and pancreas) [10]. The disease is highly burdensome with progressive multisystem nvolvement, mostly problematic due to persistent lung infections, frequent hospitalizations, and time-consuming treatment regimens taking 2 to 4 hours per day on average [11, 12]. It is a severe and progressive disease characterized by decreased physical activities and excessive dyspnea on exertion [13]. Chronically ill patients experience emotional difficulties that can sometimes even manifest themselves in anxiety and depression [14]. The study showed that individuals with chronic medical conditions have a 41% increased risk of having a psychiatric disorder [15]. Respiratory diseases have an increased risk for comorbid anxiety and depression [16]. Depression, anxiety, and cognitive impairment are common among patients with chronic obstructive pulmonary disease (COPD) and may both affect the delivery of pulmonary rehabilitation and be modified by pulmonary rehabilitation [17]. Studies show that compared with nondepressed patients, the odds are 3 times greater than depressed patients that will be noncompliant with medical treatment recommendations [18]. Symptoms of depression and anxiety have negative consequences for disease management, health-related quality of life, and health outcomes [19]. Studies measuring psychological distress in individuals with CF have found high rates of both depression and anxiety, and the prevalence of depression and anxiety ranges from 13–33% and 30% to 33% among adults, respectively [20, 21]. Depressive symptoms are prevalent among adults with CF and are associated with poorer health-related quality of life even after controlling for the lung function [14]. The study indicated that people with CF and parents who take care of children with CF are more likely to experience depression than people in the general population [22]. Since the presence of depression and anxiety has a negative influence on the quality of life, healthcare cost, and self-care, this meta-analysis contributes its own to give attention to CF patients especially to focus on prevention and screen for depression and anxiety and treat accordingly.

2. Methods and Materials

2.1. Study Design and Search Strategy. This systematic review and meta-analysis were conducted under the Preferred Reporting Items guidelines for Systematic Reviews and Meta-analyses (PRISMA) statement [23, 24]. We made the searching of articles published in the English language regardless of the year of publication that was taken from PubMed, EMBASE, MEDLINE, Cochrane, Scopus, the web of Science CINAHL, and manually on Google Scholar. The search was performed using key terms such as CF, cystic fibrosis, anxiety, depression, patient, and worldwide.

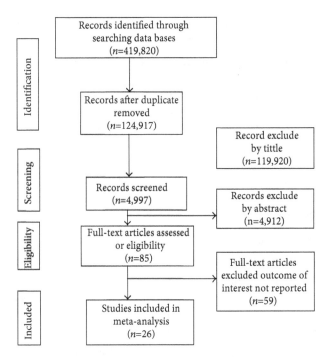

FIGURE 1: PRISMA flow diagram of study selection.

2.2. Study Selection and Eligibility Criteria

  (i) All adults who were diagnosed with CF were included

  (ii) Both published and unpublished studies conducted worldwide regardless of study design were included

2.3. Study Extraction and Quality Appraisal. The data were extracted by three independent authors (MT, TT, and NA) using a data extraction format prepared in a Microsoft Excel 2010 spreadsheet. The extracted data were the first author's name, publication year, country, region, design, sample size, sampling method, and prevalence of anxiety and depression among CF patient. The quality of each study was assessed using the modified Newcastle-Ottawa Scale (NOS) for cross-sectional studies [25]. Studies were included with a score of 5 and more on the NOS [26]. Each study's quality was evaluated independently by five authors (TT, MT, RO, GD, and TL), and any disagreements were resolved by discussion and consensus.

2.4. Publication Bias and Heterogeneity. To assess the existence of publication bias, funnel plots were used, and Egger's test was computed. A p value<0.05 was used to declare the statistical significance of publication bias. I^2 test statistics were used to check the heterogeneity of studies. I^2 test statistics of <50, $50-75\%$, and$>75\%$ were declared as low, moderate, and high heterogeneity, respectively [27].

2.5. Outcome Measure. The outcome of this review was the global prevalence of anxiety and depression among CF patient.

2.6. Data Synthesis and Analysis. STATA™ Version 14software was used to conduct the analysis. The heterogeneity test

TABLE 1: Characteristics of the included studies of anxiety in the systematic review and meta-analysis.

Authors' name	Publication year	Study area	Region	Study design	Sample	Prevalence of anxiety % (95% CI)	Prevalence of depression % (95% CI)
Quittner et al.	2014	Belgium	Europe	Cross-sectional	426	33 (28.53-37.46)	15 (11.61, 18.39)
Quittner et al.	2014	Germany	Europe	Cross-sectional	663	21 (17.90, 24.10)	10 (7.72, 12.28)
Quittner et al.	2014	Italy	Europe	Cross-sectional	741	34 (30.59, 37.18)	14 (11.50, 16.50)
Quittner et al.	2014	Spain	Europe	Cross-sectional	275	26 (20.82, 31.18)	11 (7.30, 14.70)
Quittner et al.	2014	Sweden	Europe	Cross-sectional	167	23 (16.62, 29.68)	8 (3.89, 12.11)
Quittner et al.	2014	Netherlands	Europe	Cross-sectional	515	14 (11.00, 17.00)	10 (7.41, 12.59)
Quittner et al.	2014	Turkey	Europe	Cross-sectional	52	31 (18.43, 43.57)	29 (16.67, 41.33)
Quittner et al.	2014	United Kingdom	Europe	Cross-sectional	2042	34 (31.95, 36.05)	11 (9.64, 12.36)
Quittner et al.	2014	United States	North America	Cross-sectional	1207	35 (32.31, 37.69)	9 (7.39, 10.61)
Lalic et al.	2018	Croatia	Europe	Cross-sectional	22	41 (20.45, 61.45)	18 (1.95, 34.05)
Besier and Goldbeck	2011	German	Europe	Cross-sectional	162	12.3 (7.24, 17.36)	7.4 (3.37, 11.43)
Catastini et al.	2016	Italia	Europe	Cross-sectional	528	17.2 (13.98, 20.42)	7 (4.88, 9.12)
Cronly et al.	2018	Ireland	Europe	Cross-sectional	83	25 (15.68, 34.32)	7.5 (1.83, 13.17)
Cronly et al.	2018	Ireland	Europe	Cross-sectional	64	28.1 (17.09, 39.11)	10.9 (3.26, 18.54)
Goldbeck et al.	2010	German	Europe	Cross-sectional	670	20.6 (17.54, 23.66)	9.6 (7.37, 11.83)
Modi et al.	2011	USA	North America	Cross-sectional	59	32 (20.10, 43.90)	10 (2.35, 17.65)
Olveira	2016	Spain	Europe	Cross-sectional	336	29.7 (24.81, 34.59)	12.2 (8.70, 15.70)
Quon et al.	2014	USA	North America	Cross-sectional	153	10 (5.25, 14.75)	22 (15.44, 28.56)
Yohannes et al.	2012	United Kingdom	Europe	Cross-sectional	121	33 (24.62, 41.38)	17 (10.31, 23.69)
Mursaloglu et al.	2020	USA	North America	Cross-sectional	50	17.6 (7.04, 28.16)	25.5 (13.42, 37.58)
Cepuch et al.	2007	Poland	Europe	Cross-sectional	53	25 (13.34, 36.66)	6 (-0.39, 12.39)
Graziano et al.	2020	Italia	Europe	Cross-sectional	167	46 (38.44, 53.56)	45 (37.45, 52.55)
Fainardi et al.	2011	Italia	Europe	Cross-sectional	82	40 (89.23-186.54)	18 (9.68-26.31)
Duff et al.	2014	United Kingdom	Europe	Cross-sectional	929	5 (932.15-1819.65)	10 (0.36-1.63)
Knudsen et al.	2016	Denmark	Europe	Cross-sectional	90	—	32.8 (23.1-42.4)
Riekert	2007	USA	North America	Cross-sectional	109	—	30 (21.39-38.6)

was conducted by using I–squared (I^2) statistics. The pooled prevalence of anxiety and depression among CF patient was carried out using a random-effects (DerSimonian and Laird) method. To minimize the potential random variations between studies, heterogeneity sources were analyzed using subgroup analysis and metaregression.

3. Results

3.1. Study Selection.
Initially, a total of 419,820 studies were retrieved from the databases and manual searching. From this, 124,917 duplicates were found and removed. Their title screened the remaining 119,920 articles, and abstract 4,912 irrelevant studies were removed. Eighty-five full-text articles were assessed for eligibility, and 59 of them were excluded due to not reporting the outcome of interest and low methodological quality. Finally, a total of 26 studies fulfilled the inclusion criteria and enrolled in the study (Figure 1).

3.2. Study Characteristics.
Twenty-four studies for anxiety included 9567 participants, and 26 studies for depression included 9766 [22, 28–42]. All of the included studies were cross-sectional studies, and the sample size ranged from 22 [28] to 2042 [22]. Most studies were conducted in Europe. Among the included studies, the prevalence of anxiety and depression among cystic fibrosis patient ranges from 5 [40] to 46 [38] and from 6 [39] to 45 [38], respectively (Table 1).

3.3. The Prevalence of Anxiety and Depression in Patients with Cystic Fibrosis.
The overall pooled global prevalence of anxiety and depression in patients with cystic fibrosis was 26.22% (95% CI: 22.1, 30.2) and 14.13% (95% CI: 11.25, 17.0) with a heterogeneity index (I^2) of 93.5% and 96.2%, respectively, $p < 0.001$ (Figures 2 and 3). And since the Eggers test was found significant, the final pooled prevalence was corrected for Duval and Tweedie's trim and fill analysis and was found to be 24.91 (95% CI: 20.8-28.9) for anxiety but for depression, it is similar.

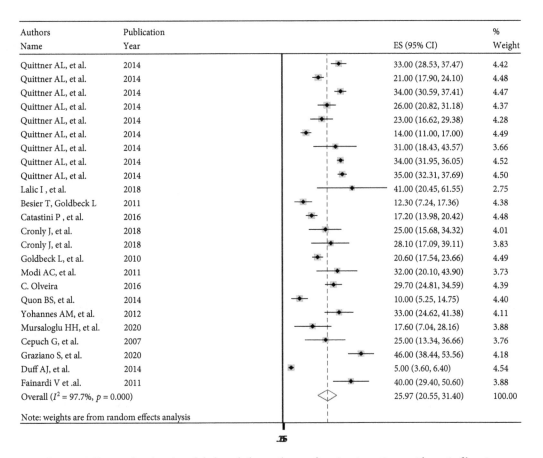

Authors Name	Publication Year	ES (95% CI)	% Weight
Quittner AL, et al.	2014	33.00 (28.53, 37.47)	4.42
Quittner AL, et al.	2014	21.00 (17.90, 24.10)	4.48
Quittner AL, et al.	2014	34.00 (30.59, 37.41)	4.47
Quittner AL, et al.	2014	26.00 (20.82, 31.18)	4.37
Quittner AL, et al.	2014	23.00 (16.62, 29.38)	4.28
Quittner AL, et al.	2014	14.00 (11.00, 17.00)	4.49
Quittner AL, et al.	2014	31.00 (18.43, 43.57)	3.66
Quittner AL, et al.	2014	34.00 (31.95, 36.05)	4.52
Quittner AL, et al.	2014	35.00 (32.31, 37.69)	4.50
Lalic I , et al.	2018	41.00 (20.45, 61.55)	2.75
Besier T, Goldbeck L	2011	12.30 (7.24, 17.36)	4.38
Catastini P , et al.	2016	17.20 (13.98, 20.42)	4.48
Cronly J, et al.	2018	25.00 (15.68, 34.32)	4.01
Cronly J, et al.	2018	28.10 (17.09, 39.11)	3.83
Goldbeck L, et al.	2010	20.60 (17.54, 23.66)	4.49
Modi AC, et al.	2011	32.00 (20.10, 43.90)	3.73
C. Olveira	2016	29.70 (24.81, 34.59)	4.39
Quon BS, et al.	2014	10.00 (5.25, 14.75)	4.40
Yohannes AM, et al.	2012	33.00 (24.62, 41.38)	4.11
Mursaloglu HH, et al.	2020	17.60 (7.04, 28.16)	3.88
Cepuch G, et al.	2007	25.00 (13.34, 36.66)	3.76
Graziano S, et al.	2020	46.00 (38.44, 53.56)	4.18
Duff AJ, et al.	2014	5.00 (3.60, 6.40)	4.54
Fainardi V et .al.	2011	40.00 (29.40, 50.60)	3.88
Overall (I^2 = 97.7%, p = 0.000)		25.97 (20.55, 31.40)	100.00

Note: weights are from random effects analysis

FIGURE 2: Forest plot showing global pooled prevalence of anxiety in patients with cystic fibrosis.

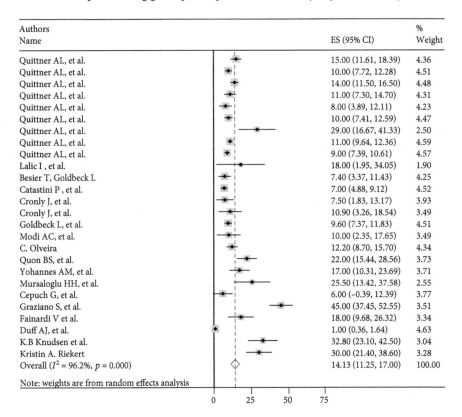

Authors Name	ES (95% CI)	% Weight
Quittner AL, et al.	15.00 (11.61, 18.39)	4.36
Quittner AL, et al.	10.00 (7.72, 12.28)	4.51
Quittner AL, et al.	14.00 (11.50, 16.50)	4.48
Quittner AL, et al.	11.00 (7.30, 14.70)	4.31
Quittner AL, et al.	8.00 (3.89, 12.11)	4.23
Quittner AL, et al.	10.00 (7.41, 12.59)	4.47
Quittner AL, et al.	29.00 (16.67, 41.33)	2.50
Quittner AL, et al.	11.00 (9.64, 12.36)	4.59
Quittner AL, et al.	9.00 (7.39, 10.61)	4.57
Lalic I , et al.	18.00 (1.95, 34.05)	1.90
Besier T, Goldbeck L	7.40 (3.37, 11.43)	4.25
Catastini P , et al.	7.00 (4.88, 9.12)	4.52
Cronly J, et al.	7.50 (1.83, 13.17)	3.93
Cronly J, et al.	10.90 (3.26, 18.54)	3.49
Goldbeck L, et al.	9.60 (7.37, 11.83)	4.51
Modi AC, et al.	10.00 (2.35, 17.65)	3.49
C. Olveira	12.20 (8.70, 15.70)	4.34
Quon BS, et al.	22.00 (15.44, 28.56)	3.73
Yohannes AM, et al.	17.00 (10.31, 23.69)	3.71
Mursaloglu HH, et al.	25.50 (13.42, 37.58)	2.55
Cepuch G, et al.	6.00 (−0.39, 12.39)	3.77
Graziano S, et al.	45.00 (37.45, 52.55)	3.51
Fainardi V et al.	18.00 (9.68, 26.32)	3.34
Duff AJ, et al.	1.00 (0.36, 1.64)	4.63
K.B Knudsen et al.	32.80 (23.10, 42.50)	3.04
Kristin A. Riekert	30.00 (21.40, 38.60)	3.28
Overall (I^2 = 96.2%, p = 0.000)	14.13 (11.25, 17.00)	100.00

Note: weights are from random effects analysis

FIGURE 3: Forest plot showing global pooled prevalence of depression in patients with cystic fibrosis.

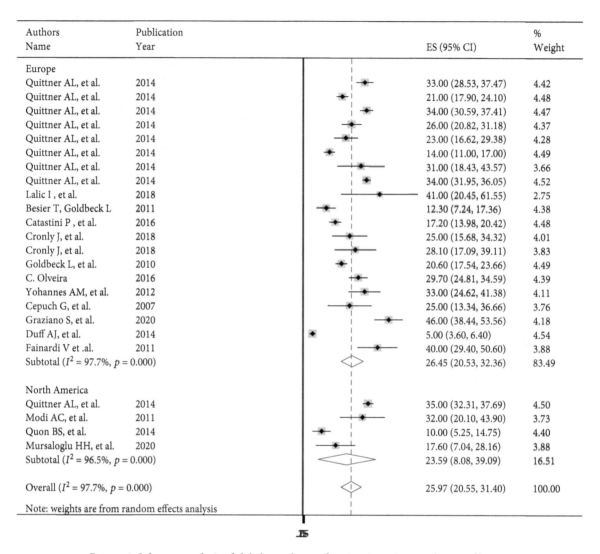

Authors Name	Publication Year		ES (95% CI)	% Weight
Europe				
Quittner AL, et al.	2014		33.00 (28.53, 37.47)	4.42
Quittner AL, et al.	2014		21.00 (17.90, 24.10)	4.48
Quittner AL, et al.	2014		34.00 (30.59, 37.41)	4.47
Quittner AL, et al.	2014		26.00 (20.82, 31.18)	4.37
Quittner AL, et al.	2014		23.00 (16.62, 29.38)	4.28
Quittner AL, et al.	2014		14.00 (11.00, 17.00)	4.49
Quittner AL, et al.	2014		31.00 (18.43, 43.57)	3.66
Quittner AL, et al.	2014		34.00 (31.95, 36.05)	4.52
Lalic I , et al.	2018		41.00 (20.45, 61.55)	2.75
Besier T, Goldbeck L	2011		12.30 (7.24, 17.36)	4.38
Catastini P , et al.	2016		17.20 (13.98, 20.42)	4.48
Cronly J, et al.	2018		25.00 (15.68, 34.32)	4.01
Cronly J, et al.	2018		28.10 (17.09, 39.11)	3.83
Goldbeck L, et al.	2010		20.60 (17.54, 23.66)	4.49
C. Olveira	2016		29.70 (24.81, 34.59)	4.39
Yohannes AM, et al.	2012		33.00 (24.62, 41.38)	4.11
Cepuch G, et al.	2007		25.00 (13.34, 36.66)	3.76
Graziano S, et al.	2020		46.00 (38.44, 53.56)	4.18
Duff AJ, et al.	2014		5.00 (3.60, 6.40)	4.54
Fainardi V et .al.	2011		40.00 (29.40, 50.60)	3.88
Subtotal ($I^2 = 97.7\%$, $p = 0.000$)			26.45 (20.53, 32.36)	83.49
North America				
Quittner AL, et al.	2014		35.00 (32.31, 37.69)	4.50
Modi AC, et al.	2011		32.00 (20.10, 43.90)	3.73
Quon BS, et al.	2014		10.00 (5.25, 14.75)	4.40
Mursaloglu HH, et al.	2020		17.60 (7.04, 28.16)	3.88
Subtotal ($I^2 = 96.5\%$, $p = 0.000$)			23.59 (8.08, 39.09)	16.51
Overall ($I^2 = 97.7\%$, $p = 0.000$)			25.97 (20.55, 31.40)	100.00
Note: weights are from random effects analysis				

FIGURE 4: Subgroup analysis of global prevalence of anxiety in patients with cystic fibrosis.

3.4. Subgroup Analysis of Anxiety. Subgroup analyses revealed a marked variation across the continents, with the lowest prevalence 23.59% (95% CI: 8.08, 39.09), $I^2 = 96.5\%$) in North America and the highest 26.77% ((95% CI: 22.5, 31.04), $I^2 = 92.8\%$) seen in Europe (Figure 4).

3.5. Subgroup Analysis of Depression. Subgroup analyses revealed a marked variation across the continents, with the highest prevalence 18.67% (95% CI: 9.82, 27.5), $I^2 = 90.2\%$) in North America and the lowest 13.27% (95% CI: -10.05, 16.5), $I^2 = 96.5\%$) seen in Europe (Figure 5).

3.6. Metaregression. Metaregression was conducted using the year of publication and sample size as a covariate to identify the source of heterogeneity. It was indicated that there is no effect of publication year and sample size on heterogeneity between studies (Tables 2 and 3).

3.7. Publication Bias. The presence of publication bias was evaluated graphically by funnel plots for both anxiety and depression. Both plots indicate paper asymmetrical. We have tested statically for the presence of small study effect and

effect of unpublished study for both anxiety and depression. The egger test for anxiety relived there is presence of small study effect with $p < 0.001$, and the Begg test indicates there is no statistical evidence for presence of unpublished studies with p value >0.05. The egger test for depression showed no small study effect with $p < 0.001$, and we have tested for the presence of unpublished study effect for depression by the begg test and since p value is >0.05, there is no statistical evidence for presence of unpublished studies (Figures 6 and 7) .

4. Discussion

Primary studies suggest that CF does have a negative impact on physical functioning aspects of quality of life. Depression and anxiety are the main factors in decreasing individual's quality of life. The prevalence of anxiety and depression among adults with cystic fibrosis patients found to be 22.2% and 42.4%, respectively [14]. In another finding, the cystic fibrosis patients have significantly worse quality of life reflecting their significantly impaired scores for physical functioning [43]. Similarly, young adult CF patients have lower scores on several measures of physical functioning

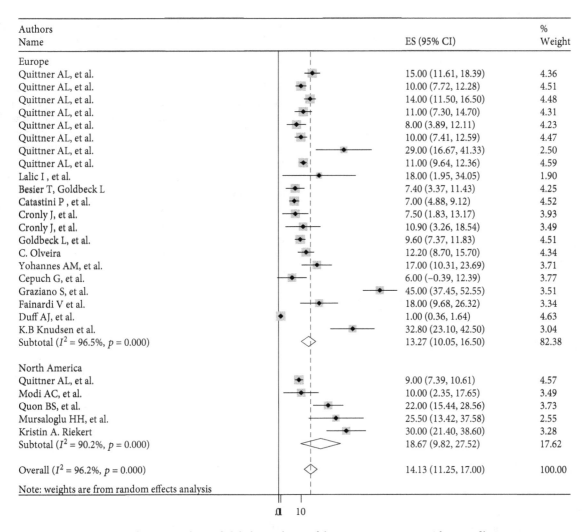

FIGURE 5: Subgroup analysis of global prevalence of depression in patients with cystic fibrosis.

TABLE 2: Metaregression analysis of factors affecting between-study heterogeneity of depression.

Heterogeneity source	Coefficients	Std. err.	p value
Publication year	0.3057765	0.6975618	0.665
Sample size	0.0058508	0.0041811	0.175

TABLE 3: Metaregression analysis of factors affecting between-study heterogeneity of anxiety.

Heterogeneity source	Coefficients	Std. err.	p value
Publication year	0.2517433	1.581655	0.875
Sample size	0.011806	0.0084867	0.179

and for general health perception, but to have similar scores for most psychosocial measures [44, 45]. Since Cystic fibrosis is a genetic disorder that damages many of the body's organs, on the top of medical treatment psychological treatment also helps to reduce anxiety and depression, improve adjustment, quality of life, and even medical outcomes, as well as knowledge, skills, and decisions regarding care.

This systematic review and meta-analysis estimated the pooled global prevalence of anxiety and depression among cystic fibrosis patients. Twenty-two studies were included in the analysis, which selected based on an inclusion criterion. To the best of our knowledge, this systematic review and meta-analysis provide a comprehensive estimation of the global pooled prevalence of anxiety and depression among cystic fibrosis patients. Depression and anxiety are more commonly observed in chronic diseases compared to the general population [46].

In this systematic review and meta-analysis, the overall pooled prevalence of anxiety and depression among cystic fibrosis patients was 26.22% (95% CI: 22.1, 30.2) and 12.66% (95% CI: 10.6, 14.6), respectively. This suggests that anxiety and depressive symptoms are common in CF patients, and it needs intensive and multifactorial approach that is required to combat the CF-related complications. Since CF is a life-threatening and incurable chronic medical disease, untreated anxiety and depression have a substantial impact on CF patients' quality of life, physical function, and healthcare utilization. Routine screening for symptoms of anxiety and depression is a worthy endeavor, and those identified with elevated clinical symptoms should be referred to

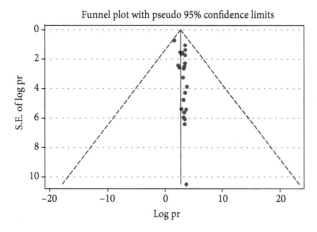

FIGURE 6: Funnel plot to test the publication bias in 24 studies of anxiety with 95% confidence limits.

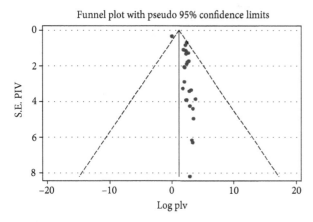

FIGURE 7: Funnel plot to test the publication bias of depression in 26 studies with 95% confidence limits.

receive appropriate treatment. This systematic review and meta-analysis have an implication for the health professional, patients, and patient's family.

In this systematic review and meta-analysis, we had the highest prevalence of anxiety among CF patients in Italia, 46% (95% CI: 38.44, 53.56), and lowest in North America, 10% (95% CI: 5.25, 14.75), whereas 45% (95% CI: 37.45, 52.55) in Italia and 6% (95% CI: -0.39, 12.39) in Poland, respectively, had prevalence of depression among CF patients. In subgroup analysis in Europe, we had 46% (95% CI: 38.44, 53.56) which has the highest prevalence of anxiety among CF patients in Italia and lowest in Germany, 12.3% (95% CI: 7.24, 17.36), whereas in Northern America, 35% (95% CI: 32.31, 37.69) and 10% (95% CI: 5.25, 14.75), respectively. For the highest prevalence of depression among CF patients in Europe, it was 45% (95% CI: 37.45, 52.55) in Italia and lowest in Poland, 6% (95% CI: -0.39, 12.39), whereas in North America, it is 25.5% (95% CI: 13.42, 37.58) and 9% (95% CI: 7.39, 10.61), respectively.

The strength of the systematic review and meta-analysis is the use of an extensive search strategy to incorporate the studies. On the other hand, studies are reported from a limited number of the country in the world and that may create underrepresentation. This systematic review and meta-

analysis presented up-to-date evidence on the global prevalence of anxiety and depression among cystic fibrosis patients.

This systematic review and meta-analysis might have faced the following limitations. First, the lack of primary studies other than Europe and northern America and may affect the generalizability of the finding. Secondly, due to there is significant heterogeneity and publication bias, the result needs to be interpreted cautiously. Thirdly, using different scales of the primary studies included in this systematic review and meta-analysis for screening depression and anxiety among CF patients might affect the pooled prevalence. Our final limitation is having difficulties in comparing our finding due to a lack of summarized and regional-wide systematic reviews and meta-analysis on the prevalence of anxiety and depression among CF patient.

5. Conclusion

The global prevalence of anxiety and depression among CF patient is common. Therefore, close monitoring of the patient, regularly screening for anxiety and depression and appropriate prevention techniques is recommended.

Abbreviations

CI:	Confidence interval
NOS:	Newcastle Ottawa Scale
OR:	Odds ratio
PRISMA:	Preferred Reporting Items for Systematic Reviews and Meta-Analyses.

Authors' Contributions

MT and TT developed the protocol and involved in the design, selection of study, data extraction, quality assessment, statistical analysis, results from interpretation, and developing the initial and final drafts of the manuscript.NA, RO, GD, and TL Involved in data extraction, quality assessment, statistical analysis, and revising subsequent drafts. All authors read and approved the final draft of the manuscript.

Acknowledgments

We would like to thank all authors of studies included in this systematic review and meta-analysis.

References

[1] American Psychiatric Association, *Diagnostic and Statistical Manual of Mental Disorders*, American Psychiatric Association, Arlington, Va, USA, 5th edition, 2013.

[2] M. Marcus, M. T. Yasamy, M. van Ommeren, D. Chisholm, and S. Saxena, *Depression: a global public health concern*, World Health Organization, 2012.

[3] World Health Organization, "World suicide prevention day 2012," 2013, http://www.who.int/mediacentre/events/annual/world_suicide_prevention_day/en/.

[4] M. O. Husain, S. P. Dearman, I. B. Chaudhry, N. Rizvi, and W. Waheed, "The relationship between anxiety, depression and illness perception In tberculosis patients in Pakistan," *Clinical Practice and Epidemiology in Mental Health*, vol. 4, no. 1, p. 4, 2008.

[5] World Health Organization, *Global Tuberculosis Control, WHO report 2013*, WHO, Geneva, 2013.

[6] WHO, "World health organization, fact sheet 2020," https://www.who.int/news-room/fact-sheets/detail/depression.

[7] GBD 2017 Disease and Injury Incidence and Prevalence Collaborators, "Global, Regional, and National Incidence, Prevalence, and Years Lived with Disability for 354 Diseases and Injuries for 195 Countries and Territories, 1990-2017: A Systematic Analysis for the Global Burden of Disease Study 2017," *The Lancet*, vol. 392, 2018.

[8] E. F. de Oliva Costa, M. M. V. Rocha, A. T. R. de Abreu Santos, E. V. de Melo, L. A. N. Martins, and T. M. Andrade, "Common mental disorders and associated factors among final-year healthcare students," *Revista da Associação Médica Brasileira*, vol. 60, no. 6, pp. 525-530, 2014.

[9] D. C. Kuo, M. Tran, A. A. Shah, and A. Matorin, "Depression and the suicidal patient," *Emergency Medicine Clinics of North America*, vol. 33, no. 4, pp. 765-778, 2015.

[10] M. A. Mall and J. S. Elborn, *ERS Monograph: Cystic Fibrosis*, European Respiratory Society, Sheffield, UK, 2014.

[11] G. S. Sawicki, C. L. Ren, M. W. Konstan et al., "Treatment complexity in cystic fibrosis: trends over time and associations with site-specific outcomes," *Journal of Cystic Fibrosis*, vol. 12, no. 5, pp. 461-467, 2013.

[12] A. L. Quittner, D. H. Barker, K. K. Marciel, and M. E. Grimley, "Cystic fibrosis: a model for drug discovery and patient care," in *Handbook of Pediatric Psychology*, M. C. Roberts and R. G. Steele, Eds., pp. 271-286, Guilford Press, New York, NY, 2009.

[13] E. J. Sims, M. Mugford, A. Clark et al., "Economic implications of newborn screening for cystic fibrosis: a cost of illness retrospective cohort study," *The Lancet*, vol. 369, no. 9568, pp. 1187-1195, 2007.

[14] K. A. Riekert, S. J. Bartlett, M. P. Boyle, J. A. Krishnan, and C. S. Rand, "The association between depression, lung function, and health-related quality of life among adults with cystic fibrosis," *Chest*, vol. 132, no. 1, pp. 231-237, 2007.

[15] K. B. Wells, J. M. Golding, and M. A. Burnam, "Chronic medical conditions in a sample of the general population with anxiety, affective, and substance use disorders," *The American Journal of Psychiatry*, vol. 146, no. 11, pp. 1440-1446, 1989.

[16] G. A. Brenes, "Anxiety and chronic obstructive pulmonary disease: prevalence, impact, and treatment," *Psychosomatic Medicine*, vol. 656, pp. 963-970, 2003.

[17] V. S. Fan and P. M. Meek, "Anxiety, depression, and cognitive impairment in patients with chronic respiratory disease," *Clinics in Chest Medicine*, vol. 35, no. 2, pp. 399-409, 2014.

[18] M. R. DiMatteo, H. S. Lepper, and T. W. Croghan, "Depression is a risk factor for noncompliance with medical treatment: meta-analysis of the effects of anxiety and depression on patient adherence," *Archives of internal medicine*, vol. 160, no. 14, pp. 2101-2107, 2000.

[19] R. Neuendorf, A. Harding, N. Stello, D. Hanes, and H. Wahbeh, "Depression and anxiety in patients with inflammatory bowel disease: a systematic review," *Journal of Psychosomatic Research*, vol. 87, pp. 70-80, 2016.

[20] G. Latchford and A. J. Duff, "Screening for depression in a single CF centre," *Journal of Cystic Fibrosis*, vol. 12, no. 6, pp. 794-796, 2013.

[21] M. D. Bethesda, "Cystic Fibrosis Foundation Patient Registry," 2012, 2012 Annual Data Report.

[22] A. L. Quittner, L. Goldbeck, J. Abbott et al., "Prevalence of depression and anxiety in patients with cystic fibrosis and parent caregivers: results of the international depression epidemiological study across nine countries," *Thorax*, vol. 69, no. 12, pp. 1090-1097, 2014.

[23] D. Moher, A. Liberati, J. Tetzlaff, D. G. Altman, and for the PRISMA Group, "Preferred Reporting Items for Systematic Reviews and Meta-analyses: the PRISMA statement," *BMJ*, vol. 339, 2009.

[24] A. Liberati, D. G. Altman, J. Tetzlaff et al., "The PRISMA Statement for Reporting Systematic Reviews and Meta-Analyses of studies that evaluate health care Interventions: explanation and elaboration," *PLoS Medicine*, vol. 6, no. 7, 2009.

[25] P. A. Modesti, G. Reboldi, F. P. Cappuccio et al., "Panethnic differences in blood pressure in Europe: a systematic review and meta-analysis," *PLoS One*, vol. 11, no. 1, p. e0147601, 2016.

[26] R. Herzog, M. J. Álvarez-Pasquin, C. Díaz, J. L. Del Barrio, J. M. Estrada, and Á. Gil, "Are healthcare workers' intentions to vaccinate related to their knowledge, beliefs and attitudes? a systematic review," *BMC Public Health*, vol. 13, no. 1, 2013.

[27] J. P. Higgins, S. G. Thompson, J. J. Deeks, and D. G. Altman, "Measuring inconsistency in meta-analyses," *BMJ*, vol. 327, no. 7414, pp. 557-560, 2003.

[28] I. Lalic, A. V. Dugac, T. Zovko et al., "Anxiety and depression in adult patients with cystic fibrosis in Croatia: results from adult CF centre," *European Respiratory Journal*, vol. 52, 2018.

[29] P. Catastini, S. di Marco, M. Furriolo et al., "The prevalence of anxiety and depression in Italian patients with cystic fibrosis and their caregivers," *Pediatric pulmonology*, vol. 51, no. 12, pp. 1311-1319, 2016.

[30] J. Cronly, A. J. Duff, K. A. Riekert et al., "Online versus paper-based screening for depression and anxiety in adults with cystic fibrosis in Ireland: a cross-sectional exploratory study," *BMJ open*, vol. 8, no. 1, 2018.

[31] L. Goldbeck, T. Besier, A. Hinz, S. Singer, and A. L. Quittner, "Prevalence of Symptoms of Anxiety and Depression in German Patients With Cystic Fibrosis," *Chest*, vol. 138, no. 4, pp. 929-936, 2010.

[32] A. C. Modi, K. A. Driscoll, K. Montag-Leifling, and J. D. Acton, "Screening for symptoms of depression and anxiety in adolescents and young adults with cystic fibrosis," *Pediatric pulmonology*, vol. 46, no. 2, pp. 153-159, 2011.

[33] C. Olveira, A. Sole, R. M. Girón et al., "Depression and anxiety symptoms in Spanish adult patients with cystic fibrosis:

associations with health-related quality of life," *General hospital psychiatry*, vol. 40, pp. 39–46, 2016.

[34] T. Besier and L. Goldbeck, "Anxiety and depression in adolescents with CF and their caregivers," *Journal of cystic fibrosis*, vol. 10, no. 6, pp. 435–442, 2011.

[35] B. S. Quon, W. D. Bentham, J. Unutzer, Y. F. Chan, C. H. Goss, and M. L. Aitken, "Prevalence of symptoms of depression and anxiety in adults with cystic fibrosis based on the PHQ-9 and GAD-7 screening questionnaires," *Psychosomatics*, vol. 56, no. 4, pp. 345–353, 2015.

[36] A. M. Yohannes, T. G. Willgoss, F. A. Fatoye, M. D. Dip, and K. Webb, "Relationship between anxiety, depression, and quality of life in adult patients with cystic fibrosis," *Respiratory care*, vol. 57, no. 4, pp. 550–556, 2012.

[37] H. H. Mursaloglu, C. Y. Yegit, A. Ergenekon et al., "Screening of depression and anxiety in cystic fibrosis patients/caregivers and evaluation of risk factors," *Authorea Preprints*, 2020.

[38] S. Graziano, B. Spanò, F. Majo et al., "Rates of depression and anxiety in Italian patients with cystic fibrosis and parent caregivers: implementation of the mental health guidelines," *Respiratory Medicine*, vol. 172, p. 106147, 2020.

[39] G. Cepuch, G. Dębska, J. Wordliczek, and H. Mazurek, "Evaluation of anxiety and depression incidence in adolescents with cystic fibrosis or malignant diseases," *Advances in Palliative Medicine*, vol. 6, no. 2, pp. 75–81, 2007.

[40] A. J. Duff, J. Abbott, C. Cowperthwaite et al., "Depression and anxiety in adolescents and adults with cystic fibrosis in the UK: a cross-sectional study," *Journal of Cystic Fibrosis*, vol. 13, no. 6, pp. 745–753, 2014.

[41] V. Fainardi, E. Iacinti, F. Longo, M. C. Tripodi, and G. Pisi, "P243 anxiety and depression in adolescents and adults with cystic fibrosis," *Thorax*, vol. 66, Suppl 4, p. A167, 2011.

[42] K. B. Knudsen, T. Pressler, L. H. Mortensen et al., "Associations between adherence, depressive symptoms and health-related quality of life in young adults with cystic fibrosis," *Springerplus*, vol. 5, no. 1, p. 1216, 2016.

[43] D. A. Pearson, A. J. Pumariega, and D. K. Seilheimer, "The development of psychiatric symptomatology in patients with cystic fibrosis," *Journal of the American Academy of Child and Adolescent Psychiatry*, vol. 30, no. 2, pp. 290–297, 1991.

[44] W. de Jong, A. A. Kaptein, C. P. van der Schans et al., "Quality of life in patients with cystic fibrosis," *Pediatric Pulmonology*, vol. 23, no. 2, pp. 95–100, 1997.

[45] M. T. Britto, U. R. Kotagal, R. W. Hornung, H. D. Atherton, J. Tsevat, and R. W. Wilmott, "Impact of recent pulmonary exacerbations on quality of life in patients with cystic fibrosis," *Chest*, vol. 121, no. 1, pp. 64–72, 2002.

[46] N. Meader, A. J. Mitchell, C. Chew-Graham et al., "Case identification of depression in patients with chronic physical health problems: a diagnostic accuracy meta-analysis of 113 studies," *The British Journal of General Practice*, vol. 61, no. 593, pp. e808–e820, 2011.

5

Assessment of Quality of Life of Epileptic Patients in Ethiopia

Esileman Abdela Muche, Mohammed Biset Ayalew ⓘ, and Ousman Abubeker Abdela ⓘ

Department of Clinical Pharmacy, School of Pharmacy, College of Medicine and Health Sciences, University of Gondar, Gondar, Ethiopia

Correspondence should be addressed to Ousman Abubeker Abdela; ousmy2009@gmail.com

Academic Editor: Tadeusz Robak

Background. Patients with epilepsy are at an increased risk of poor quality of life. *Purpose.* We aimed at assessing the quality of life and its determinants among epileptic patients at University of Gondar Referral Hospital (UoGRH), Ethiopia. *Methods.* Institution based cross-sectional study was conducted on epileptic patients on follow up at UoGRH from January 15 to April 15, 2017. Information including socio-demographic profile and diagnosis was extracted from medical records and patients. Quality Of Life In Epilepsy-10 (QOLIE-10) tool was used to measure the quality of life. Independent *t*-test and one-way analysis of variance were used to look for factors associated with quality of life. The level of statistical significance was declared at *P*-value ≤ 0.05. *Results.* A total of 354 patients were included in the study and mean age was 29.1 ± 11.7 years. The mean QOLIE-10 score was 19.85. One hundred ninety-four (54.8%) of participants had a good quality of life. Being illiterate, unemployment, and presence of co-morbid medical condition were associated with poorer quality of life. *Conclusion.* Nearly half of the participants had a poor quality of life. Patients with co-morbidity, illiteracy, and unemployment should be given special emphasis in order to improve their quality of life.

1. Introduction

The International League Against Epilepsy (ILAE) defines epilepsy as a disease of the brain defined by any of the following conditions: (i) At least two unprovoked (or reflex) seizures occurring > 24 h apart; (ii) one unprovoked (or reflex) seizure and a probability of further seizures similar to the general recurrence risk (at least 60%) after two unprovoked seizures, occurring over the next 10 years; or (iii) diagnosis of an epilepsy syndrome [1].

Epilepsy affects people of any age, gender, ethnicity, and social background, irrespective of geographic location. It is the most common chronic serious neurologic disease [2]. About 10% of the whole world population living a normal life span can expect to have at least one epileptic seizure. At least 50 million will have recurrent seizures. This could be underestimated, as partial seizures are often not recognized as such in the developing world [3]. The point prevalence of active epilepsy was 6.38 per 1,000 persons while the lifetime prevalence was 7.60 per 1,000 persons [4]. In a large community-based epidemiological study, the prevalence of epilepsy in Ethiopia was reported as 5.2 per 1000 population. The incidence was 64 per 100,000 population [5].

Growing recognition of the importance of the psychosocial effects of epilepsy has led to the need to quantify the quality of life in affected individuals. Patients with epilepsy are at increased risk of poor Quality of Life (QOL) [6, 7]. WHO defines quality of life as the perception that an individual has of his place in existence, in the context of culture and system securities in which they live, and in relation to their goals, expectations, standards, and concerns [8]. Different tools were used to standardize this concept and many studies evaluated the quality of life of epileptic patients using various types of questionnaires. QOLIE-10 questionnaire, which was used in this study, is a valid and reliable tool used to measure the QoL of patients with epilepsy which was validated by Cramer et al. [9].

People with epilepsy face a condition that can affect their QoL in multiple domains. These include physical (increased risk of injury and death), psychological (increased risk of anxiety and depression), cognitive (both epilepsy and the medications used to treat it are associated with impaired cognition), and social and occupational (epilepsy is a stigmatizing condition, and also often carries limitations on driving and employment) [10]. Hence, assessment of QoL is important in the management of epilepsy to achieve the optimal goal of therapy.

The existing studies also revealed that individuals with epilepsy suffer from a number of social, psychological and physical poor outcomes. For example, a study conducted in Ethiopia revealed that 60% of the study participants faced different problems due to their illness such as stigma (24%), inability to find a partner (31%), educational problems (17%), and problems of employment (9%)[11]. The recently released Ethiopian mental health strategic plan emphasizes the special considerations to be given to these vulnerable patient groups [12].

Though different studies have been conducted in different parts of the world including Africa, very few studies were undertaken on quality of life of epilepsy patients in Ethiopia. The evidence for the different socio-demographic characteristics like level of education, age, marital status, employment status and some clinical characteristics of epileptic patients as a factor for QoL is inconsistent [13]. The aim of this study was to determine the quality of life of epileptic patients who were taking anti-epileptic drugs and to identify factors associated with it. This study can help as an input for hospital managers' performance measurement and to improve treatment outcomes of epileptic patients. It can also be used as baseline information for researchers who need to conduct further study in the area.

2. Materials and Methods

2.1. Study Area and Period. The study was conducted at University of Gondar Referral Hospital, North-West Ethiopia. It is one of the biggest tertiary level referral and teaching hospital in the region. It provides service for an estimated 7 million population. The hospital serves as a referral center for North Gondar administrative region and the residents around. It has 400 beds in five different inpatient departments and 14 wards. Patients with Neurologic disorders get service two days per week. The service is given by two neurologists. There are around 2200 epileptic patients on follow up. Data was collected from January 15 to April 15, 2017.

2.2. Study Design and Subjects. We employed hospital-based prospective cross sectional study. Adult epileptic patients who were on follow up in UoGRH were included as a study subject. We excluded epileptic patients who were less than 18 years old, those who were on antiepileptic drugs (AEDs) for less than one year period, patients with incomplete information on their chart and involuntary and uncooperative patients.

2.3. Sample Size & Sampling Methods. The sample size was calculated using single population proportion formula, where $Z = 1.96$, $\alpha/2$, $P = 54.2\%$, taken from a study done on similar setting [14], and 5% for d (margin of error). The total sample size calculated was 381. Since the source population were <10,000 the sample was recalculated using correction formula which gave the sample size of 324. After adding 10% contingency the final sample size became 356. We used systematic random sampling to recruit participants in each data collection day. The sampling fraction (k) was calculated through dividing the number of study population available

each day by the maximum possible number of patients' that could be interviewed the same day. Every k^{th} patient was then interviewed following physician's visit.

2.4. Data Collection Instrument. Data was taken from patients' medical chart and patient interview using data extraction format; which was pretested in 18 patients (5% of calculated sample size) in Felegehiwot referral hospital. Little adjustment was made to clarify questions. QOLIE-10 questionnaire was used to assess quality of life of epileptic patients [9]. There were 10 questions about health and daily activities, one question about how much distress they feel about problems and worries related to epilepsy, and a review of what bothers them most. Two individuals who were fluent in both the English and Amharic languages translated the QOLIE-10 into Amharic version. The new Amharic version of QOLIE-10 was back-translated into English to ensure that the meaning and comprehension of the original version was retained. The Amharic version of the questionnaire was also checked for both the accuracy and meaning of the translated versions before finalized.

2.5. Data Collection Procedures. Six BSc nurses who had basic knowledge of epilepsy treatment collected the data from January 15 to April 15, 2017. Patient demographics, diagnosis, co-morbid conditions and type of drug were collected on the patient charts by using well designed data extraction format. Information needed to measure patients' quality of life was collected through face to face interview using Amharic version of QOLIE-10 questionnaire. Data collectors were trained for 2 days on the documentation and techniques of data collection. Medical chart number was documented to avoid repetition of participants. The principal investigators reviewed all filled data abstraction formats daily.

2.6. Data Processing and Analysis. Data was entered into SPSS version 20.0 for analysis. We applied double entry to check whether the data was entered correctly or not. Descriptive statistics was used for demographic details and inferential statistical tests like the *t*-test for independent variables. Analysis of variance (ANOVA) was used to compare QOL scores among various socio-demographic factors and clinical characteristics. Level of statistical significance was declared at P-value ≤ 0.05. Quality of life was considered as poor If QOLIE-10 Score for individual patient was less than the mean QOLIE-10 score for the study population.

The overall quality of life score represent the summation of all 10 item questions in the QOLIE-10 instrument. The questionnaire used has minimum score of 10 and maximum score of 50. Higher score indicate poor QoL and the lower the score the better QoL.

2.7. Ethical Consideration. We obtained letter of ethical clearance from ethical review board of school of pharmacy and letter of cooperation from UoGRH hospital. Each participant was informed about the objective of the study, procedures of selection and assurance of confidentiality. Oral consent was taken from participants before data collection. Privacy and confidentiality were ensured during patient interview and

TABLE 1: Socio-demographic characteristics of study participants, UoGRH, 2017.

Variables	Categories	Frequency (n)	Percent (%)
Age	18–25	167	47.2
	26–44	150	42.4
	>45	37	10.5
Sex	Male	216	61.0
	Female	138	39.0
Marital status	Single	224	63.3
	Married	89	25.1
	Divorced	31	8.8
	Widowed	10	2.8
Religion	Orthodox	317	89.7
	Protestant	7	1.9
	Muslim	28	7.9
	Jehovah	2	.5
Educational status	Illiterate	107	30.2
	Primary school	111	31.4
	Secondary school	84	23.7
	Diploma and above	52	14.7
Residency	Rural	145	41.0
	Urban	209	59.0
House hold income	<22$*	114	32.2
	22–66$	136	38.4
	66.1–132$	72	20.3
	132.1–220$	24	6.8
	≥220.1$	8	2.3
Occupation	Unemployed	54	15.3
	House wife	28	7.9
	Merchant or private worker	53	15.0
	Student	96	27.1
	Daily laborer	25	7.1
	Farmer	56	15.8
	Others	42	11.9
	Purchase	212	59.9

*$ = USD (United States Dollar).

TABLE 2: Clinical characteristics of study participants at UoGRH; Northwest Ethiopia, 2017.

Clinical character	Category	Frequency (n)	Percent (%)
Age at diagnosis	≤15 years old	104	29.4
	16–30 years old	194	54.8
	31–45 years old	34	9.6
	>46 years old	22	6.2
Types of seizure/ epilepsy	Focal seizure	5	1.4
	Generalized tonic-clonic epilepsy	305	86.2
	Unclassified epileptic	44	12.4
Number of AEDs	Monotherapy	291	82.2
	Two drug combination	62	17.5
	Three drug combination	1	0.3
Presence of comorbidity	Yes	36	10.2
	No	318	89.8
Duration of epilepsy	<3 years	105	29.7
	3–5 years	69	19.5
	6–10 years	89	25.1
	>10 years	91	25.7
Frequency of seizure during last follow up	No seizure	250	70.6
	1 or 2 seizure	79	22.3
	3–5 seizure	15	4.2
	>5 seizure	10	2.8
Frequency of seizure during last year	Free of seizure	129	36.4
	1–5 seizure	193	54.5
	6–10 seizure	20	5.6
	>10	12	3.4
Current status of epilepsy	Controlled	129	36.4
	Improving	199	56.2
	No change	20	5.6
	Deteriorated	6	1.7

review of patients chart. Name and address of the participants were not recorded in the data extraction formats.

3. Results

3.1. Socio-Demographic Characteristics of Study Subjects. Out of the total 356 epileptic patients enrolled, 354 of them completed the interview and included in the analysis. The mean age of participants was 29.1 ± 11.7 years with a range of 18–88 years. More than half (61%) of respondents were male, quarter of the participants (25%) were married, 209(59%) were from urban area, 218(61.6%) of respondents were below primary school in educational background and most of the participants (89.7%) were orthodox Christian in religion.

One third of participants were students, 70.6% had below 66 USD household monthly incomes. The detailed description of socio-demographic characteristics of the study participants is shown in Table 1.

3.2. Clinical Characteristics of the Study Subjects. Most of the patients (63.8%) had at least one episode of seizure a year before. The mean age of onset of epilepsy was 22 ± 12.1 years, the mean duration of epilepsy was 7.8 ± 6.4 years. Most (82.2%) of participants were on a single AED (Table 2).

3.3. Participants' Response to Quality of Life Assessment Questions. Participants mean quality of life in epilepsy-10 (QOLIE-10) score was 19.86 ± 6.91, with a minimum and maximum score of 10 and 40 respectively. Equivalent mean quality of life result was 75.36%. One hundred ninety four

TABLE 3: Response of patients for quality of life assessment questions, UoGRH, Northwest Ethiopia; 2017.

QOLIE-10 questions	All the time N (%)	Most of the time N (%)	Sometimes N (%)	Rarely N (%)	Never N (%)
Did you have enough energy for the last month?	151 (42.6)	101 (28.5)	47 (13.3)	25 (7)	30 (11.9)
Have you felt down-hearted and blue?	28 (7.9)	64 (18)	88 (24.9)	54 (15.3)	120 (33.9)
	Not at all N (%)	A little N (%)	Somewhat N (%)	A lot N (%)	A great deal N (%)
Has your epilepsy/AED caused your daily life to be terrible?	191 (54)	61 (17.2)	50 (14.1)	37 (10.5)	15 (4.2)
How much are you bothered by memory difficulty	193 (54.5)	44 (12.4)	60 (17)	40 (11.3)	17 (4.8)
How much are you bothered by work limitation?	189 (53.4)	49 (13.8)	61 (17.2)	43 (12.2)	12 (3.4)
How much are you bothered by social limitation?	214 (60.5)	41 (11.6)	39 (11)	30 (8.5)	28 (7.9)
How much are you bothered by physical effect of AED?	280 (79.1)	18 (5.1)	22 (6.2)	14 (3.9)	20 (5.6)
How much are you bothered by mental effect of AED?	236 (66.6)	40 (11.3)	34 (9.6)	24 (6.8)	20 (5.7)
How fearful are you of having seizure during the next month?	185 (52.2)	77 (21.7)	31 (8.7)	39 (11)	21 (5.9)
	Very well N (%)	Pretty good N (%)	Good = bad N (%)	Pretty bad N (%)	Very bad N (%)
How has the quality of your life been during the past 4 weeks? That is, how have things been going for you?	58 (16.4)	170 (48.0)	108 (30.5)	16 (4.5)	2 (0.6)

(54.8%) of participants had a good quality of life. Two hundred sixty one (73.7%) of participants had enough energy for most of their time, but 180(50.85%) of the patients feel down hearted or blue for at least some of their time. For more than half (54%) of patients, their epilepsy and or AEDs didnot terribly disturb their daily life (Table 3).

3.4. Factors Associated with Quality of Life. One way ANOVA analysis of QOLIE-10 scales with socio demographics and clinical characteristics showed that educational status, occupation, income, frequency of seizure during last follow up, frequency of seizure during a year before, number of AEDs and patient's perception of current status of epilepsy have significant association with quality of life.Independent *t*-test also showed that presence of co-morbidity and methods of acquiring AEDs, were significantly associated with quality of life (Table 4).

Note: independent *t*-test was done for variables with 2 categories and one way ANOVA was done for those variables with 3 or more categories.

After detecting the presence of association between some of the patients' characteristics and quality of life using one way ANOVA, then Post hock analysis was done to determine where the significant mean difference lies. Accordingly illiterates, unemployed individuals and patients with less than 22 USD monthly incomes had significantly poorer quality of life as compared to their counter parts. Patients who perceive their epilepsy status was controlled had better quality of life as

compared to patients who thought that it was improved, deteriorated or had no change (Table 5).

4. Discussion

The mean QOLIE-10 score in this study was 19.86 (75.3%). This result is in line with the study in Bangalore, India, which reported a mean quality of life of 74.9% [15]. However this finding was higher than many other studies conducted in different part of the world [14, 16–20]. This difference may be explained by the presence of high percentage of two or more AEDs use in those studies in contrast to the finding in the current study. Different literatures suggested that patients receiving two or more AEDs had poor quality of life as compared to patients on monotherapy [14, 21–24].

The higher rate of monotherapy (82.2%) reported in this study is in line with the result of previous studies done in Ethiopia. The study conducted on two hospitals in Northwest Ethiopia reported that 76.7% of epileptic patients were on monotherapy [25]. Another study in Bishoftu general hospital also reported monotherapy users to be 78.6% [26] and a study done by Birru et al. also found that 80.35% [27] of studied patients used single drug for treatment of their epilepsy. However Gurshaw et al. reported only 54.5% of studied epileptic patients in Jimma university hospital used monotherapy [28].

In this study, various socio-demographic and clinical characteristics were checked for their possible influence on quality of life. Significantly poor QoL was seen among people who

TABLE 4: Association of socio demographics and clinical characteristics with quality of life of epileptic patients, Northwest Ethiopia; 2017.

Characteristics	Category	Frequency (%)	QOLIE-10 (mean)	P-Value
Gender	Male	216 (61)	19.5926	0.371
	Female	138 (39)	20.2681	
Age		29.0 ± 11.7 (mean ± SD)		0.515
Address	Urban	209 (59)	19.5694	0.350
	Rural	145 (41)	20.2690	
Marital status	Single	224 (63.3)	19.7188	0.342
	Married	89 (25.1)	19.3933	
	Divorced	31 (8.8)	21.3226	
	Widowed	10 (2.8)	22.5000	
Educational status	Illiterate	107 (30.2)	21.6636	0.003*
	Primary school	111 (31.4)	19.7387	
	Secondary school	84 (23.7)	19.0357	
	Diploma and above	52 (14.7)	17.7115	
Religion	Orthodox	317 (89.5)	20.0365	0.793
	Protestant	7 (2)	19.7500	
	Islam	28 (7.9)	20.0000	
	Jehovah	2 (0.6)	13.0000	
Patient occupation	Unemployed	54 (15.3)	23.2778	0.003*
	House wife	28 (7.9)	20.6429	
	Merchant or private worker	53 (15.0)	18.9057	
	Student	96 (27.1)	19.3542	
	Daily laborer	25 (7.1)	19.0400	
	Farmer	56 (15.8)	19.8214	
	Others[a]	42 (11.9)	17.8095	
Monthly household income	<22 $*	114 (32.2)	21.4123	0.024*
	22–66$	136 (38.4)	19.4265	
	66.1–132$	72 (20.3)	19.3472	
	132.1–220$	24 (6.8)	17.1250	
	≥220.1$	8 (2.3)	17.7500	
Method of acquiring AED	Free	142 (40.1)	20.9718	0.013*
	Purchase	212 (59.9)	19.1085	
Age of onset	<15 years	104 (29.4)	19.4712	0.859
	16–30	194 (54.8)	19.8918	
	31–45	34 (9.6)	20.5000	
	>46	22 (6.2)	20.3636	
Types of seizure	Focal seizure	5 (1.4)	22.8000	0.469
	GTCS	305 (86.2)	19.7049	
	Unclassified epileptic	44 (12.4)	20.5682	
Duration of epilepsy (years)	<3	105 (29.7)	19.1810	0.554
	3–5	69 (19.5)	19.5652	
	5–10	89 (25.1)	20.4157	
	>10	91 (25.7)	20.3077	
Number of AEDs for treatment	Mono-therapy	291 (82.2)	19.4330	0.020*
	Two or more drug combination	63 (17.8)	21.8095	
Frequency of seizure during last follow up	No seizure	250 (70.6)	18.6240	0.001*
	1-2 seizure	79 (22.3)	21.1646	
	3–5 seizure	15 (4.2)	28.1333	
	>5 seizure	10 (2.8)	27.9000	
Frequency of seizure during last year	No seizure	129 (36.4)	17.4186	0.001*
	1–5	193 (54.5)	20.7098	
	6–10	20 (5.6)	24.8000	
	>10	12 (3.4)	24.0833	

TABLE 4: Continued.

Characteristics	Category	Frequency (%)	QOLIE-10 (mean)	P-Value
Presence of co-morbidity	Yes	36 (10.2)	22.5278	0.014*
	No	318 (89.8)	19.5535	
Patient perception of epilepsy status	Controlled	129 (36.4)	17.1938	0.001*
	Improving	199 (56.2)	20.9598	
	No change	20 (5.6)	24.7000	
	Deteriorated	6 (1.7)	24.3333	

*Significant association. GTCS: Generalized tonic clonic epilepsy. $ = USD (United States Dollar).

TABLE 5: Post-hoc analysis of demographic and clinical characteristics of patients which have significant association with quality of life in one way ANOVA, UoGRH, Northwest Ethiopia.

Characteristics	Reference category	Compared with	Mean difference	Standard error	P value	95% confidence interval	
Educational status	Illiterate	Primary school	1.92481	.92214	.038	.111	3.738
		Secondary school	2.62784	.99222	.008	.676	4.579
		Diploma and above	3.95201	1.15061	.001	1.689	6.215
Occupation	Unemployed	Merchant or private worker	4.37212	1.31080	.001	1.794	6.950
		Student	3.92361	1.15317	.001	1.655	6.191
		Daily laborer	4.23778	1.63994	.010	1.012	7.463
		Farmer	3.45635	1.29296	.008	.9133	5.999
		Others	5.46825	1.39474	.000	2.725	8.211
Income	<22$*	22–66 $	1.98581	.86855	.023	.2776	3.694
		66.1–132$	2.06506	1.02963	.046	.0400	4.090
		132.1–220$	4.28728	1.53612	.006	1.266	7.308
Patient perception of epilepsy status	Controlled	Improving	−3.76600	.74283	.000	−5.227	−2.305
		No change	−7.50620	1.57928	.000	−10.612	−4.400
		Deteriorated	−7.13953	2.74455	.010	−12.537	−1.741
	Improving	Controlled	3.76600	.74283	.000	2.305	5.227
		No change	−3.74020	1.54154	.016	−6.772	−.708
Frequency of seizure during last year	No seizure	1–5 seizure/year	−3.29124	.75071	.000	−4.767	−1.814
		5–10 seizure/year	−7.38140	1.58636	.000	−10.501	−4.261
		>10 seizure/year	−6.66473	1.99225	.001	−10.583	−2.746
Frequency of seizure during last follow up	1–5 seizure	5–10 seizure/follow up	−4.09016	1.55065	.009	−7.139	−1.040
	No seizure	1 or 2 seizure/follow up	−2.54056	.83566	.003	−4.184	−.897
		3 up to 5 seizure/follow up	−9.50933	1.72116	.000	−12.894	−6.124
		More than 5 seizure/follow up	−9.27600	2.08800	.000	−13.382	−5.169
	1 or 2 seizures	3–5 seizure/follow up	−6.96878	1.82355	.000	−10.555	−3.382
		>5 seizure/follow up	−6.73544	2.17317	.002	−11.009	−2.461

$ = USD (United States Dollar).

had no formal education. This finding is supported by many other studies [16, 29–31]. The poor QoL observed in illiterate patients may be due to the lesser knowledge they may have about the diseases and its treatment; as well as they may not easily understand instructions given from health professionals and this may result in poor adherence to medication and poorer seizure control which may finally lead to poor quality of life.

Marital status did not significantly influence QoL. Although this result is in agreement with the study done in India [15], it is contrasting with the result of the studies conducted in Malaysia, Iran and China. [31–33]. Quality of life of unemployed patients is significantly lower than those of epileptic patients who have a job. This may be because job gives mental satisfaction. Those who are unemployed get bored and face more cognitive problems. This finding is similar to the study done by Singh and Pandey [31] and Ashjazadeh et al. [32]. Mean QOLIE-10 score of patients with household monthly income <22 USD was 21.4. The score is significantly higher (lower quality of life) than for patients who got 22 USD or more per month. Therefore, income significantly affected quality of life of epileptic patients. This is consistent with the result of the study done from the US Centers for Disease Control and Prevention Managing Epilepsy Well Network [34].

Patients who have access to AEDs free of charge and those who purchase their drug out of pocket had mean QOLIE-10 score of 20.97 and 19.12 respectively. Independent t-test result showed there is significant difference in QOL score between these 2 groups. Accordingly to those who spent money to buy drug have better quality of life than who get freely. The possible explanation for this may be those who spent money to buy drugs may have better medication adherence than patients who got drugs freely.

Frequent seizure during last follow up and a year before leads to poorer quality of life score as compared to no seizure. Literatures support the finding of this study in which people with frequent seizures had significantly poorer health related QOL than those with infrequent or no seizures [15, 16, 34–36]. This finding emphasizes the importance of encouraging patients to observe symptoms of the onset of a seizure (aura, tingling, numbness, headaches, confusion, etc.), record them, and share the information with their health-care provider. Health education interventions involving medication intake, diet, regular sleep, exercise, and stress reduction can all aid in reducing seizure frequency so that patients will have better quality of life.

Patients who were taking two or more AEDs had lower quality of life as compared to patients who took single AED. Similar result was found in many other previous studies [14, 15, 21–24, 37]. Patients who perceive that their current status of epilepsy was controlled had better quality of life than patients who perceive that their epilepsy was improving, had no change or had deteriorated. In addition patients who perceived their disease is improving had better quality of life than those who perceived nothing is changed. As patients perceive their epilepsy is controlled or improving, their worry about the illness and the fear of seizure recurrence will reduce and patient will have improved quality of life. Patients who had co morbid diseases had a worse quality of life than those who have only epilepsy. Similar association was reported by Tegegne et al. [26].

Age, gender, place of residency, religion, age at diagnosis of epilepsy and duration on AEDs had no significant association with quality of life. Similar nonsignificant association of Patient's age, age at onset of epilepsy and duration of AEDs with quality of life was reported by Tegegne et al. [26]. Patients' gender did not significantly affect quality of life ($p = 0.371$). Similar result was reported by Singh and Pandey [31].

Even though the use of validated tool, excellent response rate and sufficient sample size were the strengths of this study, it is not without limitation. The cross-sectional nature of this study did not allow establishing casual relation between quality of life and the different factors associated with it. The participants were recruited from one medical center in Northwest Ethiopia. Therefore, the findings may not be generalizable to all PWE in Ethiopia. Although the concept of QOL is very broad and can be influenced by multiple variables, some other clinical and socio-demographic conditions were not addressed in the study (e.g., severity of seizures, anxiety disorders, sleep disorder, specific structural/metabolic cause of epilepsy, and family support, among others) which could affect QOL.

5. Conclusion

Nearly half of participants had poor quality of life. Presence of co-morbidity, usage of two or more AEDs, illiteracy, unemployment and monthly income of less than 22 USD were significantly associated with poor quality of life. Patients with such characteristics should be given special emphasis to improve their quality of life. Patients perception of their epilepsy status as controlled or improved, absence of seizure episode during the past 1 year period and lesser number of seizure episodes during the last follow up were significantly related with a better quality of life.

Abbreviations

AED:	Anti-epileptic drug
ANOVA:	Analysis of variance
GTCS:	Generalized tonic clonic seizure
ILAE:	The international league against epilepsy
OPD:	Outpatient department
PWE:	Patients with epilepsy
QoL:	Quality of Life
QOLIE-10:	Quality of life in epilepsy ten
SPSS:	Statistical package for social science
UoGRH:	University of gondar referral hospital
WHO:	World health organization
USD:	United States dollar.

Ethical Approval

Ethical clearance was obtained from the Ethical Review Committee of School of Pharmacy, University of Gondar. The respondents were informed about the purpose of the study and their consent to participate was obtained.

Acknowledgments

We would like to thank University of Gondar for funding this research project. We are also very grateful to the nursing staffs of chronic outpatient department of UoGRH for their cooperation in the data collection process.

References

[1] R. S. Fisher, C. Acevedo, A. Arzimanoglou et al., "Practical clinical definition of epilepsy," *Epilepsia*, vol. 55, no. 4, pp. 475–482, 2014.

[2] E. Perucca, A. Covanis, and T. Dua, "Commentary: epilepsy is a global problem," *Epilepsia*, vol. 55, no. 9, pp. 1326–1328, 2014.

[3] WHO, *Epilepsy in the WHO African Region: Bridging the Gap. The Global Campaign against Epilepsy*, WHO, Geneva, Switzerland, 2004.

[4] K. M. Fiest, K. M. Sauro, S. Wiebe, S. B. Patten, C.-S. Kwon, and J. Dykeman, "Prevalence and incidence of epilepsy a systematic review and meta-analysis of international studies," *Neurology*, vol. 88, no. 3, pp. 296–303, 2017.

[5] R. Tekle-Haimanot, L. Forsgren, and J. Ekstedt, "Incidence of epilepsy in rural central Ethiopia," *Epilepsia*, vol. 38, no. 5, pp. 541–6, 1997.

[6] A. Gholami, S. Salarilak, P. Lotfabadi, F. Kiani, A. Rajabi, and K. Mansori, "Quality of life in epileptic patients compared with healthy people," *Medical Journal of the Islamic Republic of Iran*, vol. 30, p. 388, 2016.

[7] M. P. Kerr, "The impact of epilepsy on patients' lives," *Acta Neurologica Scandinavica Supplementum*, vol. 194, pp. 1–9, 2012.

[8] A. Jacoby, D. Snape, and G. A. Baker, "Determinants of quality of life in people with epilepsy," *Neurologic Clinics*, vol. 27, no. 4, pp. 843–863, 2009.

[9] J. A. Cramer, K. Perrine, O. Devinsky, and K. Meador, "A brief questionnaire to screen for quality of life in epilepsy. The QOLIE-10," *Epilepsia*, vol. 37, no. 6, pp. 577–592, 1996.

[10] B. N. Blond, K. Detyniecki, and L. J. Hirsch, "Assessment of treatment side effects and quality of life in people with epilepsy," *Neurologic Clinics*, vol. 34, no. 2, pp. 395–410, 2016.

[11] S. Birhanu, S. Alemu, J. Asmera, and M. Prevett, "Primary care treatment of epilepsy," *Ethiopian Journal of Health Development*, vol. 16, no. 3, pp. 235–240, 2002.

[12] S. Fdroemo, *National Mental Health Strategy 2012/13-2015/16*, Federal Democratic Republic of Ethiopia Ministry of Health, Geneva, Switzerland, 2012.

[13] R. S. Taylor, J. W. Sander, R. J. Taylor, and G. A. Baker, "Predictors of health-related quality of life and costs in adults with epilepsy: a systematic review," *Epilepsia*, vol. 52, no. 12, pp. 2168–2180, 2011.

[14] M. T. Tegegne, N. Y. Muluneh, T. T. Wochamo, A. A. Awoke, T. B. Mossie, and M. A. Yesigat, "Assessment of quality of life and associated factors among people with epilepsy attending at Amanuel Mental Specialized Hospital, Addis Ababa Ethiopia," *Science Journal of Public Health*, vol. 2, no. 5, pp. 378–383, 2014.

[15] J. George, C. Kulkarni, and G. Sarma, "Antiepileptic drugs and quality of life in patients with epilepsy: a tertiary care hospital-based study," *Value in Health Regional Issues*, vol. 6, pp. 1–6, 2015.

[16] M. Anu, K. Suresh, and P. Basavanna, "A cross-sectional study of quality of life among subjects with epilepsy attending a tertiary care hospital," *Journal of Clinical and Diagnostic Research*, vol. 10, no. 12, 2016.

[17] H.-F. Chen, Y.-F. Tsai, M.-S. Hsi, and J.-C. Chen, "Factors affecting quality of life in adults with epilepsy in Taiwan: a cross-sectional, correlational study," *Epilepsy & Behavior*, vol. 58, pp. 26–32, 2016.

[18] M. Nagarathnam, B. Vengamma, S. Latheef, and K. Reddemma, "Assessment of quality of life in epilepsy in Andhra Pradesh," *NeurologyAsia*, vol. 19, no. 3, 2014.

[19] B. Norsa'adah, J. Zainab, and A. Knight, "The quality of life of people with epilepsy at a tertiary referral centre in Malaysia," *Health and Quality of Life Outcomes*, vol. 11, no. 1, pp. 111–143, 2013.

[20] C. A. E. Jovel, S. R. Salazar, C. R. Rodríguez, and F. E. S. Mejía, "Factors associated with quality of life in a low-income population with epilepsy," *Epilepsy Research*, vol. 127, pp. 168–174, 2016.

[21] A. Sinha, D. Sanyal, S. Mallik, P. Sengupta, and S. Dasgupta, "Factors associated with quality of life of patients with epilepsy attending a tertiary care hospital in Kolkata, India," *Neurology Asia*, vol. 16, no. 1, 2011.

[22] G. A. Baker, A. Jacoby, J. Gorry, J. Doughty, and V. Ellina, "Quality of life of people with epilepsy in Iran, the Gulf, and Near East," *Epilepsia*, vol. 46, no. 1, pp. 132–140, 2005.

[23] K. S. Mosaku, F. O. Fatoye, M. Komolafe, M. Lawal, and B. A. Ola, "Quality of life and associated factors among adults with epilepsy in Nigeria," *The International Journal of Psychiatry in Medicine*, vol. 36, no. 4, pp. 469–481, 2006.

[24] S. A. Pimpalkhute, C. S. Bajait, G. N. Dakhale, S. D. Sontakke, K. M. Jaiswal, and P. Kinge, "Assessment of quality of life in epilepsy patients receiving anti-epileptic drugs in a tertiary care teaching hospital," *Indian Journal of Pharmacology*, vol. 47, no. 5, p. 551, 2015.

[25] A. Getnet, S. Meseret, L. Bekana, T. Mekonen, W. Fekadu, and M. Menberu, "Antiepileptic drug nonadherence and its predictors among people with epilepsy," *Behavioural Neurology*, vol. 2016, no. 3, pp. 1–6, 2016.

[26] M. F. S. Wakjira Rishe, K. G. Belayneh, G. Thirumurgan, T. Esayas, and M. A. M. Gebremariam, "Drug use evaluation of anti-epileptic drugs in out patient epilepsy clinic of Bishoftu general hospital, East Shoa, Ethiopia," *Indo American Journal of Pharmaceutical Research*, vol. 5, no. 2, 2015.

[27] E. M. Birru, M. Shafi, and M. Geta, "Drug therapy of epileptic seizures among adult epileptic outpatients of University of gondar referral and Teaching hospital, gondar, North West Ethiopia," *Dovepress*, vol. 2016, no. 12, pp. 3213–3219, 2016.

[28] M. Gurshaw, A. Agalu, and T. Chanie, "Anti-epileptic drug utilization and treatment outcome among epileptic patients on follow-up in a resource poor setting," *Journal of Young Pharmacists*, vol. 6, no. 3, p. 47, 2014.

[29] C. B. Josephson, S. B. Patten, A. Bulloch, J. V. Williams, D. Lavorato, and K. M. Fiest, "The impact of seizures on epilepsy

outcomes: a national, community-based survey," *Epilepsia*, vol. 58, no. 5, pp. 764–771, 2017.

[30] E. Brusturean-Bota, C. A. Coadă, A. D. Buzoianu, and L. Perju-Dumbravă, "Assessment of quality of life in patients with epilepsy," *Human & Veterinary Medicine*, vol. 5, no. 3, pp. 129–134, 2013.

[31] P. Singh and A. K. Pandey, "Quality of life in epilepsy," *International Journal of Research in Medical Sciences*, vol. 5, no. 2, pp. 452–455, 2017.

[32] N. Ashjazadeh, G. Yadollahikhales, A. Ayoobzadehshirazi, N. Sadraii, and N. Hadi, "Comparison of the health-related quality of life between epileptic patients with partial and generalized seizure," *Iranian Journal of Neurology*, vol. 13, no. 2, p. 94, 2014.

[33] F.-L. Wang, X.-M. Gu, B.-Y. Hao, S. Wang, Z.-J. Chen, and C.-Y. Ding, "Influence of marital status on the quality of life of chinese adult patients with epilepsy," *Chinese Medical Journal*, vol. 130, no. 1, p. 83, 2017.

[34] M. Sajatovic, C. Tatsuoka, E. Welter, D. Friedman, T. M. Spruill, and S. Stoll, "Correlates of quality of life among individuals with epilepsy enrolled in self-management research: from the US Centers for Disease Control and Prevention Managing Epilepsy Well," *Network Epilepsy & Behavior*, vol. 69, pp. 177–180, 2017.

[35] M. Djibuti and R. Shakarishvili, "Influence of clinical, demographic, and socioeconomic variables on quality of life in patients with epilepsy: findings from Georgian study," *Journal of Neurology, Neurosurgery & Psychiatry*, vol. 74, no. 5, pp. 570–573, 2003.

[36] S. V. Thomas, S. Koshy, C. S. Nair, and S. P. Sarma, "Frequent seizures and polytherapy can impair quality of life in persons with epilepsy," *Neurology India*, vol. 53, no. 1, p. 46, 2005.

[37] F. K. Mutluay, A. Gunduz, A. Tekeoglu, S. Oguz, and S. N. Yeni, "Health related quality of life in patients with epilepsy in Turkey," *Journal of Physical Therapy Science*, vol. 28, no. 1, pp. 240–245, 2016.

6

Prevalence and Influencing Factors of Overweight and Obesity among Adult Residents of Western China

Li Zheng (ID), Feng Deng (ID), Honglin Wang (ID), Biao Yang (ID), Meng Qu (ID), and Peirong Yang (ID)

Baoji Center for Disease Control and Prevention, Baoji 721000, China

Correspondence should be addressed to Feng Deng; bjwzy68@126.com

Academic Editor: Fabrizio Stracci

Background. Overweight and obesity have become a serious health problem. There are a few data on the prevalence of overweight and obesity in Baoji city of western China, this study was conducted to investigate the epidemiologic features of overweight and obesity and explored influencing factors among Baoji adult residents. *Methods.* A cross-sectional study, including 36,600 participants aged above 15 years, was carried out in Baoji city in 2018. Each participant's weight and height were measured, and demographic and behavioral characteristics were collected using questionnaires. Data were analyzed by means of logistic regression considering 95% level of significance. *Results.* Overall, the prevalence of overweight and obesity was 30.73% and 3.11%, respectively. Male had a significantly higher prevalence of overweight (31.45% vs. 29.98%, $P < 0.05$) while female had a higher prevalence of obesity (3.50 vs. 2.74, $P < 0.001$). In the logistic regression analysis, being married or living with a partner (OR = 1.266, $P < 0.001$), unemployed or retired (OR = 1.183, $P < 0.001$), former smokers (OR = 1.116, $P < 0.05$), drinking alcohol (OR = 1.410, $P < 0.001$), sleeping more than 10 hours (OR = 1.274, $P < 0.001$), and increasing age were all significantly associated with a higher prevalence of overweight/obesity, whereas people who lived in rural areas ($R = 0.904$, $P < 0.001$) or had a sufficient leisure time physical activity per week ($R = 0.945$, $P < 0.05$) were associated with a lower prevalence. *Conclusion.* Our results demonstrate that demographic and behavioral factors play an important role in prevalence of overweight/obesity, which can support the implementation of interventions aimed at weight control and consequently prevention of related diseases in this population.

1. Introduction

Obesity has become a major public health problem; according to a recent report by the WHO, more than 1.9 billion adults were overweight, and of these over 650 million were obese, the worldwide prevalence of obesity nearly tripled between 1975 and 2016 [1]. The effect of overweight and obesity on health has been well documented in the literature; they are major risk factors for a number of chronic diseases, including diabetes, hypertension, musculoskeletal disorders, cardiovascular diseases, and some types of cancer [2].

Researchers found the prevalence of overweight and obesity varied across countries in the levels and trends with distinct regional patterns, and there were likely to be continued increases of obesity epidemic in developing countries [3]. As is known to all, China is the largest developing country, with a large economic development over the past several decades. Its rapid economic growth has provoked many changes in lifestyles involving dietary habits and physical activity, which have contributed to an increase in body weight [4]. Recent studies suggest that the prevalence of overweight and obesity in the Chinese population increased from 37.4% to 41.2% and 8.6% to 12.9% between 2000 and 2014, with an estimated increase of 0.27% and 0.32% per year, respectively [5]. Hence, prevention and control of overweight and obesity are of great urgency in China.

The rise in overweight and obesity arouse wide public concern and has led to widespread calls for regular monitoring of changes in overweight and obesity prevalence in all populations. The Chinese government has realized the importance of obesity control and issued Health China Action (2019-2030), which lists reducing the growth rate of obesity as one of its key tasks. Baoji city is located in western China, the less developed areas. To date, this is the first large representative population-based survey of chronic diseases in this area; the aims of this study were to provide the recent estimates of the prevalence of overweight and obesity and to explore potential influencing factors in western China, which will useful for policy makers in formulating policies for obesity management.

2. Methods

2.1. Subjects. Data for the present study was from the Prevalence of Major Chronic Diseases and Related Risk Factors Survey in Baoji city, western China. This was a population-based cross-sectional survey; we used a multistage cluster sampling method to select a representative sample of people aged above 15 years. The first stage covered all twelve districts and counties in Baoji city. Second, five streets (for urban areas) or towns (for rural areas) were selected from each district or county using the probability-proportional-to-size (PPS) method. Third, four neighbourhood committees (for urban areas) or villages (for rural areas) were further randomly selected from each street (for urban areas) or town (for rural areas), also using the PPS method. Fourth, in each neighbourhood committees (for urban areas) or village (for rural areas), fifty-sixty households were randomly chosen using the simple random sampling method. In the final stage, one person aged above 15 years, who was a local registered resident for more than 6 months was selected randomly from each chosen household using a Kish selection table. The ultimate target sample size was established to be 37,000, while 400 participants with missing information such as gender, age, weight, and height were excluded; therefore, 36,600 participants were included in the analysis, accounting for about 11‰ of the total adult population of Baoji city. This work was approved by Baoji Center for Disease Control and Prevention Academic Ethics Board. Written informed consent was acquired from each participant in the survey.

2.2. Data Collection. Participants were required to complete a questionnaire to collect demographic characteristics (including age, gender, location, marital status, education, and occupation) and behavioral characteristics (including smoking, drinking, sleep duration, and physical activity) through face-to-face interviews by trained medical staff. Body height and weight were measured without shoes, and in light clothing after overnight fasting, height was measured to the nearest 0.1 cm, and weight was measured to the nearest 0.1 kg.

2.3. Definition of Variables. Overweight and obesity were defined as a BMI of 24–27.9 kg/m^2 and a BMI ≥ 28 kg/m^2, respectively, by the Chinese standards [6]. Education was classified into three levels: primary school and lower (receiving only primary education or no education); middle school (including junior middle school, senior middle school, and secondary vocational schooling); and college and higher. The occupations consisted of three parts: manual worker, nonmanual worker, and unemployed and retired people. Smoking status was categorized into: current, former, or never smoker [7]. A drinker was defined as a person who had consumed more than one alcoholic drink a week during the previous year, including any form of alcohol [8]. Sleep duration was classified into four levels: <6 h, 6-8 h, 8-10 h, and >10 h; "<6 h" was defined as persons who slept less than 6 hours over 3 days a week, and those who slept more than 10 hours over 3 days a week were defined as ">10 h" [9]. Physical activity recommendations of the WHO for health were considered to be satisfied if participants reported engaging in at least 150 minutes of moderate-intensity aerobic physical activity or 75 minutes of vigorous intensity activity throughout the week or an equivalent combination of moderate and vigorous intensity activity [10]. To assess leisure time physical activity, participants were asked to report the number of exercise days in a usual week, duration of exercise per day, and exercise intensity. We classified leisure time physical activity level in this study as sufficient versus insufficient.

2.4. Statistical Analysis. Categorical variables were described as numbers and percentages. Continuous variables were presented as the mean ± standard derivation (SD). Between-group differences in participant characteristics were tested using a *t*-test for continuous variables and chi-square/Cochran-Mantel-Haenszel test for categorical variables. Separate univariate analyses were used to identify those variables associated with overweight/obesity among subjects in the populations studied. All these significant variables were included in the multivariable logistic regression models. Results of logistic regression analysis were presented together with OR and 95% confidence intervals (CI). All statistical analyses were conducted using IBM SPSS Statistics Version 19.0, and a $P \leq 0.05$ was considered statistically significant.

3. Results

3.1. Basic Characteristics. The basic characteristics of the study participants are illustrated in Table 1. A total of 36,600 participants were included in the analysis, including 18,676 (51.03%) males and 17,924 (48.97%) females and 52.33% lived in urban areas and 47.67% lived in rural areas. The mean age of 41.61 ± 16.32 years. More than three quarters (75.37%) of the residents were married or living with a partner, 60.43% had an education level of middle school, and 73.62% were manual worker. Current smokers and alcohol drinkers accounted for 17.46% and 5.84%. About 31.18% of participants had a sufficient leisure time physical activity. Compared with females, males showed higher values for height, weight, and BMI.

3.2. Prevalence of Overweight and Obesity. The overall prevalence of overweight and obesity was 30.73% and 3.11% in Baoji (Table 2). In males, 31.45% were overweight and 2.74% were obesity. Likewise, 29.98% were overweight and

TABLE 1: Descriptive characteristics of participants in Baoji, western China.

Characteristic	Male	Female	Total
Number, n (%)	18676 (51.03)	17924 (48.97)	36600 (100)
Age (years), mean (SD)	41.00 ± 16.36	42.24 ± 16.26	41.61 ± 16.32
Location, n (%)*			
Urban	9595 (51.38)	9557 (53.32)	19152 (52.33)
Rural	9081 (48.62)	8367 (46.68)	17558 (47.67)
Marriage, n (%)*			
Single	4646 (24.88)	3139 (17.51)	7785 (21.27)
Married or living with a partner	13464 (72.09)	14120 (78.78)	27584 (75.37)
Separated, divorced, or widowed	566 (3.03)	665 (3.71)	1231 (3.36)
Education, n (%)*			
Primary school and lower	3879 (20.77)	5864 (32.72)	9743 (26.62)
Middle school	12222 (65.44)	9897 (55.22)	22119 (60.43)
College and higher	2575 (13.79)	2163 (12.07)	4738 (12.95)
Occupation, n (%)*			
Manual worker	13968 (74.79)	12978 (72.41)	26946 (73.62)
Nonmanual worker	3350 (17.94)	3026 (16.88)	6376 (17.42)
Unemployed or retired	1358 (7.27)	1920 (10.71)	3278 (8.96)
Smokers, n (%)*			
Never	11301 (60.51)	16931 (94.46)	28232 (77.14)
Former	1519 (8.13)	460 (2.57)	1979 (5.41)
Current	5856 (31.36)	533 (2.97)	6389 (17.46)
Drinkers, n (%)*	1871 (10.02)	267 (1.49)	2138 (5.84)
Physical activity, n (%)			
Insufficient	12866 (68.89)	12323 (68.75)	25189 (68.82)
Sufficient	5810 (31.11)	5601 (31.25)	11411 (31.18)
Height (cm), mean (SD)*	168.98 ± 6.25	162.85 ± 5.70	165.98 ± 6.73
Weight (cm), mean (SD)*	65.53 ± 8.03	60.60 ± 7.13	63.12 ± 7.99
BMI (kg/m^2), mean (SD)#	22.95 ± 2.54	22.88 ± 2.72	22.92 ± 2.63

Data are represented as the value (percentage) or mean ± SD. BMI: body mass index; SD: standard derivation. *$p < 0.001$ when comparing male with female. #$p < 0.05$ when comparing male with female.

3.50% were obesity in females. According to the WHO BMI classification, the prevalence of overweight (BMI 25–29.9 kg/m^2) and obesity (BMI ≥ 30 kg/m^2) was 20.43% (19.51% in male, 21.40% in female) and 0.78% (0.67% in male, 0.90% in female), respectively.

As shown in Figure 1, the prevalence of overweight for male increased with age, peaking at 55~64 years (37.25%); such age trend was not seen in the prevalence of obesity. For female, a gradual increase was noted in the prevalence of overweight from the youngest age group (25.53%) up to the group aged above 65 years (36.11%), while the prevalence of obesity reached its peak at the group aged 55~64 years (5.35%) and then followed by a decline in the higher age group. Moreover, the prevalence of overweight was higher in male than in female in the group aged over 25 years, and the prevalence of obesity was higher in female than in male in the age group 15~24 and aged above 45 years.

The prevalence of overweight and obesity was higher (33.06%, 3.63%) among participants who were married or living with a partner than people who were separated, divorced, or widowed (31.84%, 2.94%) or who were single (22.31%, 1.30%). The higher prevalence of overweight or obesity was found in unemployed and retired people (35.54%, 3.63%). A lower educational level was also associated with higher prevalence of overweight and obesity. As with people residing in rural areas, participants who have a sufficient leisure time physical activity also had a lower prevalence of overweight/obesity. Overweight/obesity was also more prevalent among former smokers and drinkers. In addition, prevalence of overweight was higher (35.86%) in participants who had a ≥10-hour sleep duration, while the highest prevalence of obesity (5.86%) was found in participants with <6-hour sleep duration.

3.3. Related Factors for Overweight/Obesity. All significant factors in Table 2 added to the multivariate logistic regression model to assess the significant determinants of combined overweight and obesity (overweight/obesity), as seen in Table 3. Compared with participants aged 15-24 years, people aged 35-44 years, 45-54 years, 55-64 years, and ≥65

TABLE 2: Prevalence of overweight and obesity among various characteristics.

	Overweight		Obesity		Overweight/obesity	
	No. (%)	P value	No. (%)	P value	No. (%)	P value
Total	11248 (30.73)		1138 (3.11)		12386 (33.84)	
Gender		0.002		<0.001		0.152
Male	5874 (31.45)		511 (2.74)		6385 (34.19)	
Female	5374 (29.98)		627 (3.50)		6001 (33.48)	
Location		<0.001		0.117		<0.001
Urban	6139 (32.05)		569 (2.97)		6708 (35.03)	
Rural	5109 (29.28)		569 (3.26)		5678 (32.54)	
Age group (years)		<0.001		<0.001		<0.001
15-	1698 (22.18)		92 (1.20)		1790 (23.38)	
25-	1611 (27.68)		128 (2.20)		1739 (29.87)	
35-	2565 (32.35)		285 (3.59)		2850 (35.95)	
45-	2281 (34.44)		273 (4.12)		2554 (38.56)	
55-	1751 (35.73)		220 (4.49)		1971 (40.22)	
≥65	1342 (36.56)		140 (3.81)		1482 (40.37)	
Marriage		<0.001		<0.001		<0.001
Single	1737 (22.31)		101 (1.30)		1838 (23.61)	
Married or living with a partner	9100 (33.06)		999 (3.63)		10099 (36.61)	
Separated, divorced, or widowed	411 (31.84)		38 (2.94)		449 (36.47)	
Education		<0.001		<0.001		<0.001
Primary school and lower	3181 (32.65)		398 (4.08)		3579 (36.73)	
Middle school	6710 (30.34)		666 (3.01)		7376 (33.35)	
College and higher	1357 (28.64)		74 (1.56)		1431 (30.20)	
Occupation						
Manual	8427 (31.27)	<0.001	926 (3.44)	<0.001	9353 (34.71)	<0.001
Nonmanual	1656 (25.97)		93 (1.46)		1749 (27.43)	
Unemployed	1165 (35.54)		119 (3.63)		1284 (39.17)	
Smoker						
Never	8346 (29.56)	<0.001	874 (3.10)	0.033	9220 (32.66)	<0.001
Former	702 (35.47)		80 (4.04)		782 (39.51)	
Current	2200 (34.43)		184 (2.88)		2384 (37.31)	
Drinker		<0.001		0.062		<0.001
Yes	845 (39.52)		81 (3.79)		926 (43.31)	
No	10403 (30.19)		1057 (3.07)		11460 (33.25)	
Physical activity		<0.001		0.323		0.001
Insufficient	7892 (31.33)		768 (3.05)		8660 (34.38)	
Sufficient	3356 (29.41)		370 (3.24)		3726 (32.65)	
Sleep duration		<0.001		<0.001		<0.001
<6 h	295 (30.86)		56 (5.86)		351 (36.72)	
6-8 h	5308 (30.77)		500 (2.90)		5808 (33.67)	
8-10 h	5101 (30.23)		533 (3.16)		5634 (33.39)	
≥10	544 (35.86)		49 (3.23)		593 (39.09)	

Data are represented as value (percentage). Overweight: BMI 24-27.9 kg/m^2; obesity: BMI ≥ 28 kg/m^2; overweight/obesity: BMI ≥ 24 kg/m^2.

years had a greater correlation with developing overweight and obesity (all $P < 0.001$). Overweight/obesity seems to increase for participants who have been married or living with a partner (OR = 1.266, $P < 0.001$), unemployed and retired people (OR = 1.183, $P < 0.001$), former smokers (OR = 1.116, $P < 0.05$), drinking alcohol (OR = 1.410, $P < 0.001$), and those sleeping more than 10 hours (OR = 1.274, $P < 0.001$) and decrease with people who lived in rural areas and had a sufficient leisure time physical activity ($R = 0904$, $P < 0.001$; $R = 0.945$, $P < 0.05$).

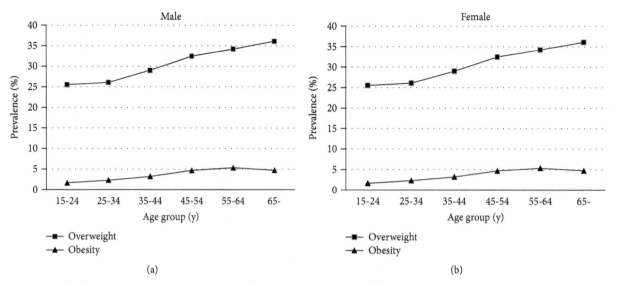

Figure 1: Prevalence of overweight and obesity by different age groups in (a) males and (b) females.

4. Discussion

Baoji is located in western China with a low level of economic development; there are few data and studies on overweight and obesity. The present study represents the first attempt to examine the prevalence and explore related factors of overweight and obesity in Baoji, using the most recent data from a large representative sample.

The prevalence of overweight and obesity was 30.73% and 3.11% in the analyzed population in Baoji; standardized prevalence by Chinese census data was 30.66% and 3.08%. The prevalence of overweight was comparable to the national level of 30.1%, while obesity was lower than the national level of 11.9% [11]. The figures reported from other regions conducted in China have varied considerably: a study in Jilin province of northeast China in 2012 indicated that the prevalence of overweight and obesity was 32.3% and 14.6% [12]; figures in Zhejiang province of eastern China in 2012 were 32.0% and 6.7% [13], while the prevalence was 25.8% and 7.9% in 2014 in Jiangxi province located in eastern China [14]. It was noted that the prevalence of obesity observed in our study population is considerably lower than the values reported in other regions, but comparable to that of Hanzhong city, northwest China [15]. Differences in the prevalence of overweight and obesity may be due to economic development level, sociodemographic variables, climate or lifestyle habits, and economic development levels [16].

Our study indicated that male has a slightly higher prevalence of overweight than female (31.45% vs. 29.98%), while a negative association was found with obesity (2.74% vs. 3.50), as found in a study including 31 countries' samples based on the International Social Survey Program (38.2% vs. 25.5%, 12.1% vs. 12.5%) [17]. However, in the multivariate analysis, it showed there was no significant gender difference of combined overweight and obesity. Yet, most literatures have found the prevalence of obesity in adults was greater for female than for male, and researchers have also identified biological, behavioral, and socioeconomic factors contributing to the differences in obesity prevalence between genders [18].

Our study found overweight/obesity was more common in urban than in rural areas (35.03% vs. 32.54%), as found in other studies [19]. Along with economic growth and the urbanization of lifestyle in China, the prevalence of overweight/obesity among both urban and rural residents has been on the rise; of particular significance, the disparity between them is narrowing. Studies from four large-scale surveys in China between 2000 and 2014 found the prevalence of overweight in the general Chinese population was 38.9% for urban residents and 34.3% for rural residents in 2000; by 2014, the prevalence was 41.4% for urban residents and 40.7% for rural residents [5]. For a large, but economically unevenly developed country like China, an appreciation of the regional distribution of obesity would be informative with respect to understanding the obesity-related health issues. The long-term trends in overweight/obesity for urban and rural residents in western China, the less developed areas, have not been characterised clearly, and it needs to be studied in the future.

It is important to note that ageing also contributes to a higher prevalence of overweight and obesity; the general prevalence reached its peak at group aged above 65 years and 55~64 years, which is consistent with a study in Beijing [20]. It also should be noted that the prevalence of obesity was higher at a younger age (35~44 years) for male, which may be related to the increasing work pressure, decreased physical activity, and unhealthy lifestyle. Another emerging challenge that should not be ignored is the change in food shopping habits induced by the fast growing online-to-offline food delivery service in China, which may decrease the amount of individual physical activity by keeping people at worksite or home and likely raise the risk of being overweight or obesity [21, 22]. Interestingly, we found the prevalence of obesity was higher in female aged above 45 years than in male, aside from the hormone changes during menopausal transition that also could be partly explained by the fact that young women paid more attention to their body

TABLE 3: Factors associated with overweight/obesity by multivariate logistic regression analysis in Baoji adults.

	Overweight/obesity	
	OR (95% CI)	P value
Age (years)		
15-25	1	
25-34	1.167 (1.056~1.290)	<0.001
35-44	1.496 (1.350~1.658)	<0.001
45-54	1.697 (1.527~1.887)	<0.001
55-64	1.828 (1.634~2.045)	<0.001
≥65	1.820 (1.611~ .055)	<0.001
Location		
Urban	1	
Rural	0.904 (0.863~0.947)	<0.001
Marriage		
Single	1	
Married or living with a partner	1.266 (1.153~1.390)	<0.001
Separated, divorced, or widowed	1.130 (0.972~1.315)	0.113
Education		
Primary school and lower	1	
Middle school	1.039 (0.982~1.100)	0.186
College and higher	1.048 (0.955~1.149)	0.322
Occupation		
Manual	1	
Nonmanual	1.009 (0.935~1.089)	0.814
Unemployed or retired	1.183 (1.092~1.282)	<0.001
Smoker		
Never	1	
Former	1.116 (1.012~1.230)	0.027
Current	1.056 (0.989~1.129)	0.102
Drinker (vs. no)	1.410 (1.283~1.550)	<0.001
Physical activity		
Insufficient	1	
Sufficient	0.945 (0.899~0.993)	0.025
Sleep duration		
<6	1	
6-8 h	0.940 (0.820~1.079)	0.381
8-10 h	0.976 (0.851~1.120)	0.729
≥10 h	1.274 (1.075~1.510)	0.005

Data are represented as OR (95% CI). Overweight/obesity: BMI ≥ 24 kg/m². OR was calculated with multivariable logistic regression analysis. OR: odds ratio; CI: confidence intervals.

weight and had a greater pressure to keep a slim figure [23]. These data implied that the overweight and obesity management in Baoji area should post 35 to 44-year-old men and postmenopausal women as the priority management groups. Multivariate analysis showed that people who were married or living with a partner were more likely to be overweight/obesity than unmarried people. Previous researches suggested that marriage was associated with weight gain and that divorce and widowhood were associated with weight loss [24, 25]. While a review indicated that marital transi-

tions are more important than marital status in predicting change in body weight, it was found that transition into marriage appears to be associated with weight gain, whereas transition out of marriage is associated with weight loss [26]. Further research is needed to illustrate the relationships between marital transitions and body weight in our study area.

The relationship between smoking and obesity is complex, and published studies have produced conflicting results. Some reported current smokers were less likely to be obese than never smokers [27]; some have shown no significant association between smoking and body mass index [28]; our study is consistent with studies that have found that former smokers were more likely to be obese [29]. These contradictory findings show that the association still requires more attention. Nowadays, recreational alcohol intake is common across the globe, and numerous studies have examined the effect of alcohol intake on obesity. Some previous studies showed no association or a negative association between alcohol intake and weight gain or obesity [30]. In contrast, we found a positive impact of drinking alcohol on overweight/obesity in line with some literatures [31, 32]. Furthermore, other studies have declared that only excessive or heavy drinking is correlated with increased body weight [33]. Apparently, available evidence on the topic is mixed and conflicting, which warrant further exploration.

Our study found a positive association of long sleep duration (>10 h) on overweight/obesity, in accordance with previous studies [34]. Yet, numerous studies showed a significant increased risk of weight gain with inadequate sleep [35]. Further studies are required to confirm such an association. Physical activity contributes to energy expenditure, prevents obesity, and reduces the risk of major NCDs and decreased all-cause mortality [36]. We found there was a lower incidence of overweight/obesity in participants with a sufficient leisure time physical activity, which is consistent with previous studies [37], while it differs from a study which reported that physical inactivity was inversely associated with overweight but not associated with obesity [17]. Moreover, some found there was no significant correlation between regular physical activity and a lower risk of overweight/obesity [19]. Such findings are probably explained by the difference in criteria used to classify participants as physically active or inactive. Our assessment of physical activity focused on leisure time domain and did not include physical activity in transportation, occupational, and household domains, which are major contributors to total physical activity. Thus, further studies are needed to elucidate the potential effect of inclusion of other types of physical activity. The Chinese government has realized the importance of obesity control and, therefore, has implemented several measures to promote participation in physical activity; figures showed these initiatives have already had some effect [5]. Nevertheless, continued nationwide or local interventions are still needed for promotion of physical activity and other healthy lifestyles.

Several limitations should be noted. First, our study was a cross-sectional design, and therefore, causal relations cannot be established. Second, dietary habits could impact on body weight or obesity, and difference in eating habits may be the main reasons for variations in overweight and obesity prevalence across regions. However, we only investigated a few defined major risk factors. In order to better control overweight and obesity, further research is warranted that includes broader factors. Third, as the study is confined to western China, the conclusions from our study cannot represent the situation in other areas in China. Despite these limitations, this is the first study to determine the prevalence of overweight and obesity and explore related factors based on a relatively large sample size in Baoji, which provides important clues for the prevention and control of local obesity.

5. Conclusions

In summary, the prevalence of overweight is almost equivalent to that of China and the prevalence of obesity is relatively lower in Baoji district. Factors significantly associated with an increased risk of overweight/obesity were older age, married condition, unemployed or retired, former smoker, drinking alcohol, and sleeping too much, while living in rural areas or having a sufficient physical activity may be a protect factor. This study provides data on current overweight and obesity prevalence and related factors in Baoji city of western China, which may guide the development of practical and effective strategies for managing and preventing overweight and obesity.

Acknowledgments

This study was supported by the Health Commission of Shaanxi Province (No. 2016D099). We acknowledge the support and help of Health Bureau and CDC of Baoji city and 12 counties as well as the participants for their contribution to the research.

References

[1] World Health Organization, "Obesity and Overweight fact sheet from the WHO," 2020, https://www.who.int/en/news-room/fact-sheets/detail/obesity-and-overweight.accessed.

[2] D. T. Chu, N. T. Minh Nguyet, T. C. Dinh et al., "An update on physical health and economic consequences of overweight and obesity," *Diabetes & metabolic syndrome*, vol. 12, no. 6, pp. 1095–1100, 2018.

[3] T. Bhurosy and R. Jeewon, "Overweight and obesity epidemic in developing countries: a problem with diet, physical activity, or socioeconomic status?," *The Scientific World Journal*, vol. 2014, Article ID 964236, 7 pages, 2014.

[4] B. M. Popkin, L. S. Adair, and S. W. Ng, "Global nutrition transition and the pandemic of obesity in developing countries," *Nutrition reviews*, vol. 70, no. 1, pp. 3–21, 2012.

[5] Y. Tian, C. Jiang, M. Wang et al., "BMI, leisure-time physical activity, and physical fitness in adults in China: results from a series of national surveys, 2000-14," *The lancet Diabetes & endocrinology*, vol. 4, no. 6, pp. 487–497, 2016.

[6] C. Chen and F. C. Lu, "The guidelines for prevention and control of overweight and obesity in Chinese adults," *Biomedical and environmental sciences: BES*, vol. 17, pp. 1–36, 2004.

[7] World Health Organization, *Guidelines for Controlling and Monitoring the Tobacco Epidemic*, World Health Organization, 1998.

[8] World Health Organization, *International Guide for Monitoring Alcohol Consumption and Related Harm*, World Health Organization, 2000.

[9] C. E. Kim, S. Shin, H. W. Lee et al., "Association between sleep duration and metabolic syndrome: a cross-sectional study," *BMC Public Health*, vol. 18, no. 1, p. 720, 2018.

[10] World Health Organization, *Global Recommendations on Physical Activity for Health*, World Health Organization, 2010.

[11] National Health Commission for Disease Control and Prevention, *Chinese residents nutrition and chronic disease status report*, People's medical publishing house, Beijing, 1st ed edition, 2015.

[12] R. Wang, P. Zhang, C. Gao et al., "Prevalence of overweight and obesity and some associated factors among adult residents of northeast China: a cross-sectional study," *BMJ open*, vol. 6, no. 7, article e010828, 2016.

[13] M. J. Jin, B. B. Chen, Y. Y. Mao et al., "Prevalence of overweight and obesity and their associations with socioeconomic status in a rural Han Chinese adult population," *PLoS one*, vol. 8, no. 11, article e79946, 2013.

[14] L. Hu, X. Huang, C. You et al., "Prevalence of overweight, obesity, abdominal obesity and obesity-related risk factors in southern China," *PLoS One*, vol. 12, no. 9, article e0183934, 2017.

[15] L. Pei, Y. Cheng, Y. Kang, S. Yuan, and H. Yan, "Association of obesity with socioeconomic status among adults of ages 18 to 80 years in rural Northwest China," *BMC public health*, vol. 15, no. 1, 2015.

[16] L. Zhang, Z. Wang, X. Wang et al., "Prevalence of overweight and obesity in China: results from a cross-sectional study of 441 thousand adults, 2012-2015," *Obesity research & clinical practice*, vol. 14, no. 2, pp. 119–126, 2020.

[17] S. Pengpid and K. Peltzer, "Associations between behavioural risk factors and overweight and obesity among adults in population-based samples from 31 countries," *Obesity research & clinical practice*, vol. 11, no. 2, pp. 158–166, 2017.

[18] F. Garawi, K. Devries, N. Thorogood, and R. Uauy, "Global differences between women and men in the prevalence of obesity: is there an association with gender inequality?," *European journal of clinical nutrition*, vol. 68, no. 10, pp. 1101–1106, 2014.

[19] Y. Gao, X. W. Ran, X. H. Xie et al., "Prevalence of overweight and obesity among Chinese Yi nationality: a cross-sectional study," *BMC public health*, vol. 11, no. 1, p. 919, 2011.

[20] L. Cai, X. Han, Z. Qi et al., "Prevalence of overweight and obesity and weight loss practice among Beijing Adults, 2011," *PLoS one*, vol. 9, article e98744, no. 9, 2014.

[21] M. Maimaiti, X. Zhao, M. Jia, Y. Ru, and S. Zhu, "How we eat determines what we become: opportunities and challenges brought by food delivery industry in a changing world in China," *European journal of clinical nutrition*, vol. 72, no. 9, pp. 1282–1286, 2018.

[22] G. N. Healy, K. Wijndaele, D. W. Dunstan et al., "Objectively measured sedentary time, physical activity, and metabolic risk: the Australian Diabetes, Obesity and Lifestyle Study (AusDiab)," *Diabetes care*, vol. 31, no. 2, pp. 369–371, 2008.

[23] Y. Wu, R. Huxley, M. Li, and J. Ma, "The growing burden of overweight and obesity in contemporary China," *CVD Prevention and Control*, vol. 4, no. 1, pp. 19–26, 2009.

[24] J. Sobal, K. L. Hanson, and E. A. Frongillo, "Gender, ethnicity, marital status, and body weight in the United States," *Obesity (Silver Spring, Md)*, vol. 17, no. 12, pp. 2223–2231, 2009.

[25] H. Samouda, M. Ruiz-Castell, V. Bocquet et al., "Geographical variation of overweight, obesity and related risk factors: findings from the European Health Examination Survey in Luxembourg, 2013-2015," *PloS one*, vol. 13, no. 6, article e0197021, 2018.

[26] L. Dinour, M. M. Leung, G. Tripicchio, S. Khan, and M. C. Yeh, "The association between marital transitions, body mass index, and weight: a review of the literature," *Journal of obesity* vol. 2012, Article ID 294974, 16 pages, 2012.

[27] B. Sakboonyarat, C. Pornpongsawad, T. Sangkool et al., "Trends, prevalence and associated factors of obesity among adults in a rural community in Thailand: serial cross-sectional surveys, 2012 and 2018," *BMC public health* vol. 20, no. 1, p. 850, 2020.

[28] Y. Kim, S. M. Jeong, B. Yoo, B. Oh, and H. C. Kang, "Associations of smoking with overall obesity, and central obesity: a cross-sectional study from the Korea National Health and Nutrition Examination Survey (2010-2013)," *Epidemiol Health*, vol. 38, article e2016020, 2016.

[29] S. Dare, D. F. Mackay, and J. P. Pell, "Relationship between smoking and obesity: a cross-sectional study of 499, 504 middle-aged adults in the UK general population," *PLoS One*, vol. 10, no. 4, article e0123579, 2015.

[30] S. Yu, L. Xing, Z. du et al., "Prevalence of obesity and associated risk factors and cardiometabolic comorbidities in rural Northeast China," *BioMed Research International*, vol. 2019, Article ID 6509083, 9 pages, 2019.

[31] K. C. Sung, S. H. Kim, and G. M. Reaven, "Relationship among alcohol, body weight, and cardiovascular risk factors in 27, 030 Korean men," *Diabetes care*, vol. 30, no. 10, pp. 2690–2694, 2007.

[32] Y. Wang, L. Pan, S. Wan et al., "Increasing prevalence of overweight and obesity in Yi farmers and migrants from 2007 to 2015 in China: the Yi migrant study," *BMC public health* vol. 18, no. 1, p. 659, 2018.

[33] S. G. Wannamethee, A. G. Shaper, and P. H. Whincup, "Alcohol and adiposity: effects of quantity and type of drink and time relation with meals," *International journal of obesity* vol. 29, no. 12, pp. 1436–1444, 2005.

[34] D. Léger, F. Beck, J. B. Richard, F. Sauvet, and B. Faraut, "The risks of sleeping "too much". Survey of a National Representative Sample of 24671 adults (INPES health barometer)," *PloS one*, vol. 9, no. 9, article e106950, 2014.

[35] K. L. Knutson, "Does inadequate sleep play a role in vulnerability to obesity?," *American journal of human biology: the official journal of the Human Biology Council*, vol. 24, no. 3, pp. 361–371, 2012.

[36] M. Q. Waleh, "Impacts of physical activity on the obese," *Primary care*, vol. 43, no. 1, pp. 97–107, 2016.

[37] F. Liu, W. Wang, J. Ma, R. Sa, and G. Zhuang, "Different associations of sufficient and vigorous physical activity with BMI in Northwest China," *Scientific reports*, vol. 8, no. 1, article 13120, 2018.

7

Variables Associated with a Urinary MicroRNAs Excretion Profile Indicative of Renal Fibrosis in Fabry Disease Patients

Sebastián Jaurretche [ID],[1,2] **Germán Perez,**[3,4] **Norberto Antongiovanni,**[5]
Fernando Perretta [ID],[6] **and Graciela Venera**[7]

[1] *Biophysics and Human Physiology, School of Medicine. Instituto Universitario Italiano de Rosario, Rosario, Santa Fe, Argentina*
[2] *Los Manantiales, Neurosciences Center, Grupo Gamma Rosario, Rosario, Santa Fe, Argentina*
[3] *Faculty of Biochemical and Pharmaceutical Sciences, Nacional University of Rosario, Rosario, Santa Fe, Argentina*
[4] *Gammalab, Grupo Gamma Rosario, Rosario, Santa Fe, Argentina*
[5] *Center for Infusion and Study of Lysosomal Diseases, Instituto de Nefrología de Pergamino, Pergamino, Buenos Aires, Argentina*
[6] *Intensive Care Unit, Hospital Dr. Enrique Erill, Belén de Escobar, Buenos Aires, Argentina*
[7] *Research Department, Instituto Universitario Italiano de Rosario, Rosario, Santa Fe, Argentina*

Correspondence should be addressed to Sebastián Jaurretche; sebastianjaurretche@hotmail.com

Academic Editor: Piotr Dziegiel

Introduction. In advanced Fabry nephropathy stages, enzyme replacement theraphy (ERT) efficacy decreases, due to its impossibility to reverse renal fibrosis. Therefore, the finding of early kidney fibrosis biomarkers in affected patients is of interest. During renal fibrosis miR-21, miR-192 and miR-433 (fibrosis promotors) are activated by transforming growth factor-β (TGF-β), and miR-29 and miR-200 family (fibrosis supressors) are inhibited by TGF-β. The aim of this study is to analyze the probability that Fabry disease (FD) patients with some clinical variables can present an urinary microRNAs excretion profile indicative of renal fibrosis through a logistic regression analysis. *Results.* A population of 34 participants was included: 24 FD patients and 10 controls. 16/24 (66.66%) FD patients presented microRNAs urinary excretion profile indicative of renal fibrosis. This profile was observed by decrease of fibrosis supresors miR-29 and miR-200 and not by increase of fibrosis promotors miR-21, miR192, and miR-433. Hypohidrosis, angiokeratomas, neuropathic pain, hearing loss, cardiac involvement, male gender, reduced αGalA activity, and renin-angiotensin-aldosterone system inhibitors treatment are associated with the appearance of amicroRNAs urinary excretion profile indicative of renal fibrosis. A probable beneficial effect on urinary microRNAs excretion profile was observed in patients receiving ERT with agalsidase beta. The correlation between parameters of renal function with each family of microRNAs was studied. The only association with statistical significance was found between miR-21 and urine albumin-creatinine ratio (p =0.021). *Conclusions.* A probable microRNAs regulation not mediated by TGF-β should be considered or TGF-β has a different effect in FD than in other nephropathies on microRNAs regulation. Typical clinical manifestations of classic FD are associated with appearance of urinary microRNAs profile indicative of renal fibrosis. FD patients express renal fibrosis biomarkers in urine prior to onset of pathological albuminuria. A direct correlation between urinary miR-21 and degree of albuminuria was observed.

1. Introduction

Fabry disease (FD, OMIM #301500) is a rare X-linked hereditary lysosomal storage disorder, caused by mutations in the GLA gene, encoding the acid hydrolase α-galactosidase-A (αGalA) enzyme, which catalyses neutral glycosphingolipids [1]. FD manifestations are consequence of glycosphingolipids accumulation in lysosomal, extralysosomal, and extracellular spaces [1, 2].

In renal tissue of affected patients, all cell types can be affected by abnormal globotriaosylceramide (Gb3) deposition from early stages of life [3]. Cellular dysfunction is believed to trigger a cascade of events including cellular death, compromised energy metabolism, small vessel injury, ion channel dysfunction, oxidative stress, impaired autophagosome maturation, toxic effect of Globotriaosylsphingosine (Lyso-Gb3), tissue ischemia, and, importantly, development of irreversible tissue fibrosis [1, 3]. Microalbuminuria is the first clinical manifestation of kidney damage that can be observed in affected patients [1]. However, irreversible renal histological lesions, including glomerulosclerosis and tubulointerstitial fibrosis, have been described in asymptomatic patients with normal estimated glomerular filtration rate (eGFR) and mild or absent proteinuria [3–6].

In Fabry nephropathy, the specific treatment effectiveness (enzyme replacement therapy: ERT) is greater if it is indicated in early stages, when irreversible histological lesions are not present. In these stages, cellular cleavage of Gb3 abnormally deposited has been reported, even in podocytes, although in this cell, the effect is dependent on accumulated dose of ERT administered [5]. In advanced renal damage stages, ERT efficacy decreases, due to its impossibility of being able to correct irreversible histological lesions, such as renal fibrosis [7, 8]. Any potential ERT benefit to ameliorate or reverse Fabry nephropathy progression is expected to take many years, especially if fibrosis is well established before ERT is started [7]. Therefore, the finding of early kidney fibrosis biomarkers in affected patients is of interest.

MicroRNAs (miRs; miRNAs) are a family of short non-coding RNAs that play important roles in posttranscriptional gene regulation. In the kidney, miRNAs play a role in the organogenesis and in the pathogenesis of several diseases, including renal fibrosis. During renal fibrosis Transforming growth factor-β (TGF-β) regulates expression of several microRNAs, such as miR-21, miR-29, miR-192, miR-200 and miR-433. MiR-21, miR-192, and miR-433 which are positively induced by TGF-β signaling play a pathological role in kidney diseases (fibrosis promotors). In contrast, both miR-29 and miR-200 families which are inhibited by TGF-β signaling protect kidneys from renal fibrosis (fibrosis supressors) [9].

Recently, we have reported that a profile of urinary microRNAs indicative of renal fibrosis is associated with decreased αGal-A activity in young FD patients with mild or absent albuminuria [10]. In this FD population, the microRNAs profile indicative of renal fibrosis was associated with miR-29 and miR-200 decreased urinary excretion [10]. In another pilot study, it was observed that FD patients show decreased urinary excretion of both miR-29 and miR-200 compared with healthy controls [11]. Both studies conclude that a microRNAs urinary excretion indicative of renal fibrosis could be present in pre-albumin stages of Fabry nephropathy.

The aim of this study is to analyze the probability that FD patients with some clinical variables can present an urinary microRNAs excretion profile indicative of renal fibrosis through a logistic regression analysis.

2. Material and Methods

2.1. Statement on Ethics.
The study was carried out in accordance with the Declaration of Helsinki for Human Research and approved by the local Ethics Committee. Written informed consent for inclusion was obtained from each participant. Adult patients who met inclusion criteria signed informed consent. Pediatric patients agreed to participate and then their legal representative or guardian signed the informed consent.

2.2. Participants Characteristics.
Patients with FD diagnosed by genetic test of any age and sex were included. Exclusion criteria: (i) patients with nephropathy by different aetiology than FD, (ii) patients who at the time of evaluation had symptoms unrelated to FD, which could alter the urinary excretion of microRNAs, and (iii) FD patients with inclusión criteria who refused to participate in the study. Elimination criteria: patients with inclusion criteria that presented some complication related to the collection process of the samples. A population of healthy subjects with similar demographic characteristics was included.

Blood samples and first morning urine were collected from the fasting participants.

All patients had a mutational study by direct sequencing and Multiplex Ligations Probe Amplification [12, 13], and quantification of αGalA enzymatic activity by fluorometric method [14]. Decreased or normal enzyme activity was considered at values < than or > than 4.0 nmol/h/l, respectively. Plasma and urine creatinine were determined by electrochemiluminescence (Roche Diagnostics). Albuminuria was determined by colorimetric method (Roche Diagnostics). The urinary albumin/creatinine ratio (uACR) was calculated to estimate 24 hour albuminuria [15]. Ratio values 0 to 30 were considered normal, 30 to 300 pathological albuminuria and > than 300 proteinuria in at least two samples. eGFR was calculated using CKD-EPI equation in adults [16] and Schwartz equation (modified in 2009) in pediatric patients [17]. To classify kidney disease, the recommendation of "Kidney Disease: Improving Global Outcomes Chronic Kidney Disease Guideline 2013 (KDIGO)" was used [18].

Peripheral nervous system (PNS) symptoms were considered by the presence of typical neuropathic pain crises and/or typical acroparesthesias and/or the demonstration of small neurological fibers damage by Quantitative Sensory Testing (QST) [1, 19]. Hypohidrosis and typical gastrintestinal (GI) symptoms were evaluated by questioning and physical examination [1, 19]. Dermatologist specialist in FD evaluated the presence of angiokeratomas [1, 19]. Hearing loss was defined by alterations of logoaudiometry test [1, 19]. Presence of cornea verticillata was evaluated by ophthalmological examination with slit lamp [1, 19]. Cardiac involvement was as follows: (1) cardiac fibrosis: presence of typical images in cardiac magnetic resonance imaging (MRI) with gadolinium and/or (2) cardiac ischemia: presence of typical changes in electrocardiogram and/or cardiac perfusion tests and/or (3) cardiac arrhythmia: presence of electrophysiological disorders in electrocardiogram; (4) left ventricular hypertrophy (LVI) assessed by tissue Doppler echocardiogram and/or cardiac MRI [1, 19]. Renal involvement was as follows: decreased eGFR and/or pathological albuminuria and/or proteinuria. Central nervous system (CNS) involvement: cerebral white matter lesions in cerebral MRI angiography and/or clinical stroke were considered by antecedents during the interrogation and physical examination and/or demonstration of lesion in cerebral MRI angiography [1, 19]. All patients studied on treatment with ERT were receiving agalsidase-beta (1mg / Kg /EOW).

In FD patients, microRNAs urinary excretion profile indicative of renal fibrosis was considered by increase of fibrosis activators miR-21, miR-192, or miR433 and/or decrease of fibrosis supressors miR29 or miR-200 compared to healthy subjects.

2.3. Urine Sample Preparation and MicroRNAs Extraction. Urine specimen was collected and sent to laboratory for processing immediately. A volume of 10 ml of urine sample was centrifuged at 3000 x g for 15 minutes. Nine ml of supernatant was discarded and the remaining milliliter was centrifuged at 15000 x g during 5 minutes. The urinary cell pellet was stored at -80°C until use.

microRNA molecules behave physicochemically different from the larger RNA molecules, and their isolation from biological samples requires validated procedures. The extraction of miRNAs was performed according to the manufacturer's protocol (NucleoSpin miRNA Plasma kits, Macherey-Nagel, Germany). This kit allows the simultaneous isolation of small RNA, large RNA and proteins in three separate fractions.

Currently, there is no available method that can assess the exact quantity or quality of small RNA and standard spectrophotometric methods to measure microRNA performance and quality are not suitable for biological samples. If the yield and concentration of miRNAs are sufficient, the evaluation of the quality of the extraction method can be performed by capillary electrophoresis or reverse transcription (RT) plus real-time polymerase chain reaction (qPCR) [20]. We evaluated the extractions by quantifying the small nucleolar RNA U6 by RT-qPCR. The reaction conditions are described below.

2.4. MicroRNAs RT-qPCR. To detect the urinary expression of miR-21, miR-29, miR-192, miR-200 families, and miR-433, reverse transcription (RT) reaction with a stem-loop primer was used [21]. Stem-loop RT primers were designed according to Chen et al. [22]. Sequence data was presented previously by us [10, 11].

The specificity of the stem-loop RT primers of each miRNA is given by an extension of six nucleotides at the 3' end; this extension is inverse and complementary to the last six nucleotides of the 3' end of the miRNA.

microRNAs were reverse transcribed using Transcriptor First Strand cDNA Synthesis Kit (Roche Diagnostics). Briefly, 5 μl total eluate was mixed with 1 μM stem-loop RT primer, 0,5 μM dNTPs, 1x RT reaction buffer, 20 U RNase inhibitor, and 10 U Transcriptor RT and made up to 20 μl with H2O. RT was performed at 16°C for 30 minutes, 42°C for 30 minutes, 60°C for 60 minutes, and 70°C for 15 minutes. The resulting cDNA was stored at -80°C until use.

FastStart Universal SYBR Green Master/ROX (Roche Diagnostics) was used for the qPCR reaction, which was performed according to the manufacturer's protocol on a StepOne Plus System (Applied Biosystems). cDNA was amplified using a miRNA-specific forward primer and the universal reverse primer [10]. The forward primers are sequence specific for each miRNA but do not contain the last six nucleotides of the 3' end of the miRNA. To improve the melting temperature, 5 to 7 nucleotides were added at the 5' end [10].

RT-qPCR was carried out in compliance with the MIQE guidelines [23]. All qPCR reactions were performed in duplicate, followed by melt curve analysis to verify their specificity and identity. Small nucleolar RNA U6 was selected as the endogenous reference control [24]. Relative microRNA expression levels were calulated using the 2-ΔΔCt method as previously described [25].

2.5. Data Analysis. Normal distribution of continuous variables was tested using the Shapiro-Wilk Test. For continuous variables, comparison of means/medians was performed using Student-t test for variables that followed a normal distribution and Mann-Whitney test/related samples Wilcoxon Signed Rank test for variables who did not. If the qualitative variable had more than two categories, an ANNOVA test was used for variables with normal distribution, and Kruskal-Wallis test was used for those without. For categorical variables, the comparison of the variables distribution between groups was done using the Chi-square or Fisher exact tests. Confidence interval was of 95%. Values of $p < 0.05$ were considered of statistical significance. Each statistical test was applied for each family of microRNA studied.

The probability that FD patients present a profile of urinary microRNAs excretion indicative of renal fibrosis was estimated with a binary logistic regression model.

The presence of this profile indicative of renal fibrosis as a dichotomous variable according to the degree of albuminuria was analyzed to evaluate its usefulness as an early biomarker of kidney damage in nonalbuminuric patients.

3. Results

A population of 34 participants was included; 24 FD patients and 10 controls. Table 1 shows the demographic characteristics of controls versus FD patients.

Twenty-three of 24 FD patients (95.83%) presented symptoms of classic FD phenotype. Twelve pediatrics FD patients (7 girls/5 boys; age: 10.33±3.93 years; eGFR: 152.33±48.39 ml/min/1.73 m²; uACR: 21.75 ± 37.13 mg/g) and 12 adult FD patients (9 females/3 males; age: 37.08±14.74 years; eGFR: 109.90±29.34 ml/min/1.73 m2; uACR: 32.93±30.86 mg/g) were included.

Figure 1 shows the relative expression levels of miRNAs in urinary sediment of controls and FD patients. 16/24 (66.66%) FD patients presented microRNAs urinary excretion profile indicative of renal fibrosis. This profile was observed by decreasing of both fibrosis suppresors (miR-29 and miR-200) and not by increase of fibrosis promotors (miR-21, miR192 and miR-433) (Figure 1).

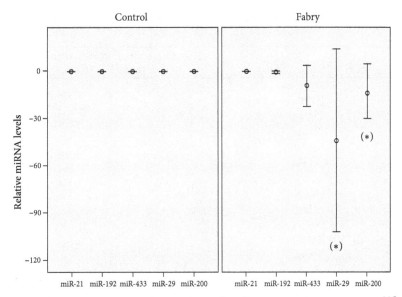

FIGURE 1: *Relative expression levels of miRNAs in urinary sediment of controls and FD patients.* Bars represent $2^{-\Delta\Delta Ct}$ values calculated by Delta-Delta Ct ($\Delta\Delta Ct$) method (Confidence interval: 95%). Expression was normalized to U6, and data are represented as means ± SEM. (*) p = < 0.005.

TABLE 1: Demographic characteristics of controls versus Fabry disease patients.

	Controls	FD patients	*p* value
N	10	24	-
Gender	4M/6F	7M/17F	-
Age*	27.00±14.77	23.70±17.26	0.602
uACR*	9.10±5.78	24.67±34.26	0.166
eGFR*	118.12±19.44	136.19±36.74	0.153
Genotype	-	E398X;R363H; L415P;R227Q; R301Q; del3&4exon; L106R;C238Y	-

(*) median ± standard desviation

References: M: male; F: females; uACR: urinary albumin/creatinine ratio; eGFR: estimated glomerular filtation rate.

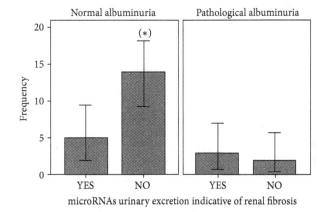

FIGURE 2: *Urinary microRNAs excretion profile indicative of renal fibrosis according to degree of albuminuria in Fabry disease patients.* Error bars indicates 95% confidence interval. (*) p = < 0.005.

A highest frequency of urinary microRNAs indicative of renal fibrosis was observed in FD patients with normal albuminuria and a lower frequency was found in FD patients with pathological albuminuria (Figure 2).

Table 2 shows the frequency of clinical manifestations and its association with urinary microRNAs indicative of renal fibrosis in FD patients.

Binary logistic regression model was able to predict the appearance of urinary microRNAs indicative of renal fibrosis in FD patients. Table 3 shows a model summary.

The correlation between uACR and eGFR with each family of microRNAs was studied. The only one association with statistical significance was found between miR-21 and uACR (p =0.021) (Figure 3). There was no statistically significant correlation between uACR and eGFR with the rest of miR studied (uACR/miR-192, p = 0.790; uACR/miR-433, p = 0.933; uACR/miR-29, p = 0.536; uACR/miR-200, p = 0.766; eFGR/miR-21, p = 0.093; eGFR/miR-192, p = 0.047; eGFR/miR-433, p = 0.122; eGFR/miR-29, p = 0.408; eGFR/miR-200, p = 0.385).

4. Discussion

Renal fibrosis is a feature of Fabry nephropathy and its early development has been reported in renal biopsies of affected patients, even with normal eGFR and without pathological albuminuria [3–7]. The time-course of kidney fibrosis is not clearly established, but emerging evidence points are early podocyte injury and fibrosis generated by epithelial cells that increase as disease progresses [3, 5, 7, 26, 27].

TABLE 2: Frequency of clinical manifestations and association with urinary microRNAs excretion profile indicative of renal fibrosis in Fabry disease patients.

	Frequency (%)	Association with microRNAs urinary excretion profile indicative of renal fibrosis. Pearson correlation (p value)
Reduced αGalA activity	9/24 (37.50)	0.548 (0.006)**
Male gender	7/24 (29.16)	0.454 (0.026)*
Neuropathic pain	13/24 (54.16)	0.414 (0.044)*
Hipohidrosis	10/24 (41.66)	0.598 (0.002)**
GI symptoms	11/24 (45.83)	0.296 (0.161)
Angiokeratomas	12/24 (50.00)	0.530 (0.008)**
Hearing loss	6/24 (25.00)	0.408 (0.048)*
Pathological Albuminuria	5/24 (20.83)	-0.29 (0.169)
Reduced eGFR	0/24 (0.00)	- (+)
Cardiac involvement	6/24 (25.00)	0.408 (0.048)*
CNS involvement	5/24 (20.83)	0.363 (0.081)
ERT treatment	9/24 (37.50)	0.365 (0.079)
RAAS inhibitors Treatment	6/24 (25.00)	0.408 (0.048)*

* The correlation is significant at the 0.05 level (bilateral)
** The correlation is significant at the 0.01 level (bilateral)
(+) Can not be calculated because the "reduced eGFR" variable is constant
References: αGalA: α-galactosidase-A; GI: gastrointestinal; eGFR: estimated glomerular filtration rate; CNS: nentral nervous system; ERT: enzyme replacement theraphy; RAAS: renin-angiotensin-aldosterone system.

The present work is an analysis of FD patients with mild nephropathy (preserved eGFR and mild or absent albuminuria) compared with healthy subjects of similar characteristics.

Our results show that miR-29 and miR-200 are decreased in urine of FD patients compared with healthy subjects while the miR-21, miR-192 and miR-433 are similarly expressed. These results, in a larger population of pediatric and adult FD patients, replicate our previous findings when only pediatric affected patients were included [10]. According to these results, a probable microRNAs regulaction not mediated by TGF-β should be considered, or that TGF-β has a different effect in FD than in other nephropathies on microRNAs regulation [10, 11].

Lyso-Gb3, a deacylated Gb3, is increased in plasma of FD patients [1]. The deleterious Lyso-Gb3 effects on podocytes and renal tubular cells have been demonstrated in both animal and human models of Fabry nephropathy [28, 29]. In podocytes, exposure to Lyso-Gb is correlated with increased expression of TGF-β and extracellular matrix components, both mechanisms associated with renal fibrosis development [28]. In renal tubular cells exposed to Lyso-Gb3, epithelial-mesenchymal transition has been described as another mechanism related to renal fibrosis [29]. The role of Lyso-Gb3 or other harmful molecules and growth factors different than TGF-β should be studied to explain this urinary microRNAs expression that appear to be different from a regulation TGF-β mediated.

In a previous pilot study on the subject, we found that miR-21, miR-29, miR-192, miR-200, and miR-433 urinary excretion was similar between healthy subjects and two FD patients subgroups: (i) women with mild FD phenotype and normal αGalA activity and (ii) women with αGalA normal and more severe phenotype who were receiving ERT [11]. In the same study, we found a urinary decrease of miR-29 and miR-200 in males of any age, with normal eGFR and without pathological albuminuria [11]. In the present work a statistical model was designed to predict the probability that FD patients with certain clinical variables may be developing a urinary microRNAs excretion profile indicative of renal fibrosis.

TABLE 3: Binary logistic regression model to predict the appearance of urinary microRNAs excretion profile indicative of renal fibrosis in Fabry disease patients.

Explanatory variable (+)	Score in the model	p value
Hipohidrosis	8.571	0.003 (∗)
Reduced αGalA activity	7.200	0.007 (∗)
Angiokeratomas	6.750	0.009 (∗)
Male gender	4.941	0.026 (∗)
Neuropathic pain	4.112	0.043 (∗)
Hearing loss	4.000	0.046 (∗)
Cardiac involvement	4.000	0.046 (∗)
RAAS inhibitors treatment	4.000	0.046 (∗)
ERT	3.200	0.074
Genotype	3.553	0.059
CNS involvement	3.158	0.076
Age	2.416	0.120
GI symptoms	2.098	0.148
Pathological albuminuria	2.021	0.155

Chi squared = 0.002; Cox y Snell R^2 = 0.720; Nagelkerke R^2 = 1.000. Global percentage correctly classified = 100%.
(+) Explanatory variables with greater capacity to predict the appearance of microRNAs urinary extretion profile indicative of renal fibrosis, classified in decreasing order.
(∗) Explanatory variables able to predict the appearance of urinary microRNAs extretion profile indicative of renal fibrosis.
References: αGalA: α-galactosidase-A; RAAS: renin-angiotensin-aldosterone system; ERT: enzyme replacement theraphy; CNS: nentral nervous system; GI: gastrointestinal.

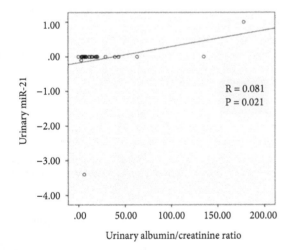

$R = 0.081$
$P = 0.021$

FIGURE 3: Linear correlation between urinary miR-21 and urinary albumin/creatinine ratio in Fabry disease patients.

In our population, we found through the regression analysis that hypohidrosis, reduced αGal-A activity, angiokeratomas, male gender, neuropathic pain, hearing loss, cardiac involvement, and renin-angiotensin-aldosterone system (RAAS) inhibitors treatment are clinical variables associated with urinary microRNAs excretion profile indicative of renal fibrosis. Except RAAS inhibitors treatment, all variables capable of predicting the appearance of urinary microRNAs indicative of renal fibrosis are typical manifestations of classic FD [19]. Classic FD (or type 1) is the most severe disease phenotype that is caused by serious deficiency of αGalA activity and tissue deposition of nonmetabolized substrates from fetal stages, with clinical manifestations since childhood and appearance of renal, cardiac, and cerebrovascular disease in affected young adult patients, all this associated with greater morbidity and mortality and shortening of life expectancy in affected patients of both genders [30].

Regarding the variables related to FD treatment, it is an expected result that ERT does not correlate with a microRNAs profile related to renal fibrosis. That is to say, a probable beneficial effect was observed in patients who receiving ERT. A paradoxical result is the correlation between RAAS inhibitors treatment and a urinary microRNAs indicative of renal fibrosis. Probably this association could be explained because the treatment with this drugs is initiated by nephrologists in presence of nephropathy (pathological albuminuria or reduced eGFR), when tissue damage is already advanced.

In our study, a significant proportion of nonalbuminuric patients had urinary microRNAs indicative of renal fibrosis. This finding could mean that FD patients express renal fibrosis biomarkers in urine prior to onset of pathological albuminuria. This could mean that urinary miRs are excreted in a similar way in FD and in other forms of chronic kidey disease (CKD), in which microRNAs urinary excretion decreases with the kidney disease progression [30].

Finally, when individual microRNAs families with other renal function parameters were analyzed, the only association found was the direct correlation between urinary miR-21 and albuminuria, although with a linear correlation of scarce significance. This is an expected finding, since miR-21 is a well-known molecule that promotes fibrosis in several CKD models of any cause. This finding should be analyzed in a greater number of patients, including a higher proportion of patients with pathological albuminuria.

Although the small size of the population studied and the cross-sectional design may represent a statistical limitation, other studies devoted to similar purposes were carried out with a similar or smaller number of patients [4, 5, 31–33].

5. Conclusions

Fibrosis supressors miR-29 and miR-200 are decreased in urine of FD patients compared with healthy subjects, while the fibrosis activators miR-21, miR-192, and miR-433 are similarly expressed. According to these results, a probable microRNAs regulation not mediated by TGF-β should be considered or TGF-β has a different effect in FD than in other nephropathies on microRNAs regulation.

Typical clinical manifestations of classic FD as hipohidrosis, angiokeratomas, neuropathic pain, hearing loss, cardiac involvement, male gender, and reduced αGalA activity are associated with the appearance of a urinary microRNAs excretion profile indicative of renal fibrosis.

A probable beneficial effect on urinary microRNAs excretion profile was observed in patients who receiving ERT with agalsidase beta.

FD patients express renal fibrosis biomarkers in urine prior to onset of pathological albuminuria but the urinary microRNAs excretion decreases with the nephropathy progression. In this sense, the profile of urinary excretion of microRNAs indicative of renal fibrosis could be useful as an early biomarker of renal fibrosis in the prealbuminuric stage but they would not be useful as biomarkers of evolution, although this hypothesis should be confirmed in longitudinal studies.

A direct correlation between urinary miR-21 and degree of albuminuria was observed. It could be hypothesized that this miR individually could be useful as a biomarker of Fabry nephropathy progression, although again, this finding should be confirmed in longitudinal studies.

Consent

No individual personal data were included in the study. All patients provided necessary consent to participate in the present study. Written informed consent was obtained from each patient or from an appropriate guardian.

References

[1] D. P. Germain, "Fabry disease," *Orphanet Journal of Rare Diseases*, vol. 5, no. 1, p. 30, 2010.

[2] H. Askari, C. R. Kaneski, C. Semino-Mora et al., "Cellular and tissue localization of globotriaosylceramide in Fabry disease," *Virchows Archiv*, vol. 451, no. 4, pp. 823–834, 2007.

[3] A. B. Fogo, L. Bostad, E. Svarstad et al., "Scoring system for renal pathology in Fabry disease: report of the international study group of fabry nephropathy (ISGFN)," *Nephrology Dialysis Transplantation* , vol. 25, no. 7, pp. 2168–2177, 2010.

[4] B. Najafian, E. Svarstad, L. Bostad et al., "Progressive podocyte injury and globotriaosylceramide (GL-3) accumulation in young patients with Fabry disease," *Kidney International*, vol. 79, no. 6, pp. 663–670, 2011.

[5] C. Tøndel, L. Bostad, K. K. Larsen et al., "Agalsidase benefits renal histology in young patients with Fabry disease," *Journal of the American Society of Nephrology*, vol. 24, no. 1, pp. 137–148, 2013.

[6] F. Perretta, N. Antongiovanni, and S. Jaurretche, "Early renal involvement in a girl with classic fabry disease," *Case Reports in Nephrology*, vol. 2017, Article ID 9543079, 4 pages, 2017.

[7] F. Weidemann, M. D. Sanchez-Niño, J. Politei et al., "Fibrosis: a key feature of Fabry disease with potential therapeutic implications," *Orphanet Journal of Rare Diseases*, vol. 8, no. 1, p. 116, 2013.

[8] A. Ortiz, A. Abiose, D. G. Bichet et al., "Time to treatment benefit for adult patients with Fabry disease receiving agalsidase β: data from the Fabry Registry," *Journal of Medical Genetics*, vol. 53, no. 7, pp. 495–502, 2016.

[9] A. C. K. Chung and H. Y. Lan, "MicroRNAs in renal fibrosis," *Frontiers in Physiology*, vol. 6, p. 50, 2015.

[10] S. Jaurretche, G. Venera, N. Antongiovanni, F. Perretta, and G. R. Perez, "Urinary excretion of microRNAs in young fabry disease patients with mild or absent nephropathy," *Open Journal of Nephrology*, vol. 8, no. 3, p. 71, 2018.

[11] S. Jaurretche, G. Venera, N. Antongiovanni, F. Perretta, and G. Pérez, "Urinary excretion profile of microRNAs related to renal fibrosis in Fabry disease patients. A pilot study," *Meta Gene*, vol. 19, pp. 212–218, 2019.

[12] C. M. Eng, L. A. Resnick-Silverman, D. J. Niehaus et al., "Nature and frequency of mutations in the alpha-galactosidase A gene that cause Fabry disease," *American Journal of Human Genetics*, vol. 53, no. 6, p. 1186, 1993.

[13] A. Schirinzi, M. Centra, C. Prattichizzo et al., "Identification of GLA gene deletions in Fabry patients by Multiplex Ligation-dependent Probe Amplification (MLPA)," *Molecular Genetics and Metabolism*, vol. 94, no. 3, pp. 382–385, 2008.

[14] Y. Li, C. R. Scott, N. A. Chamoles et al., "Direct multiplex assay of lysosomal enzymes in dried blood spots for newborn screening," *Clinical Chemistry*, vol. 50, no. 10, pp. 1785–1796, 2004.

[15] C. A. Peralta, M. G. Shlipak, S. Judd et al., "Detection of chronic kidney disease with creatinine, cystatin C, and urine albumin-to-creatinine ratio and association with progression to end-stage renal disease and mortality," *The Journal of the American Medical Association*, vol. 305, no. 15, pp. 1545–1552, 2011.

[16] S. M. Rombach, M. C. Baas, I. J. M. Ten Berge, R. T. Krediet, F. J. Bemelman, and C. E. M. Hollak, "The value of estimated GFR in comparison to measured GFR for the assessment of renal function in adult patients with Fabry disease," *Nephrology Dialysis Transplantation* , vol. 25, no. 8, pp. 2549–2556, 2010.

[17] C. Tøndel, U. Ramaswami, K. M. Aakre, F. Wijburg, M. Bouwman, and E. Svarstad, "Monitoring renal function in children with Fabry disease: comparisons of measured and creatinine-based estimated glomerular filtration rate," *Nephrology Dialysis Transplantation*, vol. 25, no. 5, pp. 1507–1513, 2009.

[18] P. E. Stevens and A. Levin, "Evaluation and management of chronic kidney disease: synopsis of the kidney disease: improving global outcomes 2012 clinical practice guideline," *Annals of Internal Medicine*, vol. 158, no. 11, pp. 825–830, 2013.

[19] A. Ortiz, D. P. Germain, R. J. Desnick et al., "Fabry disease revisited: management and treatment recommendations for adult patients," *Molecular Genetics and Metabolism*, vol. 123, no. 4, pp. 416–427, 2018.

[20] R. A. Ach, H. Wang, and B. Curry, "Measuring microRNAs: comparisons of microarray and quantitative PCR measurements, and of different total RNA prep methods," *BMC Biotechnology*, vol. 8, no. 1, p. 69, 2008.

[21] M. F. Kramer, "Stem-loop RT-qPCR for miRNAs," *Current Protocols in Molecular Biology*, vol. 95, no. 1, p. 15-10, 2011.

[22] C. Chen, D. A. Ridzon, A. J. Broomer et al., "Real-time quantification of microRNAs by stem-loop RT-PCR," *Nucleic Acids Research*, vol. 33, no. 20, p. e179, 2005.

[23] S. A. Bustin, V. Benes, J. A. Garson et al., "The MIQE guidelines: minimum information for publication of quantitative real-time PCR experiments," *Clinical Chemistry*, vol. 55, no. 4, pp. 611–622, 2009.

[24] P. Mestdagh, P. van Vlierberghe, A. de Weer et al., "A novel and universal method for microRNA RT-qPCR data normalization," *Genome Biology*, vol. 10, no. 6, p. R64, 2009.

[25] K. J. Livak and T. D. Schmittgen, "Analysis of relative gene expression data using real-time quantitative PCR and the 2−ΔΔCT method," *Methods*, vol. 25, no. 4, pp. 402–408, 2001.

[26] C. Tøndel, L. Bostad, A. Hirth, and E. Svarstad, "Renal biopsy findings in children and adolescents with fabry disease and minimal albuminuria," *American Journal of Kidney Diseases*, vol. 51, no. 5, pp. 767–776, 2008.

[27] C. Valbuena, E. Carvalho, M. Bustorff et al., "Kidney biopsy findings in heterozygous Fabry disease females with early nephropathy," *Virchows Archiv*, vol. 453, no. 4, pp. 329–338, 2008.

[28] M. D. Sanchez-Niño, A. B. Sanz, S. Carrasco et al., "Globotriaosylsphingosine actions on human glomerular podocytes: implications for Fabry nephropathy," *Nephrology Dialysis Transplantation*, vol. 26, no. 6, pp. 1797–1802, 2011.

[29] Y. J. Jeon, N. Jung, J.-W. Park, H.-Y. Park, and S.-C. Jung, "Epithelial-mesenchymal transition in kidney tubular epithelial cells induced by globotriaosylsphingosine and globotriaosylceramide," *PLoS ONE*, vol. 10, no. 8, Article ID e0136442, 2015.

[30] S. Waldek, M. R. Patel, M. Banikazemi, R. Lemay, and P. Lee, "Life expectancy and cause of death in males and females with Fabry disease: Findings from the Fabry Registry," *Genetics in Medicine*, vol. 11, no. 11, pp. 790–796, 2009.

[31] C. A. Luciano, J. W. Russell, T. K. Banerjee et al., "Physiological characterization of neuropathy in Fabry's disease," *Muscle & Nerve*, vol. 26, no. 5, pp. 622–629, 2002.

[32] B. Najafian, C. Tøndel, E. Svarstad, A. Sokolovkiy, K. Smith, and M. Mauer, "One year of enzyme replacement therapy reduces globotriaosylceramide inclusions in podocytes in male adult patients with Fabry disease," *PLoS ONE*, vol. 11, no. 4, p. e0152812, 2016.

[33] P. Phyu, A. Merwick, I. Davagnanam et al., "Increased resting cerebral blood flow in adult Fabry disease: MRI arterial spin labeling study," *Neurology*, vol. 90, no. 16, pp. e1379–e1385, 2018.

8

Pulmonary Complications Secondary to Immune Checkpoint Inhibitors

Hasan Ahmad Hasan Albitar ⓘ,[1] **Narjust Duma,**[2] **Konstantinos Leventakos,**[2] and **Alice Gallo De Moraes** ⓘ[3]

[1]*Department of Internal Medicine, Mayo Clinic, Rochester, Minnesota, USA*
[2]*Division of Medical Oncology, Mayo Clinic, Rochester, Minnesota, USA*
[3]*Division of Pulmonary and Critical Care, Mayo Clinic, Rochester, Minnesota, USA*

Correspondence should be addressed to Alice Gallo De Moraes; gallodemoraes.alice@mayo.edu

Academic Editor: Khoa Nguyen

Background. Immune checkpoint inhibitors (ICI) have changed the landscape in the treatment of a number of cancers. Immune-related adverse events (irAEs) have emerged as a serious clinical problem with the use of ICI. *Methods.* All oncology patients diagnosed with pulmonary complications secondary to ICI at Mayo Clinic Rochester from January 1, 2012 to December 31, 2018 were reviewed. Demographics, comorbidities, smoking, and oncologic history were analyzed. *Results.* A total of 10 patients developed pulmonary complications secondary to ICI. Seven patients were men (70%), and the median age at diagnosis was 61.5 (IQR 55.8-69.3) years. All patients had stage IV disease. Melanoma was the most common malignancy. Seven (70%) patients had a positive smoking history, and 6 (60%) were obese (BMI > 30). Most cases were grade 2 pneumonitis (70%). One patient with grade 4 pneumonitis required endotracheal intubation and a prolonged course of systemic corticosteroids (>30 days). Eight (80%) patients received prior radiation therapy. The median time from initiation of ICI to pneumonitis diagnosis was 3.5 months. *Conclusion.* Melanoma was the most common malignancy, the majority of patients had grade 2 pneumonitis and required treatment with steroids, and all patients affected by ICI-related pneumonitis had stage IV malignancy. Potential risk factors included smoking history, prior radiotherapy, obesity, and advance stage at the time of ICI initiation. Extrapulmonary irAEs are common in patients with pneumonitis.

1. Introduction

Programmed death 1 (PD-1) and its ligands (PD-L1 and PD-L2), in addition to cytotoxic T-lymphocyte-associated protein 4 (CTLA-4), are negative regulators of T-cell activation that play an integral role in immune homeostasis [1, 2]. The development of pharmaceutical anti-PD-1 and PD-L1 antibodies and monoclonal antibodies targeting CTLA-4 has changed the landscape in the treatment of a number of cancers and improved survival from months to complete remission in some cases [3]. However, with the development of these novel agents came a new group of distinctive immune adverse reactions, thought to be related to cytokine release, that range from transient and benign to severe and fatal [4, 5]. They are referred to as immune-related adverse events (irAEs).

Evidence shows that immune checkpoint inhibitor (ICI) use is associated with increased risk of all-grade pneumonitis compared with other conventional chemotherapeutic agents [6]. Pulmonary irAEs are of special interest because they can lead to intensive care unit (ICU) admission, endotracheal intubation, and in severe cases, death.

Commonly encountered computed tomography findings include bilateral consolidative changes and ground-glass opacities (Figure 1), predominantly in peripheral distribution but also with interlobular septal thickening in basilar distribution [7]. However, imaging findings are nonspecific and distinguishing ICI-pneumonitis from radiation-induced pneumonitis and pulmonary infections can be challenging. The cessation of ICI therapy alone is sufficient in mild pneumonitis cases and corticosteroids are typically used for treatment of more

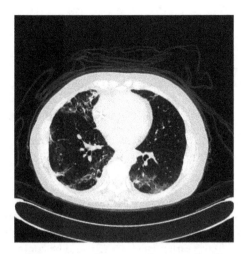

FIGURE 1: Chest computed tomography example of a case with immune-checkpoint inhibitor induced pneumonitis showing patchy bilateral areas of consolidation and ground-glass attenuation that appeared following initiation of ICI.

severe, symptomatic cases [8, 9]. Most irAEs respond to corticosteroids and resolve within 3 months [10].

Our objective in the present study is to present our center's clinical experience with ICI-induced pneumonitis, to report the baseline patient characteristics in 10 patients with ICI-induced pneumonitis and to compare the rate of these complications with the data published in previous reports.

2. Materials and Methods

2.1. Patients. Study inclusion criteria specified patient age greater than 18 years; histologically confirmed diagnosis of solid malignancy for which treatment with an ICI is approved by the US Food and Drug Administration; more than 3 months follow-up at Mayo Clinic in Rochester, Minnesota; and receipt of at least 1 dose of ICIs. Patients with hematologic malignancy, those without research consent, and patients with no close follow-up at Mayo Clinic in Rochester were all excluded.

2.2. Data Collection. Using the electronic medical record system, we identified patients with ICI-induced pneumonitis at Mayo Clinic's Rochester campus from January 1, 2012 to December 31, 2018. This study was approved by the Mayo Clinic's Institutional Review Board. Cases were reviewed by at least 1 radiologist and 1 pulmonologist and were classified and graded according to the National Cancer Institute Common Terminology Criteria for Adverse Events version 4.0 (Table 1) [11, 12].

3. Results

3.1. Baseline Patient Characteristics. Ten patients with median age of 61.5 (IQR 55.8-69.3) were identified. Baseline characteristics are summarized in Table 2.

3.2. Primary Malignancy of Patients with ICI-Induced Pneumonitis. Melanoma was the most common malignancy ($n = 5$, 50%) followed by small cell lung cancer (SCLC)

($n = 1$, 10%), spindle cell carcinoma ($n = 1$, 10%), neuroendocrine tumor of the epiglottis ($n = 1$, 10%), lung adenocarcinoma ($n = 1$, 10%), and Merkel cell carcinoma ($n = 1$, 10%). All patients with pneumonitis had stage IV cancer at the time immunotherapy was introduced. The most common sites of metastasis were liver and bones, seen in 4 patients (40%) and 6 patients (60%), respectively.

3.3. ICI Use and Pneumonitis Grade. Immune checkpoint inhibitors at the time of pneumonitis were pembrolizumab ($n = 5$, 45.5%), nivolumab ($n = 3$, 27.3%), ipilimumab ($n = 2$, 18.2%), and atezolizumab ($n = 1$, 9%), and 1 patient was on dual therapy with ipilimumab and nivolumab. Two patients (20%) had grade 1 pneumonitis; 7 (70%) had grade 2; and 1 (10%) had grade 4 pneumonitis.

3.4. Other irAEs Encountered with ICI-Induced Pneumonitis. In addition to pneumonitis, 6 patients (60%) had other irAEs. The most commonly encountered nonpulmonary irAEs were autoimmune hepatitis and colitis. Data about other irAEs are summarized in Table 3.

3.5. Outcomes after ICI Treatment. Five patients (50%) had a response after initiation of ICI therapy, 3 (30%) had disease progression, and 2 (20%) had mixed response. The median (IQR) time from initiation of ICI treatment to the pneumonitis diagnosis was 3.5 (range; 1.5-28) months. BAL was performed for 4 patients (40%) and showed inflammatory macrophage-predominant alveolitis in 3 (75%) patients. Microbiologic studies on BAL specimens for viruses, bacteria, fungi, and parasites were negative among all patients who underwent BAL.

Eight patients (80%) required systemic corticosteroids for the treatment of pulmonary and/or extrapulmonary irAEs. ICI treatment was discontinued for 8 patients (80%) and was resumed and continued for 5 (50%) after the pneumonitis cleared. One patient with grade 1 pneumonitis was continued on ICI without interruption or steroids, and 1 with grade 2 pneumonitis was treated with drug holding only. All other patients were treated with systemic corticosteroids with prednisone being the main corticosteroid used. The duration of the treatment with corticosteroids ranged from 30 to 360 days. The patient with grade 4 pneumonitis required endotracheal intubation and a prolonged course of corticosteroids (>30 days). None of the patients received any immunosuppressive treatment other than the corticosteroids.

During follow-up, 5 patients (50%) died. Early mortality rate within 1 month of pneumonitis was 10%. Among the patients who died, 1 had grade 4, and 4 had grade 2 pneumonitis. Among the 5 patients still alive at study completion, 3 patients had grade 2 and 2 patients had grade 1 pneumonitis. Cause of death was directly related to pneumonitis in 1 patient only. Details are summarized in Figure 2.

4. Discussion

The reported overall incidence of all-grade pneumonitis has ranged from 1.3% to 11% [13–16]. According to Nishino et al. [16], patients with pneumonitis most commonly present with cough (60%), dyspnea (55%), and less frequently

TABLE 1: Grades of CTCAE version 4.0.

CTCAE grade	Clinical presentation
1	Asymptomatic pneumonitis; clinical or diagnostic observations only
2	Symptomatic pneumonitis; medical intervention indicated; limited instrumental ADL
3	Severe symptoms secondary to pneumonitis; limited self-care ADL; oxygen treatment indicated
4	Life-threatening respiratory compromise; urgent intervention indicated (e.g., tracheotomy and intubation)
5	Death secondary to pneumonitis

Abbreviations: ADL: activities of daily living; CTCAE: Common Terminology of Criteria for Adverse Events. Modified from National Cancer Institute [12].

TABLE 2: Baseline characteristics of the 10 patients with pneumonitis secondary to ICI use.

Baseline characteristics	Patients, no. (%)
Age (y)	
≥65	4 (40)
<65	6 (60)
Male sex	7 (70)
Body mass index >30	6 (60)
Positive smoking history (current and prior use)	7 (70)
Cancer stage IV at time of pulmonary complications	10 (100)
Site of metastasis	
Liver	4 (40)
Bone	6 (60)
Charlson comorbidity index	
0-8	4 (40)
9-17	6 (60)
Previous radiation history	8 (80)
Chemotherapy before initiation of ICI use	
Yes	7 (70)
No	3 (30)
Medical history of COPD or emphysema	
Yes	2 (20)
No	8 (80)
Use of corticosteroid inhaler at time of pneumonitis	
Yes	1 (0)
No	9 (90)

Abbreviations: COPD: chronic obstructive pulmonary disease; ICI: immune checkpoint inhibitor.

with fever. The diagnosis of pneumonitis may represent a challenge to physicians, especially because of the similarity in presentation between ICI-induced pneumonitis, radiation pneumonitis, pneumonia, and malignant lung infiltration [17].

In this study, we presented our center's experience with ICI-induced pneumonitis and found that all patients had stage IV malignancy, melanoma was the most common malignancy, the majority of cases were grade 2 pneumonitis and that most were treated with steroids. We also found an early mortality rate of 10% which was comparable to that observed by Delaunay et al. [18] (9.4%). However, both studies showed a lower mortality rate than previous studies that reported a mortality rate of 30% to 36% [19–21]. Our study's lower mortality rate could be related to increased physician awareness and early detection and treatment of pneumonitis compared to the earlier studies and could be confounded by the low number of patients.

We also report a median time between initiation of ICI therapy and development of pneumonitis of 3.5 months, which is comparable to prior studies. According to Brahmer et al. [14], the median time to onset of treatment-related pneumonitis was 15.1 weeks. According to Borghaei et al. [22], the median time to onset of pulmonary events was 31.1 weeks. Fujimoto et al. [19] observed a median time of 1.3 months between the start of systemic anticancer treatment and the onset of pneumonitis. Similarly, Delaunay et al. [18] showed that most of their study's pneumonitis cases occurred during the first months of treatment, with a median time to onset of 2.3 months. Naidoo et al. [23] reported that the median time to onset of pneumonitis was 2.8 months.

An interesting finding in our study was that a substantial percentage of study patients with pneumonitis (60%) were obese; however, causality cannot be established using the current study design and the small number of patients. Investigators have previously shown that adipose tissue produces and releases various proinflammatory factors, including cytokines such as tumor necrosis factor-α and interleukin-6 (IL-6) [24]. Evidence also reports a positive correlation between serum IL-6 levels and body fat mass [25]. Moreover, tumor necrosis factor-α is overexpressed in the adipose tissue of obese humans [26, 27]. These cytokines trigger the production of acute-phase reactants, such as C-reactive protein, plasminogen activator inhibitor-1, and serum amyloid-A [28]. Therefore, obesity has been considered a proinflammatory state because of the increased level of inflammatory cytokines [29].

The present study has limitations. First, we recognize that the study has a small patient cohort. However, the small number of patients identified in this study is related to the fact that most patients receive their treatment at facilities elsewhere and visit Mayo Clinic for a second opinion or for restaging scans every 3 months only. This schedule limits the quality of data and decreases the possibility of recording the rate of pulmonary complications accurately because of no access to the outside records. Second, the retrospective design limits the study. However, our objective was to report our center's experience with ICI-induced pneumonitis and to report the characteristics of patients who developed

TABLE 3: Extrapulmonary irAEs*.

Other irAEs	Patients, no. (%)	Grade	Timing in relation to pneumonitis
Encountered	6 (60)		
Not encountered	4 (40)		
Type			
Hepatitis	3 (33.3)	1, 2, 1	Concurrent in all 3 cases
Colitis	2 (22.2)	2, 2	Concurrent in both cases
Sjögren syndrome	1 (11.1)	-	Prior to
Neutropenia	1 (11.1)	-	Prior to
Pericarditis and pericardial effusion	1 (11.1)	2	Concurrent
Conjunctivitis	1 (11.1)	1	Concurrent

Abbreviation: irAE: immune-related adverse event. *Some patients had more than one extrapulmonary irAE.

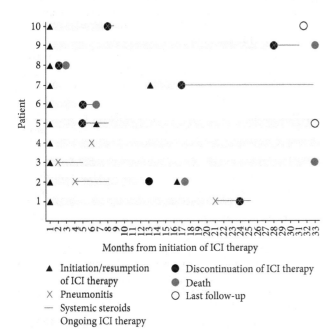

▲ Initiation/resumption of ICI therapy
● Discontinuation of ICI therapy
X Pneumonitis
● Death
— Systemic steroids
○ Last follow-up
Ongoing ICI therapy

FIGURE 2: Timeline of ICI therapy, pneumonitis, steroid therapy, and follow-up.

pneumonitis, for which a retrospective design is adequate. Third, the diagnosis of pneumonitis was determined on the basis of expert opinion after the review of imaging findings. We acknowledge that attributing causality to ICI use is always a challenge because of the lack of universal diagnostic criteria and gold standard diagnostic testing. Yet, we performed a battery of tests—including but not limited to bronchoscopy with BAL—to rule out other causes such as infections and tumor infiltration of the lungs. BAL testing was performed for 40% of our patients. This percentage is in contrast to prior studies, which did not include BAL testing in the evaluation of suspected pneumonitis cases [20, 29]. Moreover, the clinical, laboratory, radiographic, and pathologic characteristics of the study patients were reviewed extensively by experts in the field. Lastly, although we report on multiple findings in patients with pneumonitis in this study including the high rate of obesity, causality cannot be established given the current study design.

5. Conclusions

Melanoma was the most common malignancy associated with pneumonitis, the majority of patients had grade 2 pneumonitis and required treatment with steroids, and all patients affected by ICI-related pneumonitis had stage IV malignancy. Potential risk factors included smoking history, prior radiotherapy, obesity, and advance stage at the time of ICI initiation. Extrapulmonary irAEs are common in patients with pneumonitis.

Abbreviations

BAL: Bronchoalveolar lavage
COPD: Chronic obstructive pulmonary disease
ICI: Immune checkpoint inhibitor
ICU: Intensive care unit
IL-6: Interleukin-6
IQR: Interquartile range
irAE: Immune-related adverse event
SCLC: Small cell lung cancer
PD-1: Programmed death 1.

Disclosure

Pulmonary Complications Secondary to Immune Checkpoint Inhibitors was presented as an abstract at the American Thoracic Society 2019 Meeting in Dallas, Texas. This research was performed as part of employment by the Mayo Clinic in Rochester, Minnesota.

References

[1] Y. Dong, Q. Sun, and X. Zhang, "PD-1 and its ligands are important immune checkpoints in cancer," *Oncotarget*, vol. 8, no. 2, pp. 2171–2186, 2017.

[2] L. S. Walker and D. M. Sansom, "The emerging role of CTLA4 as a cell-extrinsic regulator of T cell responses," *Nature Reviews. Immunology*, vol. 11, no. 12, pp. 852–863, 2011.

[3] C. Robert, A. Ribas, O. Hamid et al., "Durable complete response after discontinuation of pembrolizumab in patients with metastatic melanoma," *Journal of Clinical Oncology*, vol. 36, no. 17, pp. 1668–1674, 2018.

[4] D. Y. Wang, J.-E. Salem, J. V. Cohen et al., "Fatal toxic effects associated with immune checkpoint inhibitors: a systematic review and meta-analysis," *JAMA Oncology*, vol. 4, no. 12, pp. 1721–1728, 2018.

[5] R. N. Schwartz, L. Stover, and J. P. Dutcher, "Managing toxicities of high-dose interleukin-2," *Oncology*, vol. 16, 11 Suppl 13, pp. 11–20, 2002.

[6] O. Abdel-Rahman and M. Fouad, "Risk of pneumonitis in cancer patients treated with immune checkpoint inhibitors: a meta-analysis," *Therapeutic Advances in Respiratory Disease*, vol. 10, no. 3, pp. 183–193, 2016.

[7] S. H. Tirumani, N. H. Ramaiya, A. Keraliya et al., "Radiographic profiling of immune-related adverse events in advanced melanoma patients treated with ipilimumab," *Cancer Immunology Research*, vol. 3, no. 10, pp. 1185–1192, 2015.

[8] J. D. Possick, "Pulmonary toxicities from checkpoint immunotherapy for malignancy," *Clinics in Chest Medicine*, vol. 38, no. 2, pp. 223–232, 2017.

[9] S. Champiat, O. Lambotte, E. Barreau et al., "Management of immune checkpoint blockade dysimmune toxicities: a collaborative position paper," *Annals of Oncology*, vol. 27, no. 4, pp. 559–574, 2016.

[10] J. S. Weber, R. Dummer, V. de Pril, C. Lebbé, F. S. Hodi, and for the MDX010-20 Investigators, "Patterns of onset and resolution of immune-related adverse events of special interest with ipilimumab: detailed safety analysis from a phase 3 trial in patients with advanced melanoma," *Cancer*, vol. 119, no. 9, pp. 1675–1682, 2013.

[11] M. Selman, A. Pardo, and T. E. King Jr., "Hypersensitivity pneumonitis: insights in diagnosis and pathobiology," *American Journal of Respiratory and Critical Care Medicine*, vol. 186, no. 4, pp. 314–324, 2012.

[12] National Cancer Institute Common Terminology Criteria for Adverse Events (CTCAE), 2018, November 2018, https://ctep.cancer.gov/protocolDevelopment/electronic_applications/ctc.htm#ctc_40.

[13] E. D. Kwon, C. G. Drake, H. I. Scher et al., "Ipilimumab versus placebo after radiotherapy in patients with metastatic castration-resistant prostate cancer that had progressed after docetaxel chemotherapy (CA184-043): a multicentre, randomised, double-blind, phase 3 trial," *The Lancet Oncology*, vol. 15, no. 7, pp. 700–712, 2014.

[14] J. Brahmer, K. L. Reckamp, P. Baas et al., "Nivolumab versus docetaxel in advanced squamous-cell non-small-cell lung cancer," *The New England Journal of Medicine*, vol. 373, no. 2, pp. 123–135, 2015.

[15] M. Nishino, A. Giobbie-Hurder, H. Hatabu, N. H. Ramaiya, and F. S. Hodi, "Incidence of programmed cell death 1 inhibitor-related pneumonitis in patients with advanced cancer: a systematic review and meta-analysis," *JAMA Oncology*, vol. 2, no. 12, pp. 1607–1616, 2016.

[16] M. Nishino, N. H. Ramaiya, M. M. Awad et al., "PD-1 inhibitor-related pneumonitis in advanced cancer patients: radiographic patterns and clinical course," *Clinical Cancer Research*, vol. 22, no. 24, pp. 6051 6060, 2016.

[17] K. S. Shohdy and O. Abdel-Rahman, "Risk of pneumonitis with different immune checkpoint inhibitors in NSCLC," *Annals of Translational Medicine*, vol. 5, no. 17, p. 365, 2017.

[18] M. Delaunay, J. Cadranel, A. Lusque et al., "Immune-checkpoint inhibitors associated with interstitial lung disease in cancer patients," *European Respiratory Journal*, vol. 50, no. 2, p. 1700050, 2017.

[19] D. Fujimoto, R. Kato, T. Morimoto et al., "Characteristics and prognostic impact of pneumonitis during systemic anti-cancer therapy in patients with advanced non-small-cell lung cancer," *PLoS One*, vol. 11, no. 12, article e0168465, 2016.

[20] R. Dhokarh, G. Li, C. N. Schmickl et al., "Drug-associated acute lung injury: a population-based cohort study," *Chest*, vol. 142, no. 4, pp. 845–850, 2012.

[21] T. Sakurada, S. Kakiuchi, S. Tajima et al., "Characteristics of and risk factors for interstitial lung disease induced by chemotherapy for lung cancer," *The Annals of Pharmacotherapy*, vol. 49, no. 4, pp. 398–404, 2015.

[22] H. Borghaei, L. Paz-Ares, L. Horn et al., "Nivolumab versus docetaxel in advanced nonsquamous non-small-cell lung cancer," *The New England Journal of Medicine*, vol. 373, no. 17, pp. 1627–1639, 2015.

[23] J. Naidoo, X. Wang, K. M. Woo et al., "Pneumonitis in patients treated with anti-programmed death-1/programmed death ligand 1 therapy," *Journal of Clinical Oncology*, vol. 35, no. 7, pp. 709–717, 2017.

[24] M. Lafontan, "Fat cells: afferent and efferent messages define new approaches to treat obesity," *Annual Review of Pharmacology and Toxicology*, vol. 45, pp. 119–146, 2005.

[25] R. H. Straub, H. W. Hense, T. Andus, J. Scholmerich, G. A. Riegger, and H. Schunkert, "Hormone replacement therapy and interrelation between serum interleukin-6 and body mass index in postmenopausal women: a population-based study," *The Journal of Clinical Endocrinology and Metabolism*, vol. 85, no. 3, pp. 1340–1344, 2000.

[26] G. S. Hotamisligil, P. Arner, J. F. Caro, R. L. Atkinson, and B. M. Spiegelman, "Increased adipose tissue expression of tumor necrosis factor-alpha in human obesity and insulin resistance," *The Journal of Clinical Investigation*, vol. 95, no. 5, pp. 2409–2415, 1995.

[27] P. A. Kern, M. Saghizadeh, J. M. Ong, R. J. Bosch, R. Deem, and R. B. Simsolo, "The expression of tumor necrosis factor in human adipose tissue. Regulation by obesity, weight loss, and relationship to lipoprotein lipase," *The Journal of Clinical Investigation*, vol. 95, no. 5, pp. 2111–2119, 1995.

[28] A. Badawi, A. Klip, P. Haddad et al., "Type 2 diabetes mellitus and inflammation: prospects for biomarkers of risk and nutritional intervention," *Diabetes, Metabolic Syndrome and Obesity: Targets and Therapy*, vol. 3, pp. 173–186, 2010.

[29] M. S. Ellulu, I. Patimah, H. Khaza'ai, A. Rahmat, and Y. Abed, "Obesity and inflammation: the linking mechanism and the complications," *Archives of Medical Science*, vol. 4, no. 4, pp. 851–863, 2017.

9

Haematological Features and Urologic Pathologies of Diabetic Subjects at Bafoussam Regional Hospital

Arsene T. Signing,[1] **Wiliane J. T. Marbou** ⓘ,[1] **Veronique P. Beng,**[2] **and Victor Kuete** ⓘ[1]

[1]*Department of Biochemistry, University of Dschang, P.O. Box 67, Dschang, Cameroon*
[2]*Department of Biochemistry, University of Yaoundé 1, Cameroun P.O. Box 812, Yaoundé, Cameroon*

Correspondence should be addressed to Victor Kuete; kuetevictor@yahoo.fr

Academic Editor: Katarzyna Zorena

Background. Diabetes mellitus is at the origin of long-term complications. *Objective.* This study is aimed at assessing the haematological features and urologic pathologies of diabetic individuals at Bafoussam Regional Hospital. *Methods.* This was a cross-sectional study conducted from August 2018 to May 2019 in Bafoussam Regional Hospital, West Cameroon. A structured questionnaire was used to gather sociodemographic data. A trained nurse measured the physical and clinical features. Fasting plasma glucose was determined using the glucose meter Accu-Chek Active system. The full blood count (FBC) was carried out using Automatic full Blood Counter, and the CD4, CD3, and CD8 T-cell counts were determined using the flow cytometry method. *Results.* There were 455 diabetic patients, and 50 nondiabetic patients were included. The mean age of diabetic patients (56.94 ± 14.33 years) was higher compared to that of nondiabetic individuals (34.76 ± 14.35 years) ($p < 0.001$). There was a significant relationship between married individuals ($\chi^2 = 79.19$, $p < 0.001$, and $df = 4$), housewife and retired ($\chi^2 = 1117.38$, $p < 0.001$, and $df = 37$), old age (40 years and above) ($\chi^2 = 79.11$, $p < 0.001$, and $df = 3$), and diabetes status. Diabetic patients had an odds of 5.52 to experience a urinary urge as compared to the controls ($p < 0.001$, 95% CI = 2.15-14.22). The majority of haematological parameters were negatively but not significantly correlated with diabetes. Binary logistic regression shows that MCV ($r = -0.251$, OR = 0.778, and 95% CI = 0.617–0.983; $p = 0.035$) and RDW-CV ($r = -0.477$, OR = 0.620, and 95% CI = 0.454–0.848; $p = 0.003$) negatively influence the probability of having diabetes. RDW-SD ($r = 0.135$, OR = 1.144, and 95% CI = 1.014–1.291; $p = 0.029$) positively influences the probability of having diabetes. *Conclusion.* This study revealed a significant haematological and urological profile difference according to diabetes status. Research and interventions targeted at diabetic population could help close gaps in diabetes complications.

1. Introduction

Diabetes is a disease that is having a significant repercussion on the socioeconomic, physical, and psychological aspects of the lives of the victims. It is a pathology characterized by an abnormal rise of the level of glucose in the blood, which is defined by a fasting glycaemia greater than or equal to 126 mg/dL (measured twice) or glycaemia greater than 200 mg/dL after a meal [1]. It has existed since antiquity but is diagnosed by polyuria alluding to abnormal diuresis in 24 hours [2]. As early as 1797, with the Englishman John Rollo, the first metabolic theories aimed at explaining diabetes were born. According to this author, excess sugar in the

urine comes from an abnormal transformation of food carbohydrates by the stomach. In 1848, Claude Bernard demonstrated the glycogenic function of the liver, and it is due to the works of Oskar Minkowski and Joseph Von Mehring that the role of the pancreas was discovered in 1886 at the University of Strasbourg [2]. The removal of the pancreas (or pancreatectomy) in dogs is followed by diabetes, this diabetes being corrected by the pancreas transplant [2].

The world population of diabetes was 360 million in 2000, and it was projected that this rate would increase to 552 million in 2030 [3]. However, new data on the global prevalence of diabetes are thrilling because recent estimates from the International Diabetes Federation indicated that

8.3% of adults (20-79 years) or 382 million people worldwide have diabetes and that number could exceed 592 million in less than 25 years [4]. Some epidemiologists predicted that the economic impact of diabetes and the number of deaths will be more than the one caused by HIV/AIDS. The prevalence of diabetes in Africa and Cameroon is 5.8% and 5% to 6%, respectively [5]. These figures make diabetes to be a public health problem, hence the need to assess all the parameters contributing to the increase in complications linked to this disease. However, the complications of this condition are not the least [4].

Indeed, diabetes is at the origin of long-term complications which can be the source of serious handicaps considerably altering the quality of life [6]. The chronic complications of diabetes include peripheral neuropathy and autonomic neuropathy, retinopathy, diabetic foot, and diabetic kidney disease [6]. The degenerative complications secondary to diabetes, having as main causes of hyperglycaemia and hyperinsulinemia, affect several organs and systems such as the cardiovascular system, eyes, nerves, limbs, and kidneys. Over time, uncontrolled accumulated blood glucose levels lead to tissue damage that can cause urologic complications in diabetic individuals. Diabetes is, therefore, an important risk factor for cardiovascular disease and one of the leading causes of blindness, kidney failure, and amputation for non-traumatic causes in the world [6]. Also, diabetes is a pathology that affects cells of the immune system and makes patients vulnerable to many infections [7]. Along the same lines, studies have shown that diabetes will increase the risk of developing infectious diseases [8]. To provide data regarding the variation of blood cell levels in diabetics, the objective of this work was to assess the distribution of the urologic pathologies and haematological characteristics of diabetes among individuals in the diabetology unit of Bafoussam Regional Hospital.

2. Materials and Methods

2.1. Study Setting. The study was conducted in Bafoussam Regional Hospital, West Cameroon. The hospital serves as a referral centre for 20 hospitals in western region districts. According to the World Population Review (2020), the total population of Bafoussam is 290768 [9].

2.2. Study Design, Period, and Sample Size. A cross-sectional study was conducted from August 01, 2018, to May 29, 2019. The source population was diabetes-confirmed individuals at the diabetology unit, and the nondiabetic individuals came to consult at the diabetes unit of Bafoussam Regional Hospital. The sample size was calculated using the single population proportion formula by considering the sample proportion as 5.8% prevalence of diabetes [5], 0.03 desired precision, 95% confidence interval (CI), and a design effect of 2. Thus, the minimum sample size (n) calculated was found to be 468. We, therefore, obtained 455 diabetic patients (41 type I diabetes and 414 type II diabetes) and 50 nondiabetic patients for a total of 505 participants. Type I diabetes and type II diabetes were considered inclusion criteria.

2.3. Ethics Considerations. Ethical clearance for this study was obtained from the Cameroon National Research Ethics Committee. We obtained a research certificate from the University of Dschang as well as a research authorization from Bafoussam Regional Hospital. All the participants were duly informed of the study goals, procedures, potential harm and benefits, and cost, as well as the finality of the study. Each patient signed an informed consent form, thereby agreeing to participate in the study. Subsequently, a questionnaire was submitted to them and the collection of samples was carried out following the scientific and ethical standards. All results were coded and kept confidential.

2.4. Exclusion Criteria. Pregnant women, tuberculosis patients, and HIV-positive patients were excluded from this study to avoid the possible impact on the anthropometric and laboratory parameters.

2.5. Demographic Data Collection. Data on demographics were collected by trained personnel through a face-to-face interview using a structured questionnaire. The study team was composed of laboratory technicians, nurses, and supervisors. Each participant was questioned for age, sex, profession, educational status, and marital status.

2.6. Physical Measurements and Clinical Features. Participants' height and weight were measured to calculate the body mass index (BMI). Clinical features were screened by a trained nurse. These clinical features include pollakiuria, dysuria, fever, burn, urinary leakage, and urge to urinate. BMI $\geq 30 \, \text{kg/m}^2$ was considered obese [10].

2.7. Biochemical Measurements. Plasma glucose (after an overnight fasting $\geq 8 \, \text{h}$) was determined using the glucose meter Accu-Chek Active system [11]. Fasting capillary blood samples were collected three times (for three consecutive hours) from a single study participant, and glucose measurement was carried out within fractions of seconds after sample collection. Then, their average was taken for analysis. The American Diabetes Association diabetes mellitus classification criteria were used for the diagnosis of diabetes. The diagnosis of DM was based on the American Diabetes Association diabetes mellitus classification criteria with fasting blood glucose of $\geq 126 \, \text{mg/dL}$ being considered positive for diabetes and fasting blood glucose (FPG) of less than $61 \, \text{mg/dL}$ to $<110 \, \text{mg/dL}$ being considered normoglycaemic [1]. An FPG level $> 126 \, \text{mg/dL}$ or a casual plasma glucose $> 200 \, \text{mg/dL}$ meets the threshold for the diagnosis of diabetes.

Furthermore, fasting venous blood was collected from each participant, using EDTA tubes for the full blood count and CD4 T-cell count. The full blood count (FBC) was carried out using Automatic full Blood Counter (*Automatic full Blood Counter ERMA*, Japan). The CD4 T-cell count of all the participants were determined using flow cytometry applied in clinical immunology by Becton Dickinson's FACSCount method [12].

2.8. Data Analysis. To examine the association between diabetes status with patients' demographic and clinical parameters, we used the chi-squared test for categorical variables and

TABLE 1: Sociodemographic characteristics of total study participants.

Sociodemographic parameters	Characteristics	Frequency ($n = 505$)	Percentage (%)
Sex	Male	215	42.57
	Female	290	57.43
Matrimonial status	Married	403	79.80
	Widow/widower	66	13.07
	Divorced	7	1.39
	Single	28	5.54
	In a relationship	1	0.20
Profession	Retired	86	17.03
	Teacher	39	7.72
	Housewife	126	24.95
	Trader	45	8.91
	Cultivator	69	13.66
	Cashier	6	1.19
	Cook	6	1.19
	Policeman	4	0.79
	Dressmaker	14	2.77
	Metalworker	2	0.40
	Nurse	12	2.38
	Resourceful	5	0.99
	Carpenter	2	0.40
	Planter	14	2.77
	Potter	2	0.40
	Engineer	3	0.59
	Driver	10	1.98
	Student	9	1.78
	Photographer	1	0.20
	Electrician	3	0.59
	Builder	3	0.59
	Mechanic	7	1.39
	Tailor	2	0.40
	Civil servant	3	0.59
	Mayor	1	0.20
	Gardener	1	0.20
	Municipal agent	3	0.59
	Hairdresser	4	0.79
	Secretary	5	0.99
	Accounting	3	0.59
	Pastor	3	0.59
	Counter	3	0.59
	Stylist	2	0.40
Educational level	GCE O-level	60	11.88
	GCE A-level	54	10.69
	First school-leaving certificate	104	20.59
	HND	8	1.58

TABLE 1: Continued.

Sociodemographic parameters	Characteristics	Frequency ($n = 505$)	Percentage (%)
	No study conducted	50	9.90
	End of primary studies without a diploma	107	21.19
	Stop high school without diplomas	59	11.68
	Bachelor	35	6.93
	Master	8	1.58
	PhD	1	0.20
	Probatory	19	3.76
Age groups	0-20	13	2.57
	21-40	76	15.05
	40-61	224	44.36
	61-90	192	38.02

GCE: General Certificate of Education; HND: Higher National Diploma.

the t-test for continuous variables. Binary logistic regression analysis was used to assess the relation between haematological features of study participants versus their diabetes status. p values < 0.05 were considered to be significant. All statistical analyses were carried out using SPSS 18.0 (release: July 30, 2009; USA) for Windows (IBM).

3. Results

3.1. Descriptive Statistics. Out of a sample of 505 research participants, 57.4% ($n = 290$) were females while 42.6% ($n = 215$) were males. With regard to the age range, 224 participants fell within the age group of 41–60 years with a percentage score of 44.4%. These were followed by those within the age range of 61–90 years with 38.0% and frequency of 192. Only 13 participants fell within the age range of 0–20 years with a percentage score of 2.6% ($n = 13$). The majority of participants ($n = 403$) were married with a percentage score of 79.8%, while the least ($n = 1$) was still cohabiting (0.2%). Majority of participants were housewives with 25.0% ($n = 126$), followed by retired civil servants with 17.0% ($n = 86$). The least among them were photographers, majors, and gardener with a percentage of 0.2% each. For the educational level, the majority of those with diabetes had CEP (first school-leaving certificate) (22.2%). Participants that ended their educational level at primary school and have no diploma followed those with CEP with 19.3% ($n = 88$). The least within the sample was a Ph.D. holder with a percentage score of 0.2 ($n = 1$) (Table 1).

3.2. Sociodemographic Characteristics of Study Participants according to the Diabetes Status. Sociodemographic features according to diabetes status are presented in Table 2. There were 455 diabetic patients (57.80% females, $n = 263$ and 42.20% males, $n = 192$) and 50 nondiabetic individuals (54%

TABLE 2: Features of participants according to diabetes status.

Sociodemographic parameters	Characteristics	Control patients ($n = 50$)	Diabetic patients ($n = 455$)	χ^2	p value
Sex	Male	23 (46)	192 (42.20)	0.26	0.606
	Female	27 (54)	263 (57.80)		
Matrimonial status	Married	22 (44)	381 (83.73)	79.19	$p < 0.001$
	Widow/widower	26 (52)	40 (8.80)		
	Divorced	2 (4)	5 (1.10)		
	Single	0 (0)	28 (6.15)		
	In a relationship	0 (0)	1 (0.22)		
Profession	Retired	3 (6)	83 (18.24)	117.37	$p < 0.001$
	Teacher	8 (16)	31 (6.81)		
	Housewife	10 (20)	116 (25.50)		
	Trader	3 (6)	42 (9.23)		
	Cultivator	4 (8)	65 (14.29)		
	Cashier	5 (10)	1 (0.22)		
	Cook	3 (6)	3 (0.66)		
	Policeman	3 (6)	1 (0.22)		
	Dressmaker	7 (14)	7 (1.54)		
	Metalworker	1 (2)	1 (0.22)		
	Nurse	2 (4)	10 (2.20)		
	Resourceful	1 (2)	4 (0.88)		
	Carpenter	0 (0)	2 (0.44)		
	Planter	0 (0)	14 (3.08)		
	Potter	0 (0)	2 (0.44)		
	Engineer	0 (0)	3 (0.66)		
	Driver	0 (0)	10 (2.20)		
	Student	0 (0)	9 (1.20)		
	Photographer	0 (0)	1 (0.22)		
	Electrician	0 (0)	3 (0.66)		
	Mason	0 (0)	3 (0.66)		
	Mechanic	0 (0)	7 (1.54)		
	Tailor	0 (0)	2 (0.44)		
	Civil servant	0 (0)	3 (0.66)		
	Mayor	0 (0)	1 (0.22)		
	Gardener	0 (0)	1 (0.22)		
	Municipal agent	0 (0)	3 (0.66)		
	Hairdresser	0 (0)	4 (0.88)		
	Secretary	0 (0)	5 (1.10)		
	Accounting	0 (0)	3 (0.66)		
	Pastor	0 (0)	3 (0.66)		
	Counter	0 (0)	3 (0.66)		
	Stylist	0 (0)	2 (0.44)		
Educational level	GCE O-level	1 (2)	59 (12.96)	32.92	$p < 0.001$
	GCE A-level	3 (6)	51 (11.20)		
	First school-leaving certificate	3 (6)	101 (22.20)		
	HND	2 (4)	6 (1.31)		
	No study conducted	11 (22)	39 (8.57)		
	End of primary studies without a diploma	19 (38)	88 (19.34)		

TABLE 2: Continued.

Sociodemographic parameters	Characteristics	Control patients ($n = 50$)	Diabetic patients ($n = 455$)	χ^2	p value
	Stop high school without diplomas	8 (16)	51 (11.20)		
	Bachelor	2 (4)	33 (7.25)		
	Master	1 (2)	7 (1.54)		
	PhD	0 (0)	1 (0.22)		
	Probatory	0 (0)	19 (4.17)		
Age groups	0-20	5 (10)	8 (1.75)		
	21-40	26 (52)	50 (10.98)	79.11	$p < 0.001$
	40-61	16 (32)	208 (45.71)		
	61-90	3 (6)	189 (41.53)		

GCE: General Certificate of Education; HND: Higher National Diploma.

females, $n = 27$ and 46% males, $n = 23$) were included. The mean age of diabetic patients (56.94 ± 14.33 years) was higher compared to that of nondiabetic individuals (34.76 ± 14.35 years) ($p < 0.001$).

At the 0.05 significance level, there was no significant difference between gender and diabetes status within the study sample ($\chi^2 = 0.27$, $p = 0.606$). Despite the differences between males and females for diabetic patients, the control of gender difference was not significant.

There was a significant ($\chi^2 = 79.19$, $p < 0.001$, and $df = 4$) relationship between married individuals and diabetes status. Among the diabetic patients, the majority (83.7%) were those who reported to having been married. These were followed by widows or widowers with a percentage score of 8.8%. At 0.05 significance level, there was a significant difference between profession of respondents and their diabetes status ($\chi^2 = 1117.38$, $p < 0.001$, and $df = 37$).

The educational level showed significant differences with diabetes status at 0.05 significance level ($\chi^2 = 32.93$, $p < 0.001$, and $df = 10$). The majority of those with diabetes had CEP (22.2%). Participants that ended their educational level at primary school and have no diploma followed those with CEP with 19.3% ($n = 88$).

The age range also differed significantly with diabetes status ($\chi^2 = 79.11$, $p < 0.001$, and $df = 3$). The majority of those with diabetes came from the age group 41–60 with a percentage score of 89.7%. In fact, the Spearman correlation analysis indicated a positive significant correlation between age and diabetes ($r = +0.96$, $p < 0.001$).

3.3. Clinical Features of the Diabetic and Nondiabetic Study Subjects. Table 3 presents the clinical features of the diabetic and nondiabetic study subjects. All the clinical parameters were significantly associated with diabetes status except for the development of fever ($\chi^2 = 0.33$, $p = 0.362$) and urinary leakage ($\chi^2 = 1.436$, $p = 0.195$). From Table 3, a majority of diabetic patients within the study population reported having had dysuria ($\chi^2 = 5.73$, $p = 0.021$, and OR = 2.39 within a 95% CI of 1.149-4.980). For the urge to urinate for example, diabetic patients had an odds of 5.52 to experience urinary urge as compared to the controls ($p < 0.001$, 95% CI = 2.15-14.22). Also, diabetic patients had an odds of 5.64 to develop obesity as compared to the controls ($p < 0.001$, 95% CI = 1.87-17.03).

3.4. t-Test Analysis to Compute the Mean Differences in Haematological Parameters between the Diabetic and Control Groups in the Study Sample. A two-independent sample t-test was run to compute the mean differences in haematological parameters between the diabetic and control groups in the study sample. Equal variances were assumed in this analysis as the differences between the haematological mean values were close enough (±1.2).

Out of the 20 haematological parameters analysed, the CD4 T-cell blood level ($p = 0.024$, 95% CI = −151.208 to -10.053), % lymphocytes ($p = 0.024$, 95% CI = −6.35 to -0.45), % monocytes ($p = 0.038$, 95% CI = −1.53 to -0.043), GR ($p < 0.001$, 95% CI = −1.72 to -0.54), HCT ($p = 0.002$, 95% CI = −4.862-1.119), RDW-CV ($p = 0.005$, 95% CI = −1.87 to -0.32), and RDW-SD ($p = 0.003$, 95% CI = −8.07 to -1.73) were significantly lower in diabetic patients compared to nondiabetic individuals. The % granulocytes ($p = 0.002$, 95% CI = −6.51 to -0.29) and MCHC ($p = 0.045$, 95% CI = 0.01 to 0.87) were significantly higher in diabetic patients compared to nondiabetic individuals (Table 4). These results reveal haematological disturbance of diabetic patients compared to nondiabetics although the difference in results is not statistically significant for the other parameters.

3.5. Relationship between Diabetes Status and Haematologic Parameters. Table 5 presents the correlation between haematologic parameters and diabetes status. The majority of haematologic parameters were negatively but not significantly correlated with diabetes. Binary logistic regression shows that MCV ($r = -0.251$, OR = 0.778, and 95% CI = 0.617–0.983; $p = 0.035$) and RDW-CV ($r = -0.477$, OR = 0.620, and 95% CI = 0.454–0.848; $p = 0.003$) negatively influence the probability of having diabetes. RDW-SD ($r = 0.135$, OR = 1.144, and 95% CI = 1.014–1.291; $p = 0.029$) positively influences the probability of having diabetes.

TABLE 3: Clinical features of the diabetic and nondiabetic study subjects.

Variable	Characteristic frequency (%)		χ^2 (p value)	OR	CI
	Type of diabetes				
	Type I	Type II			
Diabetes	41 (9.01)	414 (90.99)	NA	NA	NA
Control	0 (00)	0 (00)			
	Pollakiuria				
	Yes	No			
Diabetes	254 (55.82)	201 (44.18)	14.760 (0.001)*	0.070	0.0421–0.288
Control	42 (84)	8 (16)			
	Dysuria				
	Yes	No			
Diabetes	407 (89.45)	48 (10.55)	5.730 (0.021)*	2.390	1.149–4.980
Control	39 (78)	11(22)			
	Fever				
	Yes	No			
Diabetes	420 (92.31)	35 (7.69)	0.330 (0.362)	1.330	0.497–3.575
Control	45 (90)	5 (10)			
	Burn				
	Yes	No			
Diabetes	433 (95.16)	22 (4.84)	6.990 (0.017)*	3.204	1.294–7.931
Control	43 (86)	7 (14)			
	Urinary leakage				
	Yes	No			
Diabetes	427 (93.85)	28 (6.15)	1.430 (0.195)	0.311	0.041–2.34
Control	49 (98)	1 (2)			
	Urge to urinate				
	No	Yes			
Diabetes	254 (55.82)	201(44.18)	24.450 ($p < 0.001$)*	5.520	2.15–14.22
Control	46 (92)	4 (8)			
	Obesity				
	Yes	No			
Diabetes	301(66.15)	154 (33.85)	16.310 ($p < 0.001$)*	5.640	1.87–17.03
Control	47 (90)	3 (10)			
	Hospital attendance				
	Yes	No			
Diabetes	119 (26.15)	336 (73.85)	0.719 ($p = 0.397$)	1.348	0.67–2.70
Control	46 (92)	4 (8)			

OR = odds ratio; CI = confidence interval. *Significant at 0.05 significance level.

4. Discussion

Diabetes is the most well-known chronic metabolic disease. It is a metabolic disorder characterized by the presence of hyperglycaemia attributable to a reduction in insulin secretion or insulin action or both. Diabetes is a common condition affecting both the young and the elderly, which can lead to acute accidents of various aetiologies mainly metabolic, neurological, cardiovascular, and haematological. This study is aimed at assessing the distribution of the clinical and haematological characteristics of diabetes among individuals in the diabetology unit of Bafoussam Regional Hospital.

This study revealed that out of 505 research participants, 57.4% ($n = 290$) were females while 42.6% ($n = 215$) were males. This result can be explained by a sedentary lifestyle which is notably more accentuated in female individuals compared to males as reported by a previous study [13]. A significant relationship was observed between married

TABLE 4: Mean differences in haematological parameters between the diabetic and control groups.

Haematological parameters	Diabetes/control	Frequency	Mean	Std. deviation	Std. error mean	t-test			95% CI	
						t	df	Sig. (2-tailed)	Lower	Upper
CD4 T-cells	Diabetes	455	802.369	230.119	10.788	-2245	503	0.025	-151.208	-10.053
	Control	50	883.000	325.757	460.690					
GB (×103 cells/µL)	Diabetes	455	5.465	1.991	0.093	0.478	503	0.633	-0.432	0.711
	Control	50	5.326	1.568	0.221					
Lymphocytes (×103 cells/µL)	Diabetes	455	2.2116	0.71218	0.033	-1493	503	0.136	-0.371	0.050
	Control	50	2.3720	0.79566	0.112					
Monocytes (×103 cells/µL)	Diabetes	455	0.4570	0.16385	0.008	-1415	503	0.158	-0.084	0.013
	Control	50	0.4922	0.19436	0.027					
Granulocytes (×103 cells/µL)	Diabetes	455	2.807	1.694	0.079	1190	503	0.235	-0.191	0.777
	Control	50	2.514	1.230	0.174					
% lymphocytes	Diabetes	455	41.740	10.027	0.470	-2267	503	0.024	-6.349	-0.453
	Control	50	45.142	10.466	1.480					
% monocytes	Diabetes	455	8.852	2.511	0.117	-2079	503	0.038	-1.527	-0.043
	Control	50	9.638	2.745	0.388					
% granulocytes	Diabetes	455	49.3925	10.904	0.511	3047	503	0.002	1.762	8.162
	Control	50	44.430	11.176	15.805					
Haemoglobin	Diabetes	455	12.254	1.800	0.084	-1465	503	0.144	-0.947	0.138
	Control	50	12.659	2.293	0.324					
GR	Diabetes	455	4.762	0.628	0.029	-3743	503	0.000	-1.717	-0.535
	Control	50	5.888	6.181	0.874					
HCT	Diabetes	455	42.166	6.137	0.287	-3140	503	0.002	-4.862	-1.119
	Control	50	45.158	8.412	1.189					
MCV	Diabetes	455	88.457	6.508	0.305	1560	503	0.119	-0.430	3.753
	Control	50	86.796	11.475	1.622					
MCH	Diabetes	455	25.725	1.985	0.093	0.497	503	0.620	-0.443	0.742
	Control	50	25.576	2.366	0.334					
MCHC	Diabetes	455	29.007	1.336	0.062	2006	503	0.045	0.009	0.874
	Control	50	28.566	2.424	0.342					
RDW-CV	Diabetes	455	14.203	2.321	0.108	-2790	503	0.005	-1.872	-0.324
	Control	50	15.302	4.674	0.661					
RDW-SD	Diabetes	455	46.101	5.838	0.273	-3035	503	0.003	-8.066	-1.727
	Control	50	50.998	29.792	4.213					
PLT	Diabetes	455	238.079	77.592	3.637	0.867	503	0.386	-12.761	32.939
	Control	50	227.990	82.293	11.638					
MPV	Diabetes	455	9.981	0.77383	0.036	1307	503	0.192	-0.077	0.384
	Control	50	9.828	0.92097	0.130					
PDW	Diabetes	455	15.000	6.537	0.306	0.692	503	0.489	-1.184	2.471
	Control	50	14.356	2.056	0.290					
PCT (%)	Diabetes	455	0.232	0.069	0.003	0.703	503	0.482	-0.013	0.027
	Control	50	0.225	0.074	0.010					

CD: cluster of differentiation; FBC: full blood count; GB: white blood cells; GR: red blood cells; HCT: haematocrit; HIV: human immunodeficiency viruses; MCV: mean corpuscular volume; MCH: mean corpuscular haemoglobin; MCHC: mean corpuscular haemoglobin concentration; MPV: mean platelet volume; RDW-CV: red blood cell distribution width-coefficient of variation; RDW-SD: red blood cell distribution width-standard deviation; PCT: procalcitonin; PDW: platelet distribution width; PLT: platelet. *Significant at 0.05 significance level.

TABLE 5: Correlation of haematologic parameters and diabetes status.

Parameters	r	S.E.	Wald	df	Sig.	OR	95% CI	
							Lower	Upper
CD4 T-cells	-0.001	0.001	3.072	1	0.080	0.999	0.997	1.000
GB (×103 cells/μL)	3.317	3.259	1.036	1	0.309	27.583	0.046	16379.923
Lymphocytes (×103 cells/μL)	-2.726	3.105	0.771	1	0.380	0.065	0.000	28.769
Monocytes (×103 cells/μL)	-5.020	5.375	0.872	1	0.350	0.007	0.000	248.436
Granulocytes (×103 cells/μL)	-3.662	3.254	1.266	1	0.260	0.026	0.000	15.119
% lymphocytes	0.190	0.184	1.066	1	0.302	1.209	0.843	1.735
% monocytes	0.382	0.280	1.852	1	0.174	1.465	0.845	2.538
% granulocytes	0.290	0.193	2.248	1	0.134	1.336	0.915	1.951
Haemoglobin	0.581	0.910	0.407	1	0.523	1.787	0.300	10.635
GR	-0.169	0.821	0.043	1	0.837	0.844	0.169	4.220
HCT	-0.267	0.281	0.906	1	0.341	0.765	0.441	1.328
MCV	-0.251	0.119	4.439	1	0.035	0.778	0.617	0.983
MCH	0.801	0.440	3.313	1	0.069	2.228	0.940	5.277
MCHC	-0.494	0.708	0.488	1	0.485	0.610	0.152	2.442
RDW-CV	-0.477	0.159	8.985	1	0.003	0.620	0.454	0.848
RDW-SD	0.135	0.062	4.770	1	0.029	1.144	1.014	1.291
PLT	0.019	0.024	0.626	1	0.429	1.019	0.973	1.067
MPV	0.643	0.743	0.749	1	0.387	1.903	0.443	8.166
PDW	1.107	0.976	1.287	1	0.257	3.024	0.447	20.465
PCT (%)	-14.314	24.312	0.347	1	0.556	0.000	0.000	$3.004E14$

CD: cluster of differentiation; FBC: full blood count; GB: white blood cells; GR: red blood cells; HCT: haematocrit; HIV: human immunodeficiency viruses; MCV: mean corpuscular volume; MCH: mean corpuscular haemoglobin; MCHC: mean corpuscular haemoglobin concentration; MPV: mean platelet volume; RDW-CV: red blood cell distribution width-coefficient of variation; RDW-SD: red blood cell distribution width-standard deviation; PCT: procalcitonin; PDW: platelet distribution width; PLT: platelet. *Significant at 0.05 significance level.

individuals and diabetes status. A previous study reported that poor marital quality is associated with many different indicators of poor health such as diabetes [14]. The relationship between marital status and glycaemic control, in particular, the effect of marriage on the onset of diabetes, could probably be due to the pathophysiological and therapeutic characteristics of the disease [15]. Concerning the profession and the diabetes status, a significant difference was observed concerning housewives and retired individuals. The majority of diabetic patients were housewives, followed by retired public servants. This can be explained by the fact that these two categories of the population have a lifestyle of their own, generally characterized by a sedentary lifestyle, an unbalanced diet, travel by motorbike or vehicle even over short distances, and lack of physical activity [16]. A study from Jeddah, Saudi Arabia, indicated that nonsmoker housewives are considered the high-risk group of developing obesity among diabetic patients [17]. Regarding the level of education, the low intellectual level of our study population will justify their lack of knowledge about diabetes and its prevention methods. This may explain the fact that for our study, the majority of diabetics had a first school-leaving certificate followed by participants who completed their education level in primary school and without a diploma. This result is inconsistent with that of Agardh and colleagues in Sweden who demonstrated a considerable burden of diabetes mellitus attributed to lower educational levels in Sweden [18].

This study indicated that the majority of diabetic individuals belonged to the age group between 41 and 60 years. In fact, the Pearson correlation analysis indicated a significant positive correlation between age and diabetes. This is similar to the results obtained in other regions of sub-Saharan Africa and other developing countries such as Ghana [19]. In developed countries like the USA, the correlation was most in the patients who had over the age of 60 years [20]. This can be explained by the fact that it is the category of the socially active population that is easily exposed to certain environmental factors such as the use of alcohol and tobacco, which are the risk factor of diabetes.

About the clinical characteristics of the diabetic and nondiabetic subjects, all clinical parameters were significantly associated with diabetes, except the development of fever and urinary leakage. Diabetic patients in the study population reported having dysuria, characteristic of their type of diabetes. Diabetes status explains the fact that diabetic patients had an odds of 5.52 of experiencing a urinary urge compared to controls and also had an odds of 5.64 of developing obesity compared to controls. Diabetes and urologic pathologies are very common health problems [21]. A recent study has shown that diabetes mellitus independently increases the risk of urinary incontinence in women [22]. Urologic pathologies due to diabetes are a serious kidney-related complication of type 1 diabetes and type 2 diabetes. It affects individuals' kidneys' ability to do their usual work of removing waste products and extra fluid from your body [23].

Analysis of the means of the different haematological parameters between the diabetic group and the control group in the study sample shows that CD4 T-cell blood level, % lymphocytes, % monocytes, GR, HCT, RDW-CV, and RDW-SD were significantly lower in diabetic patients compared to nondiabetic individuals while % granulocytes and MCHC were significantly higher in diabetic patients compared to nondiabetic individuals. These results reveal the lack of immune status of diabetics compared to nondiabetics although the difference in results is not statistically significant for the other parameters. This could be explained by the difference in sample size in the two populations since a very limited number of nondiabetic patients were obtained in the context of our study. Leukocytes represent an important part of immunocompetent cells which are used for defence against infectious agents. Geerlings and Hoepelman noted a decrease in the function of polynuclear cells and monocytes/macrophages in diabetics compared to nondiabetics [24]. These results corroborate those of our study because diabetic patients had granulopenia (drop in the granulocyte level) compared to nondiabetic patients.

The correlation between the haematological parameters and the diabetes status shows that the majority of haematologic parameters were negatively but not significantly correlated with diabetes. MCV and RDW-CV negatively influence the probability of having diabetes while RDW-SD positively influences the probability of having diabetes. This is explained by the fact that diabetes affects haematological cells and functions [25].

These findings are of huge public health prominence since it helped to access the haematological features and urologic pathologies among diabetic individuals compared to nondiabetics. The small size of nondiabetic individuals constitutes one limitation of this study. The major limitation of this study is that diabetes mellitus was diagnosed using a glucose meter from capillary blood; this is not as accurate and reliable as plasma glucose estimation diagnosed using a spectrophotometer/colorimeter.

5. Conclusion

This study suggested that the mean of % lymphocytes, % monocytes, % granulocytes, GR, MCHC, RDW-CV, and RDW-SD was significantly different between the diabetic and nondiabetic patients. It also shows that the majority of haematologic parameters were negatively but not significantly correlated with diabetes. MCV and RDW-CV negatively influence the probability of having diabetes while RDW-SD positively influences the probability of having diabetes. This study also suggests that research and interventions targeted at diabetic population could help close gaps in diabetes complications.

Consent

Each participant gave written and informed consent for voluntary participation.

Authors' Contributions

ATS performed the sampling and data collection. ATS and WTJM participated in the analysis of data. ATS, WTJM, and VK drafted the manuscript. VK and VPB designed the study. VK supervised the work. All authors read the manuscript and approved the final version prior to submission.

Acknowledgments

The authors would like to thank all the staff members of the regional hospital of Bafoussam and participants for their support towards the successful completion of the study.

References

[1] American Diabetes Association, "Diagnosis and classification of diabetes mellitus," *Diabetes Care*, vol. 37, Supplement_1, pp. S81–S90, 2013.

[2] R. S. Azzedine, *Etude de quelques paramètres biologiques et physiologiques de la Néphropathie Diabétique*, Mémoire en vue l'obtention du diplôme Magister en Biol. Physiopathol. Cell, 2011.

[3] J. C. Katte, A. Dzudie, E. Sobngwi et al., "Coincidence of diabetes mellitus and hypertension in a semi-urban Cameroonian population: a cross-sectional study," *BMC Public Health*, vol. 14, no. 1, article 696, 2014.

[4] F. I. du Diabète, *Atlas du diabète*, Fédération Internationale du diabète|Diabète Québec, 8 edition, 2017, https://www.diabete.qc.ca/fr/comprendre-le-diabete/ressources/documents-utiles/atlas/.

[5] J. J. Bigna, J. R. Nansseu, J. C. Katte, and J. J. Noubiap, "Prevalence of prediabetes and diabetes mellitus among adults residing in Cameroon: a systematic review and meta-analysis," *Diabetes Research and Clinical Practice*, vol. 137, pp. 109–118, 2018.

[6] K. Papatheodorou, M. Banach, E. Bekiari, M. Rizzo, and M. Edmonds, "Complications of diabetes 2017," *Journal Diabetes Research*, vol. 2018, article 3086167, 4 pages, 2018.

[7] A. Berbudi, N. Rahmadika, A. I. Tjahjadi, and R. Ruslami, "Type 2 diabetes and its impact on the immune system," *Current Diabetes Reviews*, vol. 16, no. 5, pp. 442–449, 2020.

[8] J. Pearson-Stuttard, S. Blundell, T. Harris, D. G. Cook, and J. Critchley, "Diabetes and infection: assessing the association with glycaemic control in population-based studies," *The Lancet Diabetes & Endocrinology*, vol. 4, no. 2, pp. 148–158, 2016.

[9] "Population of cities in Cameroon," 2020, https://worldpopulationreview.com/countries/cameroon-population/cities/.

[10] F. Q. Nuttall, "Body mass index: obesity, BMI, and health: a critical review," *Nutrition Today*, vol. 50, no. 3, pp. 117–128, 2015.

[11] S.-P. Choukem, C. Sih, D. Nebongo, P. Tientcheu, and A.-P. Kengne, "Accuracy and precision of four main glucometers used in a sub-saharan african country: a cross-sectional study," *The Pan African Medical Journal*, vol. 32, article 118, 2019.

[12] B. Brando, D. Barnett, G. Janossy et al., "Cytofluorometric methods for assessing absolute numbers of cell subsets in blood," *Cytometry*, vol. 42, no. 6, pp. 327–346, 2000.

[13] M. R. Azevedo, C. L. P. Araújo, F. F. Reichert, F. V. Siqueira, M. C. da Silva, and P. C. Hallal, "Gender differences in leisure-time physical activity," *International Journal of Public Health*, vol. 52, no. 1, pp. 8–15, 2007.

[14] M. A. Whisman, A. Li, D. A. Sbarra, and C. L. Raison, "Marital quality and diabetes: results from the health and retirement study," *Health Psychology*, vol. 33, no. 8, pp. 832–840, 2014.

[15] M. Azimi-Nezhad, M. Ghayour-Mobarhan, M. R. Parizadeh et al., "Prevalence of type 2 diabetes mellitus in Iran and its relationship with gender, urbanisation, education, marital status and occupation," *Singapore Medical Journal*, vol. 49, no. 7, pp. 571–576, 2008.

[16] J. B. Echouffo-Tcheugui and A. P. Kengne, "Chronic non-communicable diseases in Cameroon - burden, determinants and current policies," *Globalization and Health*, vol. 7, no. 1, p. 44, 2011.

[17] B. Abed Bakhotmah, "Prevalence of obesity among type 2 diabetic patients: non-smokers housewives are the most affected in Jeddah, Saudi Arabia," *Open Journal of Endocrine and Metabolic Diseases*, vol. 3, no. 1, pp. 25–30, 2013.

[18] E. E. Agardh, A. Sidorchuk, J. Hallqvist et al., "Burden of type 2 diabetes attributed to lower educational levels in Sweden," *Population Health Metrics*, vol. 9, no. 1, article 60, 2011.

[19] Y. A. Amoako, D. O. Laryea, G. Bedu-Addo, H. Andoh, and Y. A. Awuku, "Clinical and demographic characteristics of chronic kidney disease patients in a tertiary facility in Ghana," *The Pan African Medical Journal*, vol. 18, article 274, 2014.

[20] J. Coresh, E. Selvin, L. A. Stevens et al., "Prevalence of chronic kidney disease in the United States," *Journal of the American Medical Association*, vol. 298, no. 17, pp. 2038–2047, 2007.

[21] J. S. Brown, H. Wessells, M. B. Chancellor et al., "Urologic complications of diabetes," *Diabetes Care*, vol. 28, no. 1, pp. 177–185, 2004.

[22] K. L. Lifford, G. C. Curhan, F. B. Hu, R. L. Barbieri, and F. Grodstein, "Type 2 diabetes mellitus and risk of developing urinary incontinence," *Journal of the American Geriatrics Society*, vol. 53, no. 11, pp. 1851–1857, 2005.

[23] V. E. Bouhairie and J. B. McGill, "Diabetic kidney disease," *Missouri Medicine*, vol. 113, no. 5, pp. 390–394, 2016.

[24] S. E. Geerlings and A. I. M. Hoepelman, "Immune dysfunction in patients with diabetes mellitus (DM)," *FEMS Immunology & Medical Microbiology*, vol. 26, no. 3–4, pp. 259–265, 1999.

[25] D. Milosevic and V. L. Panin, "Relationship between hematological parameters and glycemic control in type 2 diabetes mellitus patients," *Journal of Medical Biochemistry*, vol. 38, no. 2, pp. 164–171, 2019.

10

Referral of Patients with Nonmalignant Chronic Diseases to Specialist Palliative Care: A Study in a Teaching Hospital in Ghana

Rasheed Ofosu-Poku [1], Michael Owusu-Ansah [1], and John Antwi [2]

[1]Directorate of Family Medicine, Komfo Anokye Teaching Hospital, Kumasi, Ghana
[2]Directorate of Internal Medicine, Komfo Anokye Teaching Hospital, Kumasi, Ghana

Correspondence should be addressed to Rasheed Ofosu-Poku; alienph1215@gmail.com

Academic Editor: Tadeusz Robak

Ghana's chronic disease burden is on the rise. An essential aspect of clinical care in chronic disease management is to improve the quality of life of both patients and their families and to help them cope with the experience of life-limiting illness. Specialist palliative care services help reach this objective, especially in the context of complex psychosocial challenges and high symptom burden. It is, therefore, necessary that as many patients as possible get access to available specialist palliative care services. This paper explores the factors influencing referral of patients with nonmalignant chronic diseases for specialist palliative care. A qualitative approach was used to explore these factors from eight (8) participants—four (4) physician specialists and four (4) next of kin of patients with advanced nonmalignant chronic illness. Individual face-to-face interviews were conducted using a semistructured interview guide. Interviews were audio-recorded and data coded, themes and subthemes were identified, and thematic analysis was done. Barriers and motivators identified were categorized as either related to physicians, institution, or family. Barriers to referral were perception of the scope of palliative care, medical paternalism, lack of an institutional referral policy, poor human resource capacity of the palliative care team, and lack of awareness about the existence of specialist palliative care service. Poor economic status of the patient and family, poor prognosis, previous interaction with the palliative care team, and an appreciation of patients' expectations of the healthcare system were identified as motivators for referral. The palliative care team must therefore increase awareness among other health professionals about their services and facilitate the development and availability of a clear policy to guide and improve referrals.

1. Introduction

Chronic noncommunicable diseases (NCDs) such as cardiovascular diseases, cancer, and diabetes mellitus, account for 70% of all deaths globally [1], 75% occurring in the low- and middle-income countries (LMICs) such as Ghana [2, 3]. Morbidity and mortality from NCDs in these countries are projected to rise over the next decade, with five times as many deaths and three times disability-adjusted life years as communicable diseases by 2030 [4]. The leading causes of NCD-related deaths globally are chronic respiratory diseases, cardiovascular diseases, cancer, and diabetes mellitus, with cardiovascular diseases topping the list in Ghana [2, 5–9].

These chronic diseases have the inherent characteristic of being ominous—progressively advancing with worsening of symptoms, limiting quality of life and ability to function. Consequently, the physical, psychological, social, and spiritual facets of life of their victim are all affected remarkably [10]. To provide a holistic perspective to care, the World Health Organization recommends that palliative care be initiated along with life-prolonging therapy [11].

The World Health Organization defines palliative care as "an approach that improves the quality of life of patients and their families facing the problem associated with life-threatening illness, through the prevention and relief of suffering by means of early identification and impeccable assessment and treatment of pain and other problems, physical, psychosocial and spiritual" [11]. Thus, the overriding objective of palliative care is to enhance the quality of life of patients and their families by helping them meet their needs.

In order to integrate palliative care into the existing healthcare system, primary healthcare providers must start basic palliative care [12] but refer to specialist palliative care teams when symptoms are intractable, complex psychosocial issues arise [13], and/or the patient is likely to die within a year [14].

Palliative care development in the developed western countries such as the United States of America and the United Kingdom, as well as in East and South Africa, has advanced rapidly [15, 16]. However, its development and progress in West Africa has been rather slow [17]. In Ghana, it was not until 2003 that Ripples Health Care, a private firm, initiated a home-based palliative care service. Later, in 2006, the Ghana Palliative Care Association was formed [18].

Although it was in 2003 that Dr. Kwaku Afriyie, Ghana's then Minister of Health, raised the issue of the importance of incorporating palliative care in the nation's healthcare system, it was in 2012 that the national policy for control of NCDs highlighted the training of health professionals in palliative care in order to improve services for patients suffering from NCDs such as cancer, cardiovascular diseases, renal failure, and stroke [19, 20]. The National Cancer Control program has also devoted an entire chapter of the national strategy to palliative care, detailing how to get it properly integrated into the healthcare system towards management of patients suffering from cancer [21]. At present, specialist palliative care service in Ghana is provided by the Korle Bu Teaching Hospital (KBTH), the Tetteh Quarshie Memorial Hospital, and the Komfo Anokye Teaching Hospital (KATH).

Specialist palliative care services at KATH started in 2015, under the Family Medicine Directorate. Its models of care include in-patient consultation, out-patient clinic, and home visits. The hospital has no in-patient palliative care unit. Services provided include management of symptoms, discussing diagnosis and prognosis, negotiating goals of care, assistance with advanced care planning, end-of-life care, and bereavement support.

An essential requirement for the management of symptoms in patients with chronic diseases is the availability of syrup morphine for the management of moderate to severe pain. Morphine is imported as a powder and reconstituted into syrup by the hospital. Syrup morphine is therefore quite easily available within the hospital, albeit at a price equivalent to about 6 USD for a 100 ml bottle. Some pharmacies also have syrup morphine on sale, but at a higher price of about 15 USD for a 100 ml bottle. Apart from pharmacies in KATH, KBTH, and the country's two main cities (Kumasi and Accra), syrup morphine is hard to come by in other parts of Ghana.

Patients are seen based on referrals/consults from their respective primary physician. Most patients tend to be referred when their primary care team(s) appears to have run out of options in offering disease-modifying therapy, and patients have a few weeks to several months to live.

A review of the 2016 data on referrals to the hospital's palliative care team revealed that 49 out of fifty referrals (98%) were on account of an advanced cancer and only one (constituting 2%) was due to a nonmalignant chronic disease

(end-stage renal failure). A similar observation has been made in the literature with respect to the pattern of referrals to specialist palliative care internationally [22]. This trend leaves out all those other patients suffering from nonmalignant NCDs such as heart failure, cerebrovascular accident, diabetes mellitus, and chronic obstructive pulmonary disease.

As the hospital is a tertiary facility, patients normally present with acute phases of chronic diseases, chronic diseases challenging to manage at the primary or secondary facilities, or acute severe disease. Patients at these stages of chronic disease generally require the support of a specialist palliative care team to help meet their complex needs [13, 14]. An appreciable number of consults/referrals each month for the palliative care team's input, to help address the needs of these patients, are therefore expected.

Referrals to specialist palliative care have been associated with many benefits to the patient, family, and hospital. These benefits include increased bed turnover rate, improved patient and family satisfaction with care, reduced hospital bills and associated costs, reduced number of emergency room visits, reduced caregiver burden, improved quality of life of patients, improved transition of care from high to lower acuity settings, improved pain and symptom management, and improved communication with patient and family about end-of-life issues such as advanced directives [23–32].

The hospital not only loses the above benefits but also has a high risk of incurring financial losses because patients may take unduly long periods in the ward but relatives may not be able to pay the accumulated hospital bill. Secondly, patients requiring acute care and stabilization in the ward have to spend days at the emergency department before a bed can be secured for them in the wards.

In facilitating the hospital's vision to become a centre of excellence in the provision of specialist care [33], this gap in access to specialist palliative care for patients with nonmalignant chronic diseases needs to be investigated and appropriate solutions identified and implemented as a matter of urgency.

Identification and comprehension of the factors influencing the decision to refer patients for specialist palliative care is necessary in planning appropriate interventions for implementation. However, in view of the fact that specialist palliative care in Ghana is less than a decade old [18], and barely half a decade at the Komfo Anokye Teaching Hospital, studies investigating these factors have not been carried out yet.

This study is therefore a need of the time in order to plan appropriately towards improving access to specialist palliative care, especially for patients with nonmalignant chronic diseases. This study explores these factors from the perspective of physician specialists and relatives of patients.

2. Materials and Methods

2.1. Study Design. A qualitative exploratory study design was used. This is because palliative care is quite new in the Ghanaian context, and there is very limited existing evidence base pertaining to the setting. Secondly, the individual perspectives of participants are the focus of this study [34].

2.2. Study Site and Population. This study took place at the Komfo Anokye Teaching Hospital, Kumasi, the second leading teaching hospital in Ghana. Specialist palliative care service is run by the palliative care team under the Family Medicine Directorate. According to the daily schedule of the palliative care team, it organizes both a home visit and an in-patient consultation twice a week and an out-patient clinic once a week. By the end of October 2018, the core team was made up of two family physicians, one surgeon, and two nurses. With the exception of one nurse who had been chosen by the hospital management to lead the formation of the palliative care unit, each of them had other primary duties and worked with the palliative care team if and when it had patients.

Another of the hospital's 12 clinical directorates is the Internal Medicine Directorate. Complicated diabetes mellitus and chronic neurological and cardiovascular diseases, which are the focus in this study, are managed by this directorate.

In teaching hospitals, physician specialists head the patient's primary care team, where they act as the "gatekeepers" of the referral process [35]. Physician specialists, therefore, constitute a major group in this study. Those included in the study had practiced for at least one year as a physician specialist in the Internal Medicine Directorate.

Secondly, patients and their families have the right to access or not palliative care service following discussion and referral by primary physicians [36]. As close relatives, the closest being the next of kin, are recognized to make decisions on a client's behalf in the event of incapacitation and even act as the main support for the patient during admission, their views about palliative care are important in the referral process. They are, therefore, included as the second group of participants in this study.

2.3. Sampling Technique and Size. Purposive sampling was used to recruit physician specialists and next of kin of patients who meet the inclusion criteria. The sample size consisted of eight (8) participants—four (4) physician specialists and four (4) next of kin, as determined by data saturation—"when no new analytical information arises anymore, and the study provides maximum information on the phenomenon" [37].

2.4. Data Collection Instrument and Method. Two (2) semi-structured interview guides (one for physician specialists and the other for next of kin of patients) were developed and used to allow flexibility in exploring topics [38]. The interview guides were developed based on the objectives of the study, a review of relevant literature, and policy.

Each interview guide was reviewed by a supervisor to ensure that questions reflected the purpose of the study. They were then pretested with one participant each, a next of kin of a patient and a physician specialist. The purpose for this was threefold: to ensure the clarity of questions, to fine-tune the questions, and to provide an opportunity to practice and improve interviewing skills. The data collected during the pretest interview was not added to the study.

Following ethical approval, folders of patients on admission were reviewed to get to know patients with a diagnosis of a nonmalignant chronic disease with at least one complica-

tion. Those who were unconscious or could not communicate were excluded. A brief discussion was held with each of these selected patients to tell them about the study and to have a discussion with their next of kin. The next of kin were met in person during visiting hours, and participation in the study was discussed with them. Five out of eight consented and participated in the study.

To recruit physician specialists to participate, the principal investigator was present in the various wards of the directorate at various times of the day. Having worked in the directorate for a number of years, he knew those who fell within the inclusion criteria of the study and who among them could be most informative. Nine physician specialists were contacted in person and the study discussed with them. Of these, one declined participation on account of a busy schedule, four had busy schedules so there were challenges arranging a suitable time within the study period, and four participated in the study. These interviews were carried out in English.

Each participant was given an information leaflet and had it explained to him/her, and they each signed a consent form before their respective interviews. Individual face-to-face interviews were conducted in offices of various wards in the directorate. The purpose of employing individual face-to-face interviews was to encourage flexibility of time and venue for each participant and to encourage expression of diverse opinions [39]. Interviews lasted an average of fifteen (15) minutes, were conducted from 1st June, 2018, to 8th June, 2018, and audio-recorded with permission from the participants. At the end of each interview, the participant was thanked for their cooperation and offered no monetary reward.

2.5. Data Handling and Analysis. Interviews were transcribed verbatim and field notes added as needed. Transcripts were read by the supervisor to ensure rigor and trustworthiness. All names were replaced with pseudonyms. Signed consent forms have been kept safely in a locked cabinet and will be kept for at least five (5) years. Electronic data (transcripts and audio-recording of interviews) have been encrypted and password protected to ensure confidentiality of the study's participants.

Thematic analysis was used because of its flexibility, enabling its use in any theoretical or conceptual framework of choice, and as it allows for detailed description of data [40]. Transcripts were read and reread to gain familiarity with the data and identify the central concepts and key statements made by participants. Coding was done by assigning to sentences a phrase which conveys its purport. Codes were categorized into subthemes and subthemes into themes. Discussions were held with the supervisor to ensure that theoretical inferences are justified and personal opinions did not sway the analysis.

2.6. Methodological Rigor. Credibility was ensured through sessions with the thesis supervisor to get feedback about the quality of the data. Transferability was ensured by giving thick descriptions of the study setting and the context of the practice of specialist palliative care in the hospital. Dependability was ensured by working closely with the supervisor throughout the study and keeping an audit trail of all events and procedures followed. Detailed descriptions of the research design, data collection procedure and analysis, and basic information about study participants have been provided. Confirmability was ensured by working closely with supervisors who audited the data and inferences drawn from it. An audit trail of audio-records, transcripts, interview questions, and consent forms have also been kept for any future confirmatory audits.

2.7. Ethical Consideration. Ethical clearance was obtained from the Committee on Human Research Publication and Ethics (CHRPE) of the Kwame Nkrumah University of Science and Technology. Participants were each given an information leaflet and had it explained to them by the researcher. Those who accepted to participate completed a consent form.

In order to ensure the anonymity of respondents, they were not addressed by name during the interviews nor were their actual names used in the transcript of the interview. A code name was rather assigned to each of the participants in the transcript. Also, consent forms have been kept under lock and key, and interview transcripts and audio-records were encrypted and password protected. Participants were thanked for making time for the interview but were given no material reward as compensation.

3. Findings

3.1. Physician-Related Factors. The physician specialist interviewed had neurology and nephrology as their areas of specialization (Table 1). Table 2 illustrates the diagnosis of patients whose next of kin were interviewed. Patients' diagnoses were related to cerebrovascular accident (stroke), liver disease, and diabetes mellitus type II.

Themes and subthemes emerging from the study have been illustrated in Table 3.

3.1.1. Awareness of Specialist Palliative Care Services in the Hospital. Some physician specialists were neither aware of the hospital's ongoing specialist palliative care services nor aware of any palliative care physician specialist in the hospital. One participant said, "I don't know of anyone really in KATH who is a palliative care specialist or anything like that" (PS 4). Another physician specialist said, "We don't even have a place to send them to" (PS 2).

Another reason identified to be contributing to the level of awareness about specialist palliative care services was the lack of interaction between the palliative care team and physician specialists. One physician specialist said,

> Well, in the first place I'm aware that there is a palliative care team at the polyclinic but we hardly have any interactions. So the first step is to recognize that yes there is a palliative care team and if you want to contact the palliative care team this is their contact number, this is who is in-charge, this is how we can contact you to become part of our team. (PS 3)

Previous experience with patients and the scope of interest of physician specialists were noted to be significant in

TABLE 1: Physician Specialists and Their Areas of Specialization.

No.	Name	Specialty area
1	PS* 1	Internal medicine (with subspecialty interest in nephrology)
2	PS 2	Internal medicine (with subspecialty interest in neurology)
3	PS 3	Neurology
4	PS 4	Nephrology

*PS is a codename used for physician specialists who participated in this study.

TABLE 2: Next of Kin and Diagnosis of Patients.

No.	Name of next of kin	Diagnosis of patient
1	NOK* 1	Infarctive stroke with right hemiparesis, type II diabetes mellitus
2	NOK 2	Acute-on-chronic liver disease with stage I encephalopathy, hypertension
3	NOK 3	Cerebrovascular accident
4	NOK 4	Cerebrovascular accident

*NOK is a codename used for next of kin who participated in this study.

TABLE 3: Themes and Subthemes from Transcribed Data.

Themes		Subthemes
1	Physician related	(i) Awareness (ii) Perception about palliative care (iii) Medical paternalism (iv) "Territorial guarding"
2	Institutional factors	(i) Policy (ii) Human resource
3	Family related	(i) Awareness and acceptability (ii) Economic soundness

finding out the availability of a particular service to meet certain needs of patients. In view of his previous study in the quality of life of patients, one physician specialist had identified a family physician with specialty interest in palliative care, who he contacted when he thought a patient may needed palliative care.

> ... I actually conducted a study on quality of life and indeed quality of life is something that now has become an important outcome measure for our patients with chronic kidney disease and I've done some studies even in quality of life and to tell you plainly it's so poor. And some of the things that came out from my study... we as physicians should not only be concerned about controlling blood pressures alone but we should think about patients in terms of their mental and psychological wellbeing because most of them come depressed. I mean you wake up one morning and you are told your kidney cannot function

well and you need dialysis which is expensive...so I had a discussion with a colleague of mine who has interest in palliative that well I will be sending some cases for him to see because I get to points where they cannot afford dialysis, they are just lying on the ward and probably we are just waiting for them to die. (PS 1)

3.1.2. Perception about Palliative Care. Physician specialists held different opinions about the most appropriate time for a palliative care referral. Whereas some thought palliative care should be started at diagnosis, others were of the view that palliative care may be started when the patient is unable to afford life-prolonging therapy or available treatment is not helping.

Physician specialists inclined to neurology were of the view that palliative care must start at the time of diagnosis. One of them said,

Look ... when patients come with stroke and they are admitted, and doctors round on those patients you want a palliative care team to be part of that rounds who will be able to for instance meet with relatives and discuss prognosis in a very practical manner with them and how interventions that are palliative in nature can be instituted so that the patient even when the patient is going to die from the stroke at least the process is well managed in terms of the psychological and social implications. So from the word go, yes, palliative care team should be involved. (PS 3)

Another physician specialist said,

Umm, I think immediately the diagnosis is made. That is when. Because patients need to from the beginning be made aware what they are dealing with. They need to make life adjustments to deal with it for them and their family. They need to understand what they are dealing with. So I think that right from the beginning. (PS 2)

However, physician specialists with interest in nephrology pointed out that the triggers for a specialist palliative care referral are when prognosis is poor, the patient cannot afford available life-prolonging interventions, or available medical interventions are failing. One physician specialist was of the view that a specialist palliative care referral must be considered when the patient's condition is not improving with available medical interventions.

Of course, along the line there might be some other complications that may come on board, strokes and all that for patients with CKD, really bad electrolyte imbalances and all that which sometimes in spite of the dialysis... they do not do well eventually. So there are patients like that who in spite of the interventions will

not do well. So may be for those patients, when it's looking like in spite of our intervention things are still 'going south' then those people I think will benefit from palliative care. (PS 4)

He said once again, at the latter end of the interview,

... fine I'm in the renal clinic but we see a lot of other general cases, and for some of them its obvious things are not really going well... and they need palliative care. (PS 4).

Some physician specialists were also of the view that specialist palliative care consultation becomes necessary when a patient cannot afford the available life-prolonging therapy. That is, in their opinion, palliative care is incompatible with life-prolonging therapy and therefore cannot be considered when the patient is on interventions such as dialysis.

So I think most of them need financial assistance. And, because when you are put on dialysis and you are consistently on it for a long time I mean you can stay very long. So most patients there, I think what they need is not really palliative care but for those who cannot afford their interventions what they need is financial assistance... I think the main problem of treatment that the category of patients I have spoken about need is finances, because something can be done about their condition. For those who cannot get the things that can be done for them done, of course they can. It essentially comes down to finances. (PS 4)

Another physician specialist also said,

... now what I do is that, you know chronic kidney disease has stages so from stage 3 onwards to 5, that is when I start assessing for those I see early whether they can afford, yes and no, and how we can go around it. So I actually think sometimes depending on the background some people cope better than others. So sometimes you are talking with somebody, he is in stage 3, 4 but the coping ability is on the low side, then I think it makes sense to refer them early. (PS 1)

The perceived needs of patients and the roles their physicians perceived to be within the domain of specialist palliative care also determined the possibility of the involvement of specialist palliative professionals in the care of patients. To the physician specialists, the roles of specialist palliative care professionals include communication, patient and family support, symptom management, and advanced care planning.

One physician specialist, referring to the role of communication in palliative care, said,

What would have been ideal will be to have a multidisciplinary team, not only made up of neurologists but having nurses, physiotherapists, occupational therapist, nutritionist, psychologist and palliative specialist who will be able to manage patients when they come so that it's not just a matter of prescribing drugs but there is this aspect of social care where the relatives are involved and they are informed about potential outcomes of strokes and about how palliation can be administered for those who we know may not survive the stroke and even for those who are going to live with permanent disabilities some of which may involve some of them being in bed almost for the rest of their life. (PS 3)

Another physician specialist discussed his view of the role of specialist palliative care in supporting patients and family as follows:

Um definitely, because most of these things are not curative. They are things they have to live with for the end of their life. So they need a lot of support all through to the end. So, I mean, definitely, the way I understand palliative care, … allowing them to endure their life, making use of what they have till the end. And that is basically what they need in addition to rehabilitation. (PS 2)

Symptom management and advanced care planning were identified to be roles of palliative care professionals, and thus, needs, which when identified, may encourage physician specialists to refer patients for palliative care. One physician specialist said,

… so I had a discussion with a colleague of mine who has interest in palliative that well I will be sending some cases for him to because I get to points where they cannot afford dialysis, they are just lying on the ward and probably we are just waiting for them to die. So then in that case a bit of pain control here, a bit of how to make them comfortable, how probably to help them to write their last their wills. (PS 1)

A system in which healthcare professionals make available little information to patients and their family, and thus make all the decisions for them, make them only passive members of the healthcare team. This may result in delayed or nonreferral of patients who may otherwise benefit from specialist palliative care. One participant said,

I think it all depends on the doctor. If the doctor says you have to do something about it, why not. What do I know about it to say? Even if we have to bring him every week, I can put

him in a car and bring him. So even if it's one or two days, when you finish seeing him, I can take him back. (NOK 3)

When asked if he may wish to suggest palliative care to the patient's doctor, one participant remarked,

For some of them if you say this to them, he may get angry. Or am I telling lies? 'If you think I cannot take care of you then go.' And that will also cause you a problem. (NOK 2)

3.2. Institutional Factors. The unavailability of an institutional or working guideline, either of the hospital, department, or teams, was identified to be a major factor influencing palliative care referral practices. In response to the question of whether any protocol or guidelines were available to guide referral to specialist palliative care, one physician specialist said,

Not that I know of. And indeed for nephrology, I think I can speak more of, we do not have a clear protocol. Like I said, it's on as and when basis. So I think I assess my patients and I think this is what they need, so I just refer them for the appropriate, yeah. (PS 1)

Hinting at the unavailability of adequate human resource to meet the need for specialist palliative care, one physician specialist said,

It's [referring to specialist palliative care] a budding area so even if you want to be aggressive the human resource is not there, I mean. Hopefully, if you come out to help on the nursing side to help the colleagues who are physicians to be able to, to you know build it well. But as it stands, you know it's a new area and it's not every time they are around so we also have to bear with it. (PS 1)

One issue raised by a physician specialist was that various health professionals appear to be working in isolation with each guarding their respective "territories."

…what is currently happening is we have a very disjointed post-stroke care where the patients come to neurology clinic and are seen and they have to go to physiotherapy for physiotherapy needs to be done and then if they have a nutritional care need they have to go and see a nutritionist. So it's disjointed. But if we have a comprehensive clinic where when a patient comes all these can be provided. Then that will be able to work. But people work in territories and people do not feel comfortable sometimes you encroaching on their territory, so that's one of the things that we need to overcome. (PS 3)

3.3. Family-Related Factors

3.3.1. Awareness and Acceptability of Specialist Palliative Care Services. When asked whether they had ever heard of the expression "palliative care," all next of kin interviewed responded in the negative. After explaining to them what palliative care is and the services provided by specialist palliative care professionals, they expressed acceptance of specialist palliative care services for their respective family members who were on admission. One respondent said,

> Yes I will be interested and willing. You mentioned quite a number of services, about how we can take care of her. And I do not know those things I can do, so I think I should be able to see you so that you teach me so that the patient can also get better and I will also get better, I like it. (NOK 1)

3.3.2. Family-Related Barriers. One concern raised was the possible cost of palliative care services. In response to whether he would engage or be interested in the services of palliative care professionals if the patient's primary physician discussed referral with him, one respondent said,

> So do you render the service for free? I will be interested if I think I have the necessary support, made the needed preparation and can afford [touches pocket]. (NOK 4)

Distance from one's place of residence to the hospital was also identified as a potential barrier of access to specialist palliative care services. One respondent said,

> What about if I am from far away? I hope you get what I mean? From what we are discussing, it is like the person is from Kumasi here, even if it is far it cannot be as far as Nkawie, Bibiani, Enchi. Enchi is the place where we came from. (NOK 2)

Another respondent said,

> Where the house is, one has to walk let us say between here and the gate. So even if he is discharged, last time they were saying they will let him do physio, so when we are bringing him from the house, for me when he is discharged I have to leave and go back to work. So just look at this woman [patient's wife], can she carry this man over a distance of 200meters before coming to pick a car? It is impossible, it will not work. (NOK 3)

3.4. Suggestions. The development of protocols or guidelines on when to refer a patient for palliative care and what the role they will play in the management of the patient was suggested by physician specialists as a way of improving referral practices. One physician specialist said,

> I think the first step will be for the neurology team and the palliative care team to sit down together and devise a protocol and then each one knows the contribution they are going to make to the patient and then putting those ideas together in setting up a protocol so that it's clear that okay this is what I can do for the patient. So at this point I will do A, B and C, and at this point you do AB, A and C. So I think that's the first step for the two teams to sit down together and devise a protocol or a guideline. (PS 2)

Another physician specialist said,

> My suggestion is that I think we have to work together and they can also give us some input on how to go about it. You know then they let us know if you have a patient who fits a particular criteria A, B, C, D, okay let us have a look at this patient and we can advise. On the other hand, you have a patient who probably as per criteria is stable for you to manage then manage until this stage and you can refer to us. (PS 1)

Another suggestion given by physician specialists was that the palliative care team should get more vocal about their field by increasing awareness through presentations and interactions with colleagues from various departments. For instance, one physician specialist said,

> I am a specialist I have been here for quite some time and I did not know so... I do not think people really know that you can get a consult for someone to be seen... like the way we do consults from other departments. So I think that's the first step. Or may be to make people aware because a lot of patients, fine I'm in the renal clinic but we see a lot of other general cases, and for some of them its obvious things are not really going well... and they need palliative care. So I think that's the first step. People should know that there is a palliative care specialist around. (PS 4)

Another physician specialist also said,

> And maybe they should be a bit more vocal, they should come out, do presentations, lets know what it's really about... so my suggestion is they come out more, let other departments or people really know their importance so when the patient is getting to the stage of hospice and all, we know we have to call somebody. (PS 1)

One next of kin suggested that each ward must have a palliative care focal person who will identify patients who need specialist palliative care and obtain a referral for them.

> So what I was thinking was that, you should discuss with them so that they get to know, so that for each ward one of your members can be there. (NOK 2)

4. Discussion of Findings

4.1. Physician-Related Factors. The study found that having knowledge about the existence of specialist palliative care services in an institution, knowing a colleague who has interest in palliative care, and previous clinical experience or interactions with specialist palliative care professionals were associated with increased likelihood of referrals from primary physicians to specialist palliative care professionals. This finding supports those of a multisite qualitative study in the United States in which lack of knowledge about the availability of palliative care services was a barrier to referral to specialist palliative care professionals [41]. A study by Opoku in 2014 among healthcare professionals and members of the general public in Ghana similarly found the unavailability of palliative care services as a barrier to provision of palliative care [17]. Also, in a study examining professional caregivers' experiences with palliative care for noncancer patients, they were found to have a "vague understanding of palliative care" and thus had difficulties identifying palliative care needs or initiating a conversation about palliative care [42]. In Nigeria, Onyeka and Iloanusi in 2014, describing their achievement in establishing palliative care in Enugu, have highlighted poor knowledge of palliative care among physicians as a contributory factor to low referrals previously recorded [43].

Another factor emerging from interaction with physician specialists, which had a direct effect on the possibility of the referral of patients to specialist palliative care, was their perception of the concept of palliative care. The findings centered on the appropriate time for a consult to specialist palliative care and the role of specialist palliative care professionals in the care of patients.

Physician specialists with interest in neurology, the majority of whose patients are suffering from stroke, pointed out the most appropriate time for involvement of the specialist palliative care team to be immediately when the diagnosis is made. However, those with interest in nephrology were of the view that specialist palliative care referral becomes necessary when prognosis is poor in spite of disease-modifying therapy being delivered or when the patient/family is in financial difficulties and hence cannot afford such therapy as dialysis. Although their responses seem to vary, one common issue is that acute stroke is life limiting/threatening, and like advanced chronic kidney disease, it may have a poor prognosis. Thus, both groups were of the view that poor prognosis was a trigger for specialist palliative care referral. This finding reflects the study among professionals caring for heart failure patients in which some health professionals believed that the right time to involve specialist palliative care is when disease-modifying therapy stops and prognosis is poor [44]. Similarly, in a study describing factors which predict the referral of cancer patients for specialist palliative care in Uganda, poor performance state (ECOG (Eastern Cooperation Oncology Group) 3 or 4)—a prognostic measure on the care of cancer patients—was the "only significant predictor of referral" [45].

The need to control physical symptoms, discuss diagnosis and prognosis with the patient and the family, provide them support, help them reintegrate into society following illness, and help them plan and manage affairs in the event of death were identified as reasons why physician specialists will contemplate the involvement of specialist palliative care professionals. This finding supports the findings of the study by Kavalieratos et al. [44] in which most healthcare providers based referral on reasons such as prognosis, symptom presence, care coordination, and advanced care planning. The study in Ghana exploring factors that affect provision of palliative care similarly found that the need for symptom management and holistic support were major reasons for initiating palliative care [17].

The above finding that patient's needs may trigger referral brings into perspective the fact that where a primary care provider feels confident in addressing an identified need, the patient is less likely to be referred for specialist palliative care. This inference is supported by the findings of a study among hematologists in which their confidence and comfort in addressing certain identified needs significantly influenced referral to specialist palliative care professionals [46]. Another study conducted by Low et al. [45] describing the referral pattern to specialist palliative care in Uganda further supports this inference. Their study showed that most physicians felt confident in dealing with a wide array of issues related to palliative care such as symptom management and basic communication and so referred patients for specialist palliative care when other needs of patients related to end-of-life care arose for which they were less confident. Thus, patients referred for specialist palliative care in their study were referred quite late, with a median survival of 5 days postreferral recorded [45].

Another factor identified in this study was that various professionals tend to work in isolation, "guarding their territories." That is, some physicians do not permit other physicians to see their patients for various reasons, for instance, to prevent contradictory information from being communicated to patients and their relatives. A similar observation was made in a previous study in which some primary physicians avoided referral of their patients to specialist palliative care out of fear that palliative care professionals may present a "dismal" prognostic picture to patients and thus affect their willingness to continue to receive disease-modifying therapy [31]. Low et al. in 2018 similarly found in their survey that about 60% of doctors felt patients and family are more likely to lose hope and get depressed when end-of-life issues are discussed [45].

This study also found that close relatives of patients had left the entire burden of decision making about the plan of care for their loved ones on the primary physician. This reflects a feeling of inadequacy on the part of a patient's family about the progress of disease and options available. Such a state is indicative of the extent to which relations of patients are not abreast with care and are not deemed important in making decisions about the care of the patients. Following a review of several studies, Devlin and Maida in 2017 have highlighted the threat medical paternalism poses to specialist palliative care referral [47]. In addition, Adwedaa in 2015 had discussed how this practice of keeping information and making decisions on behalf of the patient and the family is common among doctors in

Ghana [48]. It appears that doctors in Ghana keep information away from patients and their family in order to prevent them from losing hope, or they believe they know what is in the best interest of the patient and the family.

4.2. Institutional Factors. Another contributory factor to low referrals of patients for specialist palliative care is the lack of institutional or departmental policies and guidelines. Physician specialists were unanimous on the point that there were no guidelines for referral to specialist palliative care and recommended that clear guidelines are essential in ensuring access to specialist palliative care for their patients. This finding corroborates a study in Australia in which the availability of a team-based policy was a major motivator for referral to specialist palliative care [49]. In a recent study in Uganda in which the median period of survival after referral to specialist palliative care was found to be 5 days, the lack of a clear referral protocol was found to be a major contributory factor to the poor referral pattern [45].

This study also found that the unavailability of the required human resource capacity to meet the specialist palliative care needs of patients in the hospital may affect referrals. A study in Korea exploring doctor's perception and referral barriers towards palliative care similarly found the unavailability of resources for specialist palliative care such as nurses and doctors with relevant training as the second most commonly reported barrier [50]. Likewise, in Low et al.'s study in Uganda, referring doctors expressed concerns about the lack of adequate staff working with the specialist palliative care team and felt the team's poor staff strength cannot match the demand if referrals were to be made for all patients who need specialist palliative care [45].

4.3. Family-Related Factors. One finding emerging from this study is the unawareness of the concept of palliative care by relatives of patients. When patients or their close relations have no idea of a healthcare service, it is unlikely that they may raise a discussion about it during their interaction with their primary physicians. Especially in the context of patients suffering from nonmalignant chronic diseases, the use of the expressions like "palliation" or "palliative care" by health professionals is less common as compared to those with malignancies (cancers). It is, therefore, not abnormal for relatives of patients suffering from nonmalignant chronic diseases to have never heard the expression "palliative care." This finding reinforces a nationwide survey of hospice and palliative care programs in the United States in which lack of awareness about palliative care by close relatives was rated as a major barrier to palliative care referral for noncancer patients [51].

Another concern expressed by close relatives of patients is the potential cost of services and the distance from their place of residence to the hospital and the stress involved. This may cause patients and their relatives not to turn in a referral to specialist palliative care. A study in a predominantly rural area in Norway similarly found that patients with lower socioeconomic status were unable to have follow-up sessions of palliative radiotherapy on account of the cost implications for treatment and transportation to the facility [52]. Another

study exploring barriers to palliative care in Ghana also found the inability to pay for palliative care services as hampering the provision of specialist palliative care services [17].

Relatives of patients were receptive of the concept of palliative care after it had been explained to them and were interested in having palliative care professionals care for and guide them in the care of their loved ones. A qualitative grounded theory on the experiences of patients and caregivers with palliative care, in which participants expressed feeling a sense of holistic support, supports this finding [53]. Further corroborating the above finding of this study is a review of the palliative care service received by adult cancer patients receiving home-based care in Ibadan. Although patients had died at the time the study was conducted, relatives expressed profound gratitude to the palliative care team for their care and support [54]. However, the study by Lee et al. in 2012 reported the refusal of patients and their relatives as a significant barrier to specialist palliative care [50].

5. Conclusion

This study indicates that close relatives of patients are receptive of the concept of palliative care and are interested in benefiting from their services. However, they are generally unaware of its existence and are unable to initiate the discussion with their physicians because they think the physician knows best or may get angry and neglect the patient. As advocates for the welfare of the patient and relatives, nurses must assess patients and relatives and discuss involvement of specialist palliative care professionals with their respective physicians when needed. This, therefore, requires that not only should nurses be able to carry out a holistic assessment of patient and family, but that they should also be knowledgeable about palliative care and the triggers for specialist palliative care referral.

This study also revealed that close relatives of patients anticipate challenges with distance between their place of residence and the hospital, making the task of taking a patient to the hospital for review quite challenging. Another potential barrier to specialist palliative care revealed by relatives of patients was their financial constraints. The Ministry of Health must, therefore, formulate appropriate policies to ensure that training of specialist palliative care professionals is ongoing and that they are fairly distributed throughout the country for equitable access. To reduce the financial constraints on patients and families requiring specialist palliative care, the Ministry of Health must work towards ensuring that specialist palliative care consultation and essential medications used in palliative care are covered by the National Health Insurance Scheme.

Another major barrier is unawareness of available specialist palliative care services by physician specialists. The palliative care team must therefore carry out sensitization and interactive seminars with physicians, nurses, and other health professionals in the hospital to tell them about the services offered by the team and how they can be reached.

The unavailability of clear referral guidelines to specialist palliative care is also a major barrier. The hospital must therefore devote resources to the formulation of referral guidelines from various specialty areas to specialist palliative care.

This study focuses on physician specialists and close relatives of patients only, using a qualitative approach. It cannot be denied that nurses and the patients themselves are important members of the healthcare team, and the importance of their perspective cannot be overemphasized. Further studies could also explore these factors from their perspective using both a qualitative approach for an in-depth understanding of the factors and a quantitative approach to determine its scope.

Secondly, this study focuses only on the Internal Medicine Specialty. However, it is likely that not all patients suffering from cancer who require a referral to specialist palliative care receive it. So it is that, based on the peculiar needs of patients in other directorates such as Child Health, Emergency Medicine, Surgery, and Obstetrics and Gynaecology, some patients may require specialist palliative care but do not get referred. Further studies can look into these areas as well so that the majority of patients have their physical and psychosocial needs addressed through a healthcare system whose structures are evidence-based and proactive.

Additional Points

Study Limitations. As diabetes mellitus and cardiovascular diseases are among those nonmalignant chronic diseases which form part of this study's focus, we wished to interview physician specialists with interest in endocrinology and cardiology as well. However, on account of their busy schedule and the limited time available for data collection, they could not be included.

Acknowledgments

I am grateful to the Faculty of the Ghana College of Nurses and Midwives, especially Dr. Prince Appiah-Yeboah and Ms. Dzigbordi Kpikpitse, as well as the Internal Medicine Directorate of the Komfo Anokye Teaching Hospital, particularly Dr. Elliot Koranteng Tannor, for their support, guidance, constructive critique, and encouragement throughout the study.

References

[1] World Health Organization (WHO), *Media centre: Noncommunicable diseases*, World Health Organisation, 2017.

[2] WHO, *Global Status Report on Noncommunicable Diseases*, World Health Organization, Switzerland, 2014.

[3] WHO, *Noncommunicable Diseases Progress Monitor 2017*, World Health Organization, 2017.

[4] WHO, *Global Health Observatory (GHO) data: Premature NCD deaths*, World Health Organisation, 2018.

[5] WHO, *Cancer: Key facts*, WHO, 2018.

[6] WHO, *Cardiovascular diseases (CVDs): Key facts*, WHO, 2018.

[7] WHO, *Chronic respiratory diseases*, WHO, 2018.

[8] WHO, "Diabetes: Key facts," WHO, 2018.

[9] WHO, *Ghana: WHO statistical profile*, WHO, 2015.

[10] K. Megari, "Quality of life in chronic disease patients," *Health Psychology Research*, vol. 1, no. e27, pp. 141–148, 2013.

[11] WHO, *Cancer: WHO Definition of Palliative Care*, World Health Organisation, 2018.

[12] C. L. Ahia and C. M. Blais, "Primary palliative care for the general internist: integrating goals of care discussions into the outpatient setting," *The Ochsner Journal*, vol. 14, no. 4, pp. 704–711, 2014.

[13] T. E. Quill and A. P. Abernethy, "Generalist plus specialist palliative care—creating a more sustainable model," *New England Journal of Medicine*, vol. 368, no. 13, pp. 1173–1175, 2013.

[14] J. Downar, R. Goldman, R. Pinto, M. Englesakis, and N. K. J. Adhikari, "The "surprise question" for predicting death in seriously ill patients: a systematic review and meta-analysis," *Canadian Medical Association Journal*, vol. 189, no. 13, pp. E484–E493, 2017.

[15] J. Seymour and B. Cassel, "Palliative care in the USA and England: a critical analysis of meaning and implementation towards a public health approach," *Mortality*, vol. 22, no. 4, pp. 275–290, 2017.

[16] J. Y. Rhee, E. Garralda, E. Namisango et al., "An analysis of palliative care development in Africa: a ranking based on region-specific macroindicators," *Journal of Pain and Symptom Management*, vol. 56, no. 2, pp. 230–238, 2018.

[17] J. K. Opoku, "Health and care development: an exploration of factors that hamper better palliative care in sub-Saharan Africa," *European Journal of Biology and Medical Science Research*, vol. 2, no. 4, pp. 1–16, 2014.

[18] M. K. Gyakobo, E. A. Opare-Lokko, D. N. N. Nortey et al., *Developing a Model Palliative Care Service: The Korle Bu Experience*, Stellenbosch University, 2015.

[19] Ghana News Agency, *Palliative care needed for terminal ill health*, GhanaWeb, 2003.

[20] Ghana Ministry of Health, *National Policy for the Prevention and Control of Chronic Non-Communicable Diseases in Ghana*, Ministry of Health, Ghana, 2012.

[21] Ghana Ministry of Health, *National Strategy for Cancer Control in Ghana*, Ministry of Health, Ghana, 2011.

[22] K. Beernaert, J. Cohen, L. Deliens et al., "Referral to palliative care in COPD and other chronic diseases: a population-based study," *Respiratory Medicine*, vol. 107, no. 11, pp. 1731–1739, 2013.

[23] B. Kapp, C. Mireles, S. Sanchez-Reilly, J. Healy, and S. Lee, "Benefits of palliative care in the MICU (S781)," *Journal of Pain and Symptom Management*, vol. 51, no. 2, pp. 452-453, 2016.

[24] J. A. Greer, *Study Confirms Benefits of Early Palliative Care for Advanced Cancer*, National Cancer Institute, 2016.

[25] N. S. M. Ann and M. J. Deodhar, "Respite model of palliative care for advanced cancer in India: development and evaluation of effectiveness," *Journal of Palliative Care and Medicine*, vol. 5, no. 5, pp. 1–4, 2015.

[26] R. Roy, "Role of palliative care department in modifying ICU admissions for patients with advanced cancer: a study," *Journal of Clinical Oncology*, vol. 30, pp. 10-11, 2017.

[27] J. B. Cassel, "Palliative care's impact on utilization and costs: implications for health services research and policy," in *Meeting the Needs of Older Adults with Serious Illness. Aging Medicine*, A. Kelley and D. Meier, Eds., Humana Press, New York, NY, USA, 2014.

[28] P. H. Chong, J. A. de Castro Molina, K. Teo, and W. S. Tan, "Paediatric palliative care improves patient outcomes and reduces healthcare costs: evaluation of a home-based program," *BMC Palliative Care*, vol. 17, no. 1, pp. 11–18, 2018.

[29] M. P. Davis, J. S. Temel, T. Balboni, and P. Glare, "A review of the trials which examine early integration of outpatient and home palliative care for patients with serious illnesses," *Annals of Palliative Medicine*, vol. 4, no. 3, pp. 99–121, 2015.

[30] S. M. Enguidanos, D. Cherin, and R. Brumley, "Home-based palliative care study: site of death, and costs of medical care for patients with congestive heart failure, chronic obstructive pulmonary disease, and cancer," *Journal of Social Work in End-of-Life & Palliative Care*, vol. 1, no. 3, pp. 11-12, 2017.

[31] D. Kavalieratos, J. Corbelli, D. Zhang et al., "Association between palliative care and patient and caregiver outcomes: a systematic review and meta-analysis," *JAMA*, vol. 316, no. 20, pp. 2104–2114, 2016.

[32] C. L. Smoak, *The Effect of Inpatient Palliative Care Consultations on Hospital Readmission Rates for those with Alzheimer's Disease*, Proquest LLC, 2015.

[33] KATH, "About us/our history," 2016, November 2017, http://www.kathhsp.org/about.html.

[34] J. Sutton and Z. Austin, "Qualitative research: data collection, analysis, and management," *The Canadian Journal of Hospital Pharmacy*, vol. 68, no. 3, pp. 226–231, 2015.

[35] G. Greenfield, K. Foley, and A. Majeed, "Rethinking primary care's gatekeeper role," *BMJ*, vol. 354, no. i4803, 2016.

[36] Ghana Health Service, "The patient's charter," 2017, March 2018, http://www.ghanahealthservice.org/ghs-subcategory.php?cid=2&scid=46.

[37] A. Moser and I. Korstjens, "Series: practical guidance to qualitative research. Part 3: sampling, data collection and analysis," *The European Journal of General Practice*, vol. 24, no. 1, pp. 9–18, 2018.

[38] S. Jamshed, "Qualitative research method-interviewing and observation," *Journal of Basic and Clinical Pharmacy*, vol. 5, no. 4, pp. 87-88, 2014.

[39] Centre for Community Health and Development, "Section 12. Conducting interviews," in *Community Tool Box*, pp. 1–8, University of Kansas, Lawrence, KS, 2017.

[40] V. Braun and V. Clarke, "Using thematic analysis in psychology," *Qualitative Research in Psychology*, vol. 3, no. 2, pp. 77–101, 2006.

[41] Y. Schenker, M. Crowley-Matoka, D. Dohan et al., "Oncologist factors that influence referrals to subspecialty palliative care clinics," *Journal of Oncology Practice*, vol. 10, no. 2, pp. e37–e44, 2014.

[42] C. A. Mousing, H. Timm, K. Lomborg, and M. Kirkevold, "Barriers to palliative care in people with chronic obstructive pulmonary disease in home care: a qualitative study of the perspective of professional caregivers," *Journal of Clinical Nursing*, vol. 27, no. 3-4, pp. 650–660, 2018.

[43] T. Onyeka and N. Iloanusi, "Palliative care in Enugu, a success story," *Asia-Pacific Journal of Clinical Oncology*, vol. 10, 2014.

[44] D. Kavalieratos, E. M. Mitchell, T. S. Carey et al., ""Not the 'Grim Reaper Service'": an assessment of provider knowledge, attitudes, and perceptions regarding palliative care referral barriers in heart failure," *Journal of the American Heart Association*, vol. 3, no. 1, article e000544, 2014.

[45] D. Low, E. C. Merkel, M. Menon et al., "End-of-life palliative care practices and referrals in Uganda," *Journal of Palliative Medicine*, vol. 21, no. 3, pp. 328–334, 2018.

[46] B. Wright and K. Forbes, "Haematologists' perceptions of palliative care and specialist palliative care referral: a qualitative study," *BMJ Supportive & Palliative Care*, vol. 7, no. 1, pp. 39–45, 2014.

[47] M. Devlin and V. Maida, "The demon in deeming," *Canadian Family Physician*, vol. 63, pp. 191–193, 2017.

[48] E. Adwedaa, "Respect for patient autonomy: a patient perspective," *Postgraduate Medical Journal of Ghana*, vol. 4, no. 1, 2015.

[49] E. Kirby, A. Broom, P. Good, J. Wootton, and J. Adams, "Medical specialists' motivations for referral to specialist palliative care: a qualitative study," *BMJ Supportive & Palliative Care*, vol. 4, no. 3, pp. 277–284, 2014.

[50] J.-R. Lee, J. K. Lee, S. Hwang, J. E. Kim, J. I. Chung, and S. Y. Kim, "Doctor's perception and referral barriers toward palliative care for advanced cancer patients," *The Korean Journal of Hospice and Palliative Care*, vol. 15, no. 1, pp. 10–17, 2012.

[51] A. M. Torke, L. R. Holtz, S. Hui et al., "Palliative care for patients with dementia: a national survey," *Journal of the American Geriatrics Society*, vol. 58, no. 11, pp. 2114–2121, 2010.

[52] C. Nieder, J. Norum, O. Spanne, I. Bilberg, G. Vagstad, and A. Dalhaug, "Does distance to treatment centre influence the rate of palliative radiotherapy in adult cancer patients?," *Anticancer Research*, vol. 29, no. 7, pp. 2641–2644, 2009.

[53] B. Hannon, N. Swami, G. Rodin, A. Pope, and C. Zimmermann, "Experiences of patients and caregivers with early palliative care: a qualitative study," *Palliative Medicine*, vol. 31, no. 1, pp. 72–81, 2017.

[54] N. E. Omoyeni, O. A. Soyannwo, O. O. Aikomo, and O. F. Iken, "Home-based palliative care for adult cancer patients in Ibadan—a three year review," *ecancermedicalscience*, vol. 8, no. 490, pp. 1–7, 2014.

Usefulness of qSOFA and ECOG Scores for Predicting Hospital Mortality in Postsurgical Cancer Patients without Infection

Silvio A. Ñamendys-Silva (ID),[1,2,3] Emerson Joachin-Sánchez,[1]
Aranza Joffre-Torres,[1] Bertha M. Córdova-Sánchez (ID),[1] Guadalupe Ferrer-Burgos,[1]
Octavio González-Chon,[2] and Angel Herrera-Gomez[1]

[1]Department of Critical Care Medicine, Instituto Nacional de Cancerología, Mexico City, Mexico
[2]Department of Critical Care Medicine, Medica Sur Clinic & Foundation, Mexico City, Mexico
[3]Department of Critical Care Medicine, Instituto Nacional de Ciencias Médicas y Nutrición Salvador Zubirán, Mexico City, Mexico

Correspondence should be addressed to Silvio A. Ñamendys-Silva; snamendys@incan.edu.mx

Academic Editor: Shahinaz Gadalla

Background. The quick sequential organ failure assessment (qSOFA) and the Eastern Cooperative Oncologic Group (ECOG) scale are simple and easy parameters to measure because they do not require laboratory tests. The objective of this study was to compare the discriminatory capacity of the qSOFA and ECOG to predict hospital mortality in postsurgical cancer patients without infection. *Methods*. During the period 2013–2017, we prospectively collected data of all patients without infection who were admitted to the ICU during the postoperative period, except those who stayed in the ICU for <24 hours or patients under 18 years. The ECOG score during the last month before hospitalization and the qSOFA performed during the first hour after admission to the intensive care unit (ICU) were collected. The primary outcome for this study was the in-hospital mortality rate. *Results*. A total of 315 patients were included. The ICU and hospital mortality rates were 6% and 9.2%, respectively. No difference was observed between the qSOFA [AUC=0.75 (95% CI = 0.69-0.79)] and the ECOG scores [AUC=0.68 (95%CI =0.62-0.73)] (p=0.221) for predicting in-hospital mortality. qSOFA greater than 1 predicted in-hospital mortality with a high sensitivity (100%) but low specificity (38.8%); positive predictive value of 26.3% and negative predictive value of 93.1% compared to 74.4% of specificity, 55.1% of sensitivity%; positive predictive value of 18% and negative predictive value of 94.2% for an ECOG score greater than 1. Multivariable Cox regression analysis identified two independent predicting factors of in-hospital mortality, which included ECOG score during the last month before hospitalization (HR: 1.46; 95 % CI:1.06-2.00); qSOFA calculated in the first hours after ICU admission (OR: 3.17; 95 % CI: 1.79–5.63). *Conclusion*. No difference was observed between the qSOFA and ECOG for predicting in-hospital mortality. The qSOFA score performed during the first hour after admission to the ICU and ECOG scale during the last month before hospitalization were associated with in-hospital mortality in postsurgical cancer patients without infection. The qSOFA and ECOG score have a potential to be included as early warning tools for hospitalized postsurgical cancer patients without infection.

1. Introduction

The introduction of new treatments for cancer and advances in intensive care have improved the outcomes of critically ill cancer patients. Patients with cancer may require admission to the intensive care unit (ICU) after surgery [1]. The quick sequential organ failure assessment (qSOFA) [2] and the Eastern Cooperative Oncologic Group (ECOG) scale [3] are simple and easy parameters to measure because they do not require laboratory tests. The qSOFA consists of three clinical

elements, hypotension (systolic blood pressure ≤100 mmHg), tachypnea (respiratory rate ≥22 minute^{-1}), and alteration in mental status (Glasgow Coma Score ≤13 points) (total score ranges between 0 and three) [2]. The qSOFA was derived from data of symptomatic patients; thus, it is not a screening tool for sepsis [4]. Patients with acute medical illness, such as acute coronary syndrome, hypovolemic shock, or trauma, may have a qSOFA ≥ 2. The qSOFA has been used to predict mortality in patients without suspected infection [5, 6]. The ECOG is used by oncohematologists and intensivists for decision making for cancer patients [1, 7–9]. The performance status impairment classified according to the ECOG has prognostic value in general critically ill patients [7] and critically ill cancer patients [8]. The ECOG has six categories (total score ranges between 0 and five):

(a) Score of 0: indicating that the patient is fully active, able to carry on all pre-disease performance without restriction

(b) Score of 1: indicating restriction in physically strenuous activity, but the patient is still ambulatory and able to carry out work of a light or sedentary nature (e.g., light house work; office work)

(c) Score of 2: indicating that the patient is ambulatory and capable of all self-care but unable to carry out any work activities. Up and about more than >50 % of waking hours

(d) Score of 3: indicating that the patient is capable of only limited self-care and is confined to the bed or chair more than >50 % of waking hours

(e) Score of 4: indicating that the patient is completely disabled, cannot carry on any self-care: totally confined to the bed or chair

(f) Score of 5: indicating death

The performant status impairment in the week before hospital admission has been associated with increased hospital mortality in the critically ill patients [7].

The objective of this study was to compare the discriminatory capacity of the qSOFA [2] and ECOG [3] to predict hospital mortality in postsurgical cancer patients without infection.

2. Methods

This observational study was performed in the ICU of the Instituto Nacional de Cancerología (INCan), Mexico City. The Bioethics Committee of INCan approved this study, and the need for informed consent was waived (Rev/03/2013). During the period 2013-2017, we collected data of all patients without infection who were admitted to the ICU during the postoperative period, except those who stayed in the ICU for <24 hours or patients under 18 years. Demographic and clinical data were collected during the first day of the ICU stay, including the ECOG score during the last month before hospitalization, type of tumor, cancer status, need for mechanical ventilation (MV), length of invasive MV, length of stay in the ICU, length of stay in the hospital, and ICU and in-hospital mortality. The qSOFA was performed during the first hour after admission to the ICU. The qSOFA was determined by assigning one point for each of the following variables: Glasgow coma scale <15 before surgery, systolic blood pressure ≤100 mm Hg, or respiratory rate ≥22/min [2]. Each patient's length of stay in the hospital was measured based on the number of days between their admission and discharge from the INCan. The disease status was categorized into the following: recently diagnosed (prior to treatment or administration of first line of treatment),

active disease (disease progression or during second- and third-line treatment), and complete remission.

2.1. Statistical Analysis. The primary outcome (the dependent variable) for this study was the in-hospital mortality rate. Continuous variables are expressed as the means ± standard deviation or as medians and interquartile ranges for skewed distributions. Categorical variables are expressed as percentages. To assess the performances of the qSOFA and the ECOG scores to predict in-hospital mortality, we calculated the sensitivity, specificity, negative predictive value, positive predictive value, positive likelihood ratio, and negative likelihood ratio. The area under the receiver operating characteristic curve (AUC) was used to evaluate the ability of the qSOFA and ECOG scores to discriminate between patients who lived and those who died. Comparison of the AUC was performed using the methodology suggested by Hanley and McNeil [10]. Cox proportional hazards univariate and multivariate analyses (forward selection) were used to identify factors with potential prognostic significance for in-hospital mortality. The final Cox model was assessed for potential interactions. The results were reported using hazard ratios (HRs) and the corresponding 95% confidence intervals (95% CIs). Survival curves were estimated using the Kaplan-Meier method. A two-sided p value <0.05 was used to determine statistical significance.

3. Results

A total of 315 patients were included. The mean age of the patients was 50.6 ± 15.9 years, and 59% (186) were female. There were 195 patients (61.9%) who required invasive MV during their stay in the ICU, with a median duration of two days (1-4 days), and the median length of stay in the ICU was 2 days (1-4 days). Sixty-eight (21.6%) patients had a gynecological malignancy, while the other most common primary cancer sites were the gastrointestinal (16.2%) and sarcoma (14.3%). In terms of cancer status, 50.8% were newly diagnosed, 48.8% had disease progression, and 0.3% had complete remission of disease. Table 1 reports the main clinical characteristics. The ICU and hospital mortality rates were 6% and 9.2%, respectively. For patients with qSOFA scores less than 2, the hospital mortality rate was 7.36% vs 35.7% for patients with a qSOFA score of 2 or higher (absolute difference, 28.3%; 95% CI, 13%-47.7%, p<0.001). For patients with ECOG scores less than 2, the hospital mortality rate was 6.1% vs 21.9% for patients with a ECOG score of 2 or higher (absolute difference, 15.8%; 95% CI, 6.8%-26.1%, p<0.001). No difference was observed between the qSOFA [AUC=0.75 (95% CI = 0.69-0.79)] and the ECOG scores [AUC=0.68 (95%CI =0.62-0.73)] (p=0.221) for predicting in-hospital mortality (Figure 1). Table 2 reports the sensitivity, specificity, positive predictive value, and negative predictive value for the qSOFA and ECOG scores for predicting in-hospital mortality. qSOFA greater than 1 predicted in-hospital mortality with a high sensitivity (100%) but low specificity (38.8%); positive predictive value of 26.3% and negative predictive value of 93.1% compared to 74.4% of specificity,

TABLE 1: Clinical characteristics of critically ill patients without infection who were admitted to the ICU during the postoperative period (n = 315).

Characteristics	Finding
Age, years, mean ± SD	50.6 ± 15.9
Gender (female), n (%)	186(59)
Length of stay in ICU (days), median (IQR)	2 (1–4)
Length of stay in the hospital (days), median (IQR)	8(6-15)
Quick sequential organ failure assessment (qSOFA), n(%)	
qSOFA=0	111(35.2)
qSOFA=1	166(52.7)
qSOFA=2	37(11.3)
qSOFA=3	1(0.3)
Eastern Cooperative Oncologic Group (ECOG), n (%)	
ECOG=0	88(27.9)
ECOG=1	138(43.8)
ECOG=2	50(15.9)
ECOG=3	29(9.2)
ECOG=4	10(3.2)
ICU mortality, n (%)	19(6)
Hospital mortality, n (%)	29 (9.2)

TABLE 2: Sensitivity, specificity, positive predictive value, negative predictive value, positive likelihood ratio, and negative likelihood ratio for quick sequential organ failure assessment (qSOFA) and Eastern Cooperative Oncologic Group (ECOG) for in-hospital mortality.

Finding	qSOFA				ECOG			
	>0	>1	>2	>3	>0	>1	>2	>3
Sensitivity, %	100.0	34.4	0	0	89.6	55.1	24.1	10.3
Specificity, %	38.8	90.21	99.6	100.0	29.7	74.4	88.8	97.5
Positive predictive value, %	14.2	26.3	0	0	11.5	18.0	17.9	30.0
Negative predictive value, %	100	93.1	90.8	90.8	96.6	94.2	92.0	91.5
Positive likelihood ratio	1.63	3.52	0.0	0.0	1.2	2.16	2.16	4.2
Negative likelihood ratio	0.0	0.73	1.00	1.00	0.35	0.60	0.85	0.23

55.1% of sensitivity%; positive predictive value of 18% and negative predictive value of 94.2% for an ECOG score greater than 1 (Table 2). Multivariable Cox regression analysis identified two independent predicting factors of in-hospital mortality, which included ECOG score during the last month before hospitalization (HR: 1.46; 95 % CI: 1.06-2.00) and qSOFA calculated in the first hours after ICU admission (HR: 3.17; 95 % CI: 1.79–5.63) (Table 3). Survival probabilities in postsurgical cancer patients without infection, according to the qSOFA and ECOG scale, are shown in Figures 2 and 3.

4. Discussion

The main findings of this study are that no difference was observed between the qSOFA and ECOG for predicting in-hospital mortality. Both the qSOFA and ECOG scale demonstrated a poor to fair level of discrimination for in-hospital mortality. The qSOFA has been used to predict mortality in patients without suspected infection [5, 6]. Singer et al. [5] reported the utility of qSOFA for assessing the outcome of adult emergency department (ED) patients without suspected infection. The qSOFA score at the time of ED admission (within 2 minutes or less) demonstrated an AUC=0.70 (95% CI=0.65-0.74), suggesting fair accuracy for mortality prediction. Jawa et al. [6] reported the ability of the qSOFA to predict outcomes in blunt trauma patients presenting to the ED. The qSOFA score calculated from the initial vital signs in the ED demonstrated an AUC of 0.73 [95% CI 0.69-0.76]. Similarly, in our cohort of critically ill cancer patients without infection the qSOFA score demonstrated a fair level of discrimination for in-hospital mortality prediction. The performance status impairment classified according to the ECOG has prognostic value in general critically ill patients [7] and critically ill cancer patients [8]. The ECOG scale could account for factors that cannot be accounted for by critical care severity scores. Park et al. [9] reported a significant trend for increasing hospital mortality as the ECOG score became higher. The qSOFA is not part of the new sepsis definitions; a critically ill patient or cancer patient may have a qSOFA ≥2 without infection or sepsis: for example, acute coronary syndrome, hypovolemic shock, or trauma. The qSOFA and ECOG score of 2 or higher could identify the critical point at which critically ill cancer patients without infection exhibit the highest risk of death during

TABLE 3: Univariable and multivariable analysis of factors associated with in-hospital mortality.

Variable	Hazard ratio	95% CI	p	Hazard ratio	95% CI	p
		Univariate			Multivariate	
Age, years	1.02	0.99-1.04	0.062			
Gender, female	1.05	0.50-2.22	0.881			
ECOG, points	1.60	1.15-2.21	0.004	1.46	1.06-2.00	0.018
qSOFA, points	3.14	1.86-5.31	<0.001	3.17	1.79-5.63	<0.001
Length of stay in the ICU, days	0.95	0.87-1.04	0.301			

Abbreviations: CI=confidence interval, ICU=Intensive Care Unit, ECOG=Eastern Cooperative Oncology Group, and qSOFA= quick sequential organ failure assessment.

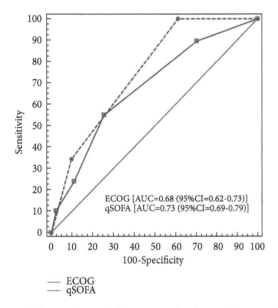

ECOG [AUC=0.68 (95%CI=0.62-0.73)]
qSOFA [AUC=0.73 (95%CI=0.69-0.79)]

— ECOG
----- qSOFA

FIGURE 1: Comparisons of the areas under the receiver operating characteristic curves for the prediction of in-hospital mortality of the quick sequential organ failure assessment (qSOFA) and the Eastern Cooperative Oncologic Group (ECOG) scale.

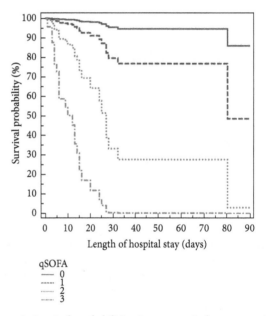

qSOFA
— 0
----- 1
······ 2
-·-·- 3

FIGURE 2: Survival probabilities in postsurgical cancer patients without infection, according to the quick sequential organ failure assessment (qSOFA) scale.

hospitalization. The qSOFA and ECOG scores are simple and easy to measure; they can be used as generic tools to predict clinically important outcomes for critically ill cancer patients likely to be admitted to the ICU regardless of whether infection is suspected. A strength of this study is that it presents the outcomes of postsurgical cancer patients without infection admitted to ICU. To the best of our knowledge, this study is the first to compare the predictive accuracy of the qSOFA and ECOG scales to predict the outcomes of critically ill cancer patients without infection. However, our study has some limitations in that it only included cancer patients without infection who were admitted to the ICU during the postoperative period and represents the experience of a single center.

5. Conclusion

No difference was observed between the qSOFA and ECOG for predicting in-hospital mortality. The qSOFA score performed during the first hour after admission to the ICU and ECOG scale during the last month before hospitalization were associated with in-hospital mortality in postsurgical cancer patients without infection. The qSOFA and ECOG score have a potential to be included as early warning tools for hospitalized postsurgical cancer patients without infection.

Abbreviations

qSOFA:	Quick sequential organ failure assessment
ECOG:	Eastern Cooperative Oncologic Group
ICU:	Intensive Care Unit
INCan:	Instituto Nacional de Cancerología
MV:	Mechanical ventilation
AUC:	Area under the receiver operating characteristic curve
HR:	Hazard ratio
ED:	Emergency department.

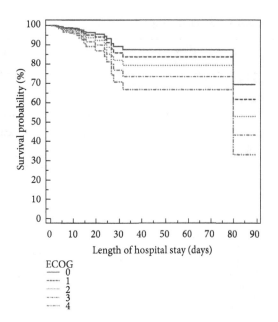

FIGURE 3: Survival probabilities in postsurgical cancer patients without infection, according to the Eastern Cooperative Oncologic Group (ECOG) scale.

Authors' Contributions

Ñamendys-Silva had full access to all of the data in the study and takes responsibility for the integrity of the data and the accuracy of the data analysis. All authors contributed to the study concept and design as well as acquisition, analysis, or interpretation of data. All authors partook in drafting of the paper. Ñamendys-Silva was responsible for the critical revision of the paper for important intellectual content and the statistical analysis as well as the study supervision. Herrera-Gomez, Córdova-Sánchez, and Ferrer-Burgos undertook the administrative, technical, or material support.

References

[1] S. A. Ñamendys-Silva, E. P. Plata-Menchaca, E. Rivero-Sigarroa, and A. Herrera-Gómez, "Opening the doors of the intensive care unit to cancer patients: a current perspective," *World Journal of Critical Care Medicine*, vol. 4, no. 3, pp. 159–162, 2015.

[2] M. Singer, C. S. Deutschman, C. W. Seymour et al., "Third international consensus definitions for sepsis and septic shock (Sepsis-3)," *The Journal of the American Medical Association*, vol. 315, pp. 801–810, 2016.

[3] M. M. Oken, R. H. Creech, D. C. Tormey et al., "Toxicity and response criteria of the eastern cooperative oncology group," *American Journal of Clinical Oncology*, vol. 5, no. 6, pp. 649–655, 1982.

[4] M. Singer and M. Shankar-Hari, "QSOFA, cue confusion," *Annals of Internal Medicine*, vol. 168, no. 4, pp. 293–295, 2018.

[5] A. J. Singer, J. Ng, H. C. Thode, R. Spiegel, and S. Weingart, "Quick SOFA scores predict mortality in adult emergency department patients with and without suspected infection," *Annals of Emergency Medicine*, vol. 69, no. 4, pp. 475–479, 2017.

[6] R. S. Jawa, J. A. Vosswinkel, J. E. McCormack et al., "Risk assessment of the blunt trauma victim: the role of the quick sequential organ failure assessment score (qSOFA)," *The American Journal of Surgery*, vol. 214, no. 3, pp. 397–401, 2017.

[7] F. G. Zampieri, F. A. Bozza, G. M. Moralez et al., "The effects of performance status one week before hospital admission on the outcomes of critically ill patients," *Intensive Care Medicine*, vol. 43, no. 1, pp. 39–47, 2017.

[8] S. A. Ñamendys-Silva, M. O. González-Herrera, J. Texcocano-Becerra, and A. Herrera-Gómez, "Clinical characteristics and outcomes of critically ill cancer patients with septic shock," *QJM: An International Journal of Medicine*, vol. 104, no. 6, pp. 505–511, 2011.

[9] C.-M. Park, Y. Koh, K. Jeon et al., "Impact of Eastern Cooperative Oncology Group Performance Status on hospital mortality in critically ill patients," *Journal of Critical Care*, vol. 29, no. 3, pp. 409–413, 2014.

[10] J. A. Hanley and B. J. McNeil, "A method of comparing the areas under receiver operating characteristic curves derived from the same cases," *Radiology*, vol. 148, no. 3, pp. 839–843, 1983.

12

Association of CCL2, CCR5, ELMO1 and IL8 Polymorphism with Diabetic Nephropathy in Malaysian Type 2 Diabetic Patients

Mohd Jokha Yahya ⓘ,[1] **Patimah binti Ismail,**[2]
Norshariza binti Nordin ⓘ,[1] **Abdah binti Md Akim,**[1] **Wan Shaariah binti Md. Yusuf,**[3]
Noor Lita binti Adam,[3] **and Maryam Jamielah Yusoff**[1]

[1]*Department of Biomedical Sciences, Faculty of Medicine and Health Sciences, Universiti Putra Malaysia, Malaysia*
[2]*Department of Human Development and Growth, Faculty of Medicine and Health Sciences, Universiti Putra Malaysia, Malaysia*
[3]*Department of Medicine (Endocrinology & Nephrology), Hospital Tuanku Ja'afar, Malaysia*

Correspondence should be addressed to Mohd Jokha Yahya; mohdjokhayahya@gmail.com

Academic Editor: Vita Dolzan

The unique variants or biomarkers of individuals help to understand the pathogenesis as well as the potential risk of individuals or patients to diabetic nephropathy (DN). The aim of this study was to investigate the association of a genetic polymorphism of monocyte chemoattractant protein-1 (CCL2-rs3917887), chemokine receptor 5 (CCR5-rs1799987), engulfment and cell mortality (ELMO1-rs74130), and interleukin-8 (IL8-rs4073) with the development of DN among Malaysian type 2 diabetes mellitus (T2DM) patients. More than one thousand diabetic patients were examined and a total of 652 T2DM patients were tested comprising 227 Malays (nonnephrotic=96 and nephrotic=131), 203 Chinese (nonnephrotic=95 and nephrotic=108), and 222 Indians (nonnephrotic=136 and nephrotic=86). DNA Sequenom mass ARRAY was employed to identify polymorphisms in CCL2, CCR5, ELMO1, and IL8 genes. DNA was extracted from the secondary blood samples taken from the T2DM patients. The alleles and genotypes were tested using four genetic models and the best mode of inheritance was chosen. CCR5 rs1799987 (G>A) showed strong association with the development of diabetic nephropathy only among the Chinese with OR=6.71 (2.55-17.68) 95% CI while IL8 rs4073 (T>A) showed association with nephropathy only among the Indians with OR=1.57 (0.66-3.71) 95% CI. The additive model was the best model for the mode of inheritance of all the genes. The contribution of genetic variants differs across ethnic groups or background. Further studies which involve environmental risk factors should be taken into consideration.

1. Introduction

The most common modifiable risk factors for most chronic diseases include, but not limited to, dyslipidemia, hypertension, and glycemic control while factors such as age, race, and genetic profile are generally unmodifiable [1–3].

Diabetes nephropathy (DN) has become a major determinant of morbidity and mortality in diabetic patients worldwide in addition to being the most common cause of end-stage renal disease (ESRD) [4]. Though the main causes of DN are hemodynamic and metabolic factors, it has recently been suggested that DN is an inflammatory process involving immune cells [5]. For instance, hyperglycemia, free fatty acids (FFA), and obesity may activate nuclear factor

κB (NF-κB) through protein kinase C (PKC) and reactive oxygen species (ROS) to rapidly stimulate the expression of cytokines which stimulate some genes that promote the development of DN [6]. Thus, the pathogenesis of DN via increased vascular inflammation and fibrosis has implicated inflammatory cells, cytokines, and profibrotic growth factors such as transforming growth factor-β (TGF-β), monocyte chemoattractant protein-1 (MCP-1), interleukin-1 (IL-1), interleukin-6 (IL-6), and interleukin-18 (IL-18), among others [7]. The activation of PKC, oxidative stress, and advanced glycation end products (AGEs) due to the diabetic state also increases the production of cytokines such as TNF-α and interleukins, which stimulate the production of MCP-1, also known as CCL2. PKC also directly induces the production of NF-ţB which promotes the production of proinflammatory proteins and extracellular matrix turnover such as thrombospondin 1, chemokine CCL2, osteopontin, fibronectin, decorin, plasminogen activator inhibitor 1, and aldose reductase [8].

CCR5 is a β-chemokine receptor expressed on the surface of the monocytes for its ligands or known as regulated on activation of normal T cell expressed and secreted (RANTES) on mesangial cells. It is normally involved in the migration of monocytes, NK cells, and some T-cells to the inflammation site [9, 10]. An SNP of CCR5 (G59029A) gene is also registered as rs1799987. Its gene is located on the short arm of chromosome 3 (3p21.31) [11] at the promoter region. Though there are conflicting and inconclusive reports on the association of CCR5 gene promoter polymorphism with the risk of DN, the polymorphism in CCR5 might affect individual susceptibility to DN [12]. The gene, however, has been reported to have an association to nephropathy in T2DM among the Japanese and Asian Indian population [13–16]. Some polymorphisms of CCR5 gene have been reported to affect the severity of multiple autoimmune and infectious diseases through mediating inflammatory responses [17]. According to Nazir et al. [10], CCR5 rs1799987 is the most studied genetic variant in inflammatory cytokines with the genetic variant rs1799987 in CCR5 gene A allele being the risk factor for diabetic nephropathy. The G allele of rs1799987, however, is considered as a protective allele [18]. CCL2 is also recognized as monocyte chemoattractant protein-1 (MCP-1) is the strongest known chemotactic factor for monocytes and is upregulated in DN. The CCL2 gene is located on chromosome 17q11.1–q21.1. The insertion-deletion sequence located in intron 1 (AGCTCTCCTTCTC/-) is registered as rs3917887 and was found to be significantly correlated to TDM2 among the North and South Indian population [13]. The blockade of CCL2/CCR2 signaling by RS102895 reportedly ameliorates diabetic nephropathy by improving blood glucose levels and preventing CCL2/CCR2 signaling from altering renal nephrin and VEGF expressions through blocking macrophage infiltration, inflammation, and oxidative stress in type 2 diabetic mice [19].

Interleukin-8 is a potent chemokine inducing chemotaxis which recruits and activates acute inflammatory cells such as neutrophils, basophils, and T lymphocytes [20, 21]. The IL8 urinary level was found to be increased in T2DM patients with nephropathy in stage 1 and stage 2 [22]. The high level of IL-8 is due to the IL8 T-251A polymorphism (rs4073) on chromosome 4q12–13 that lies at the regulatory region also known as a promoter that affects the gene expression [23]. Ahluwalia et al. [13] have reported an association between nephropathy and IL-8 gene polymorphism in North and South Indians.

Engulfment And Cell Motility 1 (ELMO1) is a protein consisting of 720 amino acids. It is encoded by the ELMO1 gene on chromosome 7p14 with 22 exons. ELMO1 encodes for one of the ELMO proteins which promotes phagocytosis and cell migration by interacting with the cytokinesis protein. Polymorphisms in ELMO1 are strongly associated with susceptibility to DN [24, 25]. ELMO1 variants have been studied; the most strongly associated, however, is rs741301

among the Chinese population [26], African Americans [27], and Japanese [28].

In general, the roles of the aforementioned four proinflammatory genes in the development of DN have been established in some races. Therefore, this study is aimed at investigating the association of a genetic polymorphism of CCL2-rs3917887, CCR5-rs1799987, ELMO1-rs74130, and IL8-rs4073 with the development of DN among Malaysian type 2 diabetes mellitus (T2DM) patients.

2. Materials and Methods

This study employed a case-control design using cases with nephropathy and without nephropathy control groups of T2DM patients. The study was approved by the National Medical Research Register (NMRR) of the Ministry of Health Malaysia (KKM) with the reference number: (2) DLM.KKM/NIHSEC/08/0804/P12-519). The study also conforms to the items of the Declaration of Helsinki. All the subjects gave a written and signed informed consent. The subjects were recruited from the outpatients of the Medical Clinic of Hospital Tuanku Ja'afar Seremban (HTJS), Negeri Sembilan, Malaysia. The same patient cohort participated in another study for oxidative stress-related polymorphisms by Yahya et al. [29].

2.1. Sampling Method. From over 1000 T2DM patients' records screened from the medical outpatient department in HTJS, only 820 subjects were found to be suitable for the research with only 652 eventually selected with 203, 227, and 222 Chinese, Malays, and Indians, respectively. The selection of the subjects was based on the inclusion criteria for nephropathy (case) and nonnephropathy (control) following expert opinions of the specialists in the endocrinology and nephrology clinics. Only interested patients with signed consent were allowed to participate in this research. The exclusion criteria for both the case and control include biologically related patients, those with age onset ≤ 35 years, diabetes duration ≤ 10 years, normal fasting glucose level, nondiabetic and normal albumin excretion rate, patients without renal symptoms with a duration of < 10 years of diabetes, unclear cause of renal damage, and ESRD or Non-ESRD of T1DM patients as well as patients with glycated hemoglobin (HbA1c) <6.5%.

2.2. DNA Extraction and Genotyping. The samples used were secondary blood samples of T2DM patients who routinely visit the clinic. The samples were taken with ethylenediaminetetraacetic acid (EDTA) anticoagulant vacutainer tubes and stored at −20°C for further extraction and analysis. Both the patients' demography and most recent biochemical results were obtained from the patients' records and laboratory information system (LIS) in the Department of Pathology, respectively. Commercial DNA extraction kit (QIAGEN, USA) was used for the genomic DNA extraction while Sequenom Mass ARRAY iPLEX platform was employed for the SNPs genotyping. The derivation of the primer was done based on the work of Ahluwalia et al. (2011). Table 1 shows

TABLE 1: The sequence of primers and size of the PCR products used for the genotyping.

No	SNP	Forward	Reverse	PCR Products (bp)	Tm (°C)
1	rs1799987	ACGTTGGATGATACGGGGAGAGTGGAGAAA	ACGTTGGATGCCAACTTTAAATGTAGAGGG	95	47.0
2	rs3917887	ACGTTGGATGCCTATGCTGTAAAATGGGTA	ACGTTGGATGGTCCGTCTTAATGACACTTG	117	45.4
3	rs4073	ACGTTGGATGCTGAAGCTCCACAATTTGGT	ACGTTGGATGGCCACTCTAGTACTATATCTG	118	45.2
4	rs741301	ACGTTGGATGCAGTTCCCATGGTGGTTATC	ACGTTGGATGGAACTCTTCAAGCTCAATAG	110	46.1

TABLE 2: Comparison of clinical characteristic across the races.

SNP	Nephropathy				Without Nephropathy			
	Malay	Chinese	Indian	p-value df=2	Malay	Chinese	Indian	p-value df=2
Albumin excretion rate (g/24hr)	1363.18±136.00	1952.50±144.30	1756±155.44	0.77	25.83±2.10	23.00±5.70	26.67±1.9	0.61
Glycated hemoglobin (%)	8.67±2.34	9.19±2.31	7.79±2.08	<0.01*	9.07±1.97	9.45±2.56	8.30±1.63	<0.01*
Fasting blood glucose (mmol/L)	9.91±3.3	9.60±2.10	9.8±0.137	0.17	9.86±3.70	8.6±3.70	8.78±3.69	0.61
Total cholesterol (mmol/L)	6.42±1.37	6.58±1.19	6.48±1.42	0.11	4.84±1.01	4.26±1.13	4.74±1.23	0.021
HDL cholesterol (mmol/L)	1.02±0.39	1.01±0.24	1.16±0.25	0.13	1.22±0.26	1.11±0.24	1.29±0.26	0.14
LDL cholesterol (mmol/L)	2. 45±1.25	2.69±1.05	2.61±1.25	0.22	2.82 ±1.10	2.53±0.90	2.60±1.06	0.11
Triglycerides (mmol/L)	1.85±0.80	1.72±0.64	1.55±0.67	0.12	2.07±1.81	1.36±0.80	1.87±0.87	0.16

*P <0.05 shows significant difference.

the sequence of primers and size of the PCR products used for the genotyping.

2.3. Statistical Analysis. The Statistical Package for the Social Sciences version 17.0 (SPSS17.0) was used for all the statistical genetic analyses. Descriptive and inferential statistics were used to compare between the cases and controls for the frequencies of alleles and genotypes. One-way analysis of variance (ANOVA) was also used to test the differences between the clinical data. The conformation of the controls to Hardy-Weinberg Equilibrium (HWE) and the variants distributions were tested using Pearson's Chi-square goodness-of-fit test. Conventional Pearson's Chi-square test for independence with 2df was used for the genotype frequencies for each SNP to determine their associations with T2DM nephropathy. The statistical significance was set at p<0.05 (two-tailed). The Fisher Exact tests 2 × 3 and 2 × 2 were performed only when more than 20% of the cells had expected values less than 5 and when more than 20% of the cells had expected values less than 10, respectively. Three types of the model using Chi-square with 1 df as well as Cochran-Armitage trend test were also used to determine the significant SNPs. Odds ratio (OR) with corresponding 95% confidence interval (CI) was employed for the strength of association or the risk of developing diabetic nephropathy. VassarStats was used to calculate the OR. And the model with the least p-value was chosen to determine the mode of inheritance.

3. Results

3.1. Characteristics of T2DM Sampling Subjects. The Malays, Chinese, and Indians in this study were 227, 203, and 222, respectively, making a total of 652 T2DM patients. As reported earlier by Yahya et al. [29], the age ranges of the Malay, Chinese and Indian T2DM subjects were 32–83, 36–89, and 35–86 years old, respectively, while the mean ages were 59.0±8.23, 63.28±11.56, and 61.33±10.1, respectively.

In line with the aim of this study to only observe the effects of polymorphism as risk factors, the development of nephropathy was, therefore, not staged among the T2DM nephropathy patients and the basis of selection was mainly with the AER more than 300 mg/24hr. In the clinical demographics of the subjects in this study (data not shown), all

the races showed similar characteristics where the significant difference between the case and control was observed in AER, total cholesterol, and HDL (p<0.05). The biochemical observation among the races is shown in Table 2. There was no difference in duration of diabetes, glycated hemoglobin, fasting blood glucose, LDL, and triglycerides level (p>0.05) in the T2DM subjects case and control.

The statistical analysis by one-way ANOVA did not indicate a significant difference in the chemistry results (p>0.05) except for the glycated hemoglobin (HbA1c) concentration (p<0.01). The Chinese had the worst glycemic control in both case and control. There is a significant difference in glycemic control value among the races. The sampling was not randomly chosen; therefore the results might not reflect the true population clinical status among the races. Samples were selectively chosen to fulfill criteria of the research interest and might cause bias results.

3.2. Genotyping of Polymorphisms. All the polymorphisms were done by the mass array, and the homozygous and heterozygous genotype were interpreted by the observation of peaks produced in the chromatogram. The results are shown in Tables 3, 4, and 5.

3.3. Chi-Square Test of Genotype and Allele Association. In this study, all controls were tested for HWE and the results showed that all the controls were in the HWE with p>0.05 as shown in Table 6. Pearson's Chi-square test for independence was done to determine the association between variants and nephropathy (Table 7). The outcome of the Chi-square at df=2 with p<0.05 was accepted as a statistically significant association (a difference in genotype frequency between the case and control) of nephropathy with the gene polymorphism of the genotype and allele. Fisher Exact test probability was tested when more than 20% of the cells had the expected value < 5.

3.4. Dominant and Recessive Model. The association of the above genotypes was then stratified against the dominant and recessive model as shown in Table 7. Only the rs1799987 showed significant association in both dominant (p=9.2x10^{-5}) and recessive (p=0.0021) models among the Chinese only.

TABLE 3: Genotype distribution and frequencies in case and control.

SNP	Malay						Chinese						Indian					
	Case			Control			Case			Control			Case			Control		
	major/ major	major/ minor	minor/ minim	major/ major	major/ minor	minor/ minor	major/ major	major/ minor	minor/ minor	major/ major	major/ minor	minor/ minor	major/ major	major/ minor	minor/ minor	major/ major	major/ minor	minor/ minor
CCR5 rs1799987	GG=47 (35.9)	AG=69 (52.7)	AA=15 (11.5)	GG=43 (44.8)	AG=42 (43.8)	AA=11 (11.5)	GG=25 (23.1)	AG=58 (53.7)	AA=25 (23.1)	GG=47 (49.5)	AG=41 (43.2)	AA=7 (7.4)	GG=29 (33.7)	AG=44 (51.2)	AA=13 (15.1)	GG=48 (35.3)	AG=70 (51.5)	AA=18 (13.2)
CCL2 rs3917887	II=42 (32.1)	DI=57 (43.5)	DD=32 (24.4)	II=32 (33.3)	DI=47 (44.0)	DD=17 (20.7)	II=20 (18.5)	DI=69 (63.9)	DD=19 (17.6)	II=26 (27.4)	DI=57 (54.7)	DD=17 (17.9)	II=33 (38.8)	DI=40 (47.1)	DD=12 (14.1)	II=41 (31.2)	DI=62 (51.7)	DD=17 (14.1)
IL8 rs4073	TT=45 (34.4)	TA=66 (50.4)	AA=20 (15.3)	TT=45 (34.4)	TA=66 (50.4)	AA=14 (15.3)	TT=43 (39.8)	TA=57 (52.8)	AA=8 (7.4)	TT=35 (36.8)	TA=50 (52.6)	AA=10 (10.5)	TT=23 (26.7)	TA=51 (59.3)	AA=12 (14.0)	TT=60 (44.1)	TA=56 (41.2)	AA=20 (14.7)
ELMO1 rs741301	AA=50 (38.2)	AG=58 (44.3)	GG=23 (17.6)	AA=82 (36.1)	AG=108 (47.6)	GG=37 (16.3)	AA=40 (37.0)	AG=51 (47.2)	GG=17 (15.7)	AA=42 (44.2)	AG=44 (46.3)	GG=9 (9.5)	AA=33 (38.4)	AG=45 (52.3)	GG=8 (9.3)	AA=57 (41.9)	AG=59 (43.4)	GG=20 (14.7)

Genotype data are presented as a number of subjects (%).

TABLE 4: Allele distribution and frequencies in case and control.

SNP	Malay				Chinese				Indian			
	Case		Control		Case		Control		Case		Control	
CCR5 rs1799987	G=163 (62.2)	A=99 (37.8)	G=128 (66.7)	A=64 (33.3)	G=108 (50)	A=108 (50)	G=102 (71.1)	A=55 (28.9)	G=102 (59.3)	A=70 (40.7)	G=166 (61)	A=106 (39.0)
CCL2 rs3917887	I=99 (45.0)	D=121 (55.0)	I=111 (57.8)	D=81 (42.2)	I=109 (50.5)	D=107 (49.5)	I=104 (54.7)	D=86 (45.3)	I=62 (36.9)	D=106 (63.1)	I=144 (60.0)	D=96 (40.0)
IL8 rs4073	T=156 (59.4)	A=106 (40.6)	T=122 (63.5)	A=70 (36.5)	T=156 (68.0)	A=73 (32.0)	T=120 (63.2)	A=70 (36.8)	T=97 (56.4)	A=75 (43.6)	T=176 (64.7)	A=96 (35.3)
ELMO1 rs741301	A=158 (60.3)	G=104 (36.7)	A=114 (59.4)	G=78 (40.6)	A=131 (60.6)	G=85 (39.4)	A=128 (67.4)	G=62 (32.6)	A=111 (64.5)	G=61 (35.5)	A=173 (63.6)	G=99 (36.4)

Allele data are presented as a number of subjects (%).

TABLE 5: Differences in the frequencies of allele distribution among the races.

SNP	Control						P value χ^2 df=2	Case						P value χ^2 df=2
	Malay		Chinese		Indian			Case		Control		Indian		
CCR5 rs1799987	G=128 (66.7)	A=64 (33.3)	G=102 (71.1)	A=55 (28.9)	G=166 (61)	A=106 (39.0)	0.432 1.68	G=163 (62.2)	A=99 (37.8)	G=108 (50)	A=108 (50)	G=102 (59.3)	A=70 (40.7)	0.023* 7.57
CCL2 rs3917887	I=111 (57.8)	D=81 (42.2)	I=104 (54.7)	D=86 (45.3)	I=144 (60.0)	D=96 (40.0)	1.200 0.549	I=99 (45.0)	D=121 (55.0)	I=109 (50.5)	D=107 (49.5)	I=62 (36.9)	D=62 (63.1)	<0.001* 28.24
IL8 rs4073	T=122 (63.5)	A=70 (36.5)	T=120 (63.2)	A=70 (36.8)	T=176 (64.7)	A=96 (35.3)	0.9371 0.13	T=156 (59.4)	A=106 (40.6)	T=156 (68.0)	A=73 (32.0)	T=97 (56.4)	A=75 (43.6)	0.004* 6.56
ELMO1 rs741301	A=114 (59.4)	G=78 (40.6)	A=128 (67.4)	G=62 (32.6)	A=173 (63.6)	G=99 (36.4)	0.2671 2.34	A=158 (60.3)	G=104 (36.7)	A=131 (60.6)	G=85 (39.4)	A=111 (64.5)	G=61 (35.5)	0.641 0.89

*p <0.05 indicates the significant difference of allele distribution in the population.

3.5. Cochran-Armitage Trend Test. For best understanding of the mode of inheritance and to calculate the additive model association, the association was tested for trend using Cochran-Armitage trend test (C-ATT). From Table 8, the best model fit for all the variants was the additive. The best model was chosen based on the least p-value compared to the other models.

The OR of the associated polymorphisms is skewed towards increasing risk of nephropathy for T2DM patients among the Malaysian. The exposure to the tested polymorphisms is not absolute as there are many other related polymorphisms that need to be incorporated.

From Table 9, individuals with homozygous SNP of rs1799987, CCR5, have the strongest association to nephropathy in T2DM (p=1.0×10^{-5}) with OR=6.71, 95% CI 2.55-17.68) but this is only among the Chinese. The weakest association would be the rs4073, IL8 (p= with OR=1.57, 95% CI 0.66-3.71) that is only applicable among the Indians, odd ratio (OR), 95% CI.

4. Discussion

4.1. Genetic Association and Correlation. In this study, four polymorphisms of four different genes were tested to confirm variants that might be the risk factors to increase the susceptibility to DN among Malaysians. Among the four proinflammatory genes studied, only the CCR5 and IL-8 were significant among the Chinese and Indians, respectively.

In the present study, CCR5 59029 A allele has a significant and strong association with nephropathy in T2DM Malaysian Chinese only. Evidently, 50% of A allele carriers were found in the case group while only 28.9% of the carriers were found in the control group. The CCR5 59029A-genotype has been shown to be associated with increased CCR5 expression. According to the literature, CCR5 59029A increased CCR5 expression as observed in peripheral blood mononuclear cells in individuals [30], suggesting that the genotype could regulate CCR5 gene expression. The infiltration of monocytes and macrophages is reportedly increased as the glomerulosclerosis progresses [31, 32]. As CCR5 expression increases, the recruitment of monocytes and differentiation of these cells to macrophage in glomeruli will also be induced in manifolds. In the present study, none of the statistic models shows any association (p>0.05) among the Malays and Indians. The result is in agreement with the Caucasians studies in Irish T1DM [33] and T2DM in Danish, Finnish, and French [34]. The allelic frequency is significantly different between different ethnic groups. An SNP that is essentially benign in one ethnic group can be very problematic in another. This can be due, for example, to differences in the frequencies of other

TABLE 6: Hardy Weinberg Equilibrium test for the control and case.

SNP	Malay						Chinese						Indian					
	Control			Statistic		df	Control			Statistic		df	Control			Statistic		df
	major/major	major/minor	minor/minor	χ^2	p-value		major/major	major/minor	minor/minor	χ^2	p-value		major/major	major/minor	minor/minor	χ^2	p-value	
CONTROL																		
CCR5 rs1799987	GG=43 (44.8)	AG=42 (43.8)	AA=11 (11.5)	0.023	0.8795	1	GG=47 (49.5)	AG=41 (43.2)	AA=7 (7.4)	0.229	0.6313	1	GG=48 (35.3)	AG=70 (51.5)	AA=18 (13.2)	0.916	0.3385	1
CCL2 rs3917887	II=32 (33.3)	DI=47 (44.0)	DD=17 (20.7)	0.001	0.9745	1	II=26 (27.4)	DI=57 (54.7)	DD=17 (17.9)	2.229	0.1354	1	II=41 (31.2)	DI=62 (51.7)	DD=17 (14.1)	0.700	0.4028	1
IL8 rs4073	TT=45 (34.4)	TA=66 (50.4)	AA=14 (15.3)	1.960	0.1615	1	TT=35 (36.8)	TA=50 (52.6)	AA=10 (10.5)	1.629	0.2018	1	TT=60 (44.1)	TA=56 (41.2)	AA=20 (14.7)	1.319	0.2508	1
ELMO1 rs741301	AA=82 (36.1)	AG=108 (47.6)	GG=37 (16.3)	0.021	0.8848	1	AA=42 (44.2)	AG=44 (46.3)	GG=9 (9.5)	0.271	0.6027	1	AA=57 (41.9)	AG=59 (43.4)	GG=20 (14.7)	0.540	0.4624	1
CASE																		
CCR5 rs1799987	GG=47 (35.9)	AG=69 (52.7)	AA=15 (11.5)	1.895	0.1686	1	GG=25 (23.1)	AG=58 (53.7)	AA=25 (23.1)	0.5926	0.4414	1	GG=29 (33.7)	AG=44 (51.2)	AA=13 (15.1)	0.309	0.0788	1
CCL2 rs3917887	II=42 (32.1)	DI=57 (43.5)	DD=32 (24.4)	2.036	0.1536	1	II=20 (18.5)	DI=69 (63.9)	DD=19 (17.6)	8.340	0.0039*	1	II=33 (38.8)	DI=40 (47.1)	DD=12 (14.1)	0.001	0.9748	1
IL8 rs4073	TT=45 (34.4)	TA=66 (50.4)	AA=20 (15.3)	0.273	0.0601	1	TT=43 (39.8)	TA=57 (52.8)	AA=8 (7.4)	3.477	0.0622	1	TT=23 (26.7)	TA=51 (59.3)	AA=12 (14.0)	3.641	0.0564	1
ELMO1 rs741301	AA=50 (38.2)	AG=58 (44.3)	GG=23 (17.6)	0.741	0.3893	1	AA=40 (37.0)	AG=51 (47.2)	GG=17 (15.7)	0.012	0.9117	1	AA=33 (38.4)	AG=45 (52.3)	GG=8 (9.3)	1.761	0.1845	1

p>0.05 shows consistency with HWE. Genotype data are presented as a number of subjects (%).

TABLE 7: Association of polymorphism in T2DM with and without nephropathy.

| | | Malay | | | | Chinese | | | | Indian | | | |
| | | Multiplicative model | | Dominant Model Major vs. others (df=1) | Recessive Model Minor vs. others (df=1) | Multiplicative model | | Dominant Model Major vs. others (df=1) | Recessive Model Minor vs. others (df=1) | Multiplicative model | | Dominant Model Major vs. others (df=1) | Recessive Model Minor vs. others (df=1) |
		Genotype (df=2)	Allele (df=1)			Genotype (df=2)	Allele (df=1)			Genotype (df=2)	Allele (df=1)		
CCR5	χ^2	2.012	0.955	1.840	0.0001	19.012	18.645	15.304	9.478	0.172	0.131	0.058	0.155
rs1799987	p	0.3656	0.3284	0.1749	0.9920	7.4×10^{-5}*	1.6×10^{-5}*	9.2×10^{-5}*	0.0021*	0.9176	0.7174	0.8096	0.6938
CCL2	χ^2	1.545	6.735	0.041	1.478	2.460	0.740	2.259	0.003	0.511	0.399	0.468	0.0001
rs3917887	p	0.4618	0.0094	0.8395	0.2241	0.2923	0.3897	0.1328	0.9563	0.7745	0.5276	0.4939	0.9920
IL8	χ^2	1.321	0747	1.266	0.200	0.671	1.1384	0.189	0.608	7.865	3.073	0.024	0.173
rs4073	p	0.5165	0.3874	0.2605	0.6547	0.7150	0.2859	0.6638	0.4355	0.0196*	0.0796	0.8769	0.6775
ELMO1	χ^2	1.369	0.040	0.561	0.359	2.203	1.976	0.011	1.080	2.282	0.040	0.274	1.396
rs741301	p	0.5043	0.8414	0.4538	0.5491	0.332	0.1598	0.9165	0.2986	0.3195	0.8414	0.6007	0.2374

*P <0.05 indicates an association of polymorphisms and disease in a different mode of inheritance.

TABLE 8: Cochran-Armitage trend testing.

| | | Malay | | | | Chinese | | | | Indian | | |
		Multiplicative df=1	Additive df=1	Dominant df=1	Recessive df=1	Multiplicative df=1	Additive df=1	Dominant df=1	Recessive df=1	Multiplicative df=1	Additive df=1	Dominant df=1	Recessive df=1
CCR5 rs1799987	χ^2	-	-	-	-	19.012	53.983	9.478	15.303	-	-	-	-
	p					$7.4\times10^{-5*}$	$1.0\times10^{-15*}$	0.0021^*	0.00009^*				
IL8 rs4073	χ^2	-	-	-	-	-	-	-	-	3.073	7.769	0.024	6.793
	p					-	-	-	-	0.0796^*	0.0053^*	0.8768	0.0092^*

The mode of inheritance is best presented with the least **p-value***.

TABLE 9: The odd ratio of polymorphism in association with T2DM and nephropathy.

	Malay				Chinese				Indian			
	Allele	Genotype			Allele	Genotype			Allele	Genotype		
	Multiplicative Model a vs. A	Additive Model AA vs aa / Aa vs aa	Dominant Model AA vs. Aa + aa	Recessive Model AA + Aa vs. aa	Multiplicative Model a vs. A	Additive Model AA vs aa / Aa vs aa	Dominant Model AA vs. Aa + aa	Recessive Model AA + Aa vs. aa	Multiplicative Model a vs. A	Additive Model AA vs aa / Aa vs aa	Dominant Model AA vs. Aa + aa	Recessive Model AA + Aa vs. aa
CCR5 rs1799987 (G/A)	-	-	-	-	2.46 (1.62-3.71)	6.71 (2.55-17.68) 2.52 (0.99-6.39)	0.31 (0.12-0.56)	3.79 (1.56-9.22)	-	-	-	-
IL8 rs4073 (T/A)	-	-	-	-	-	-	-	-	1.42 (0.96-2.10)	1.57 (0.66-3.71) 0.66 (0.29-1.48)	0.46 (0.26-0.83)	0.94 (0.43-2.04)

ODD Ratio (OR), 95% CI. A: the major allele; a: the minor allele or increased risk.

SNPs as well as epigenetic differences such as methylation due to diet.

The proinflammatory chemokine IL8 is important in the regulation of the inflammatory response. The A allele in the regulatory region upregulates the gene expression and increases IL8 levels [20]. IL8 is detectable in the urine when the plasma level is high [35]. It has been earlier reported that rs4073 is associated with the development of DN among T2DM in the North and South Indian populations [13]. In the present study, among the Malaysians, only the Indians showed a significant association of rs4073 but not the Malays and Chinese. This may be due to the same ancestral origin of the Indians. The association was significantly observed in the

risk of T2DM nephropathy with weak association among the Malaysian Indians.

4.2. CCL2 rs3917887 D>I. CCL2 is upregulated and directly involved in the pathogenesis of DN [36]. This research examined the insertion/deletion of the CCL2 gene for association with DN but showed no significant association among Malaysians. The result disagrees with the finding of Ahluwalia et al. [13] among the North and South Indians. Though there was no significant association of rs3917887 with T2DM nephropathy among the Malays, Chinese, and Indians, the Indians had the highest percentage of deleted microsatellites carriers in the case subjects (63.1%) compared to the control (40.0%). The differences of deleted microsatellites carriers' frequency among the Malays in case (55.0%) and control (42.2%) were similar to the Chinese's case (49.5%) and control (45.3%).

4.3. ELMO1 rs741301 A>G. SNP rs741301 increases the production of ELMO1 which promotes phagocytosis, with excessive production of extracellular protein (type 1 collagen and fibronectin), and diminishes cell adherence [24, 28, 37], thereby causing the development and progression of T2DM glomerulosclerosis. The control sample of Shimazaki et al. [28] was not in HWE as noted by Sulgi et al. [38], due to systematic differential bias in genotyping or population stratification within their samples. The same association was also found among the Chinese [26] and African Americans [27]. In the present study, there was no significant statistical association of rs741301 with T2DM nephropathy when the genotype was initially tested by conventional Chi^2 test with df=2. Both control and case are in the HWE (p>0.05). Therefore, a null hypothesis was statistically accepted when tested with the other three models. Similar observation of no association was reported by [39]. Therefore SNP rs741301 is not a contributing risk factor to T2DM nephropathy among the Malaysian population.

5. Conclusion

An inflammatory process involving immune cells plays significant roles in the development and pathogenesis of DN among T2DM. Among the four genetic polymorphisms evaluated in the present study (CCL2-rs3917887, CCR5-rs1799987, ELMO1-rs74130, and IL8-rs4073), rs4073 (T>A) of IL8 is associated with the Indians only while rs1799987 (G>A) of CCR5 was associated with Chinese. The additive model was the best model for the mode of inheritance of all the genes. Nevertheless, the contribution of genetic variants differs across ethnic groups or background.

Acknowledgments

The authors express sincere appreciation to the Ministry of Health Malaysia for providing the research grant and the Department of Pathology, Blood Bank, and Medical Clinic of Hospital Tuanku Ja'afar for the technical support. The authors also acknowledge that the same patient cohort participated in another study for oxidative stress-related polymorphisms (in press article).

References

[1] I. A. Ahmed, M. A. Mikail, and M. Ibrahim, "Baccaurea angulata fruit juice ameliorates altered hematological and biochemical biomarkers in diet-induced hypercholesterolemic rabbits," *Nutrition Research*, vol. 42, pp. 31–42, 2017.

[2] M. Ibrahim, M. A. Mikail, I. A. Ahmed et al., "Comparison of the effects of three different Baccaurea angulata whole fruit juice doses on plasma, aorta and liver MDA levels, antioxidant enzymes and total antioxidant capacity," *European Journal of Nutrition*, pp. 1–12, 2017.

[3] M. Ibrahim, I. A. Ahmed, M. A. Mikail et al., "Baccaurea angulata fruit juice reduces atherosclerotic lesions in diet-induced Hypercholesterolemic rabbits," *Lipids in Health and Disease*, vol. 16, no. 1, article no. 134, 2017.

[4] U. A. A. Sharaf El Din, M. M. Salem, and D. O. AbdulAzim, "Diabetic nephropathy: Time to withhold development and progression - A review," *Journal of Advanced Research*, vol. 8, no. 4, pp. 363–373, 2017.

[5] M. Tziastoudi, I. Stefanidis, G. M. Hadjigeorgiou, K. Stravodimos, and E. Zintzaras, "A systematic review and meta-analysis of genetic association studies for the role of inflammation and the immune system in diabetic nephropathy," *Clinical Kidney Journal*, vol. 10, no. 3, pp. 293–300, 2017.

[6] A. Mima, "Inflammation and Oxidative Stress in Diabetic Nephropathy: New Insights on Its Inhibition as New Therapeutic Targets," *Journal of Diabetes Research*, vol. 2013, Article ID 248563, 8 pages, 2013.

[7] A. A. Elmarakby and J. C. Sullivan, "Relationship between oxidative stress and inflammatory cytokines in diabetic nephropathy," *Cardiovascular Therapeutics*, vol. 30, no. 1, pp. 49–59, 2012.

[8] A. P. Sanchez and K. Sharma, "Transcription factors in the pathogenesis of diabetic nephropathy," *Expert Reviews in Molecular Medicine*, vol. 11, article e13, 2009.

[9] A. I. Ahmed, N. A. Osman, M. NasrAllah, and M. M. Kamal, "The association between diabetic nephropathy and polymorphisms in PPAR947: Pro12Ala and CCR5948; 32 genes in type 2 diabetes," *The Egyptian Journal of Internal Medicine*, vol. 25, no. 1, pp. 10–14, 2013.

[10] N. Nazir, K. Siddiqui, S. Al-Qasim, and D. Al-Naqeb, "Meta-analysis of diabetic nephropathy associated genetic variants in inflammation and angiogenesis involved in different biochemical pathways," *BMC Medical Genetics*, vol. 15, no. 1, 2014.

[11] M. Zare-Bidaki, M. Karimi-Googheri, G. Hassanshahi, N. Zainodini, and M. Kazemi Arababadi, "The frequency of CCR5 promoter polymorphisms and CCR5 Δ 32 mutation in Iranian populations," *Iranian Journal of Basic Medical Sciences*, vol. 18, no. 4, pp. 312–316, 2015.

[12] Z. Zhang, X. Zhang, J. Dong et al., "Association of chemokine ligand 5/chemokine receptor 5 gene promoter polymorphisms with diabetic microvascular complications: A meta-analysis," *Journal of Diabetes Investigation*, vol. 7, no. 2, pp. 212–218, 2016.

[13] T. S. Ahluwalia, M. Khullar, M. Ahuja et al., "Common variants of inflammatory cytokine genes are associated with risk of nephropathy in type 2 diabetes among Asian Indians," *PLoS ONE*, vol. 4, no. 4, 2009.

[14] A. Mokubo, Y. Tanaka, K. Nakajima et al., "Chemotactic cytokine receptor 5 (CCR5) gene promoter polymorphism (59029A/G) is associated with diabetic nephropathy in Japanese patients with type 2 diabetes: A 10-year longitudinal study," *Diabetes Research and Clinical Practice*, vol. 73, no. 1, pp. 89–94, 2006.

[15] K. Nakajima, Y. Tanaka, T. Nomiyama et al., "Chemokine receptor genotype is associated with diabetic nephropathy in Japanese with type 2 diabetes," *Diabetes*, vol. 51, no. 1, pp. 238–242, 2002.

[16] P. Prasad, A. K. Tiwari, K. M. P. Kumar et al., "Association of TGFβ1, TNFα, CCR2 and CCR5 gene polymorphisms in type-2 diabetes and renal insufficiency among Asian Indians," *BMC Medical Genetics*, vol. 8, article 20, 2007.

[17] J. Li, Y. Peng, H. Liu, and Q. Wu, "The association between CCR5 Δ32 polymorphism and susceptibility to breast cancer," *Oncotarget*, vol. 8, no. 47, pp. 82796–82802, 2017.

[18] A. L. Mooyaart, E. J. J. Valk, L. A. Van Es et al., "Genetic associations in diabetic nephropathy: a meta-analysis," *Diabetologia*, vol. 54, no. 3, pp. 544–553, 2011.

[19] S. S. Jin, L. E. Soo, K. G. Tae et al., *Blockade of CCL2/CCR2 signalling ameliorates diabetic nephropathy in db/db mice*, vol. 28, 2013.

[20] D. E. Corina, E. A. Amalia, M. Neagu, and I. Nicolae, *Interleukin 8 And Diabetic Nephropathy*, vol. 7, 2015.

[21] R. Shanmuganathan, K. Ramanathan, G. Padmanabhan, and B. Vijayaraghavan, "Evaluation of Interleukin 8 gene polymorphism for predicting inflammation in Indian chronic kidney disease and peritoneal dialysis patients," *Alexandria Journal of Medicine*, vol. 53, no. 3, pp. 215–220, 2017.

[22] K. Tashiro, I. Koyanagi, and A. Saitoh, "Urinary levels of monocyte chemoattractant protein-1 (MCP-1) and interleukin-8 (IL-8), and renal injuries in patients with type 2 diabetic nephropathy," *Journal of Clinical Laboratory Analysis*, vol. 16, no. 1, pp. 1–4, 2002.

[23] T. C. Dakal, D. Kala, G. Dhiman, V. Yadav, A. Krokhotin, and N. V. Dokholyan, "Predicting the functional consequences of non-synonymous single nucleotide polymorphisms in IL8 gene," *Scientific Reports*, vol. 7, no. 1, article no. 6525, 2017.

[24] C. K. Hathaway, A. S. Chang, R. Grant et al., "High Elmo1 expression aggravates and low Elmo1 expression prevents diabetic nephropathy," *Proceedings of the National Acadamy of Sciences of the United States of America*, vol. 113, no. 8, pp. 2218–2222, 2016.

[25] K. R. Sharma, K. Heckler, S. J. Stoll et al., "ELMO1 protects renal structure and ultrafiltration in kidney development and under diabetic conditions," *Scientific Reports*, vol. 6, 2016.

[26] Y. H. Wu, Y. Wang, M. Chen et al., "Association of ELMO1 gene polymorphisms with diabetic nephropathy in Chinese population," *Journal of Endocrinological Investigation*, vol. 36, no. 5, pp. 298–302, 2013.

[27] T. S. Leak, P. S. Perlegas, S. G. Smith et al., "Variants in intron 13 of the ELMO1 gene are associated with diabetic nephropathy in African Americans," *Annals of Human Genetics*, vol. 73, no. 2, pp. 152–159, 2009.

[28] A. Shimazaki, Y. Kawamura, A. Kanazawa et al., "Genetic variations in the gene encoding ELMO1 are associated with susceptibility to diabetic nephropathy," *Diabetes*, vol. 54, no. 4, pp. 1171–1178, 2005.

[29] M. J. Yahya, P. Ismail, N. Nordin et al., "CNDP1, NOS3, and MnSOD Polymorphisms as Risk Factors for Diabetic Nephropathy among Type 2 Diabetic Patients in Malaysia," *Journal of Nutrition and Metabolism*, Article in Press.

[30] A. Joshi, E. B. Punke, M. Sedano et al., "CCR5 promoter activity correlates with HIV disease progression by regulating CCR5 cell surface expression and CD4 T cell apoptosis," *Scientific Reports*, vol. 7, no. 1, 2017.

[31] A. K. H. Lim, "Diabetic nephropathy—complications and treatment," *International Journal of Nephrology and Renovascular Disease*, vol. 7, pp. 361–381, 2014.

[32] S. Niu, Z. Bian, A. Tremblay et al., "Broad Infiltration of Macrophages Leads to a Proinflammatory State in Streptozotocin-Induced Hyperglycemic Mice," *The Journal of Immunology*, vol. 197, no. 8, pp. 3293–3301, 2016.

[33] K. A. Pettigrew, A. J. McKnight, C. C. Patterson, J. Kilner, D. M. Sadlier, and A. P. Maxwell, "Resequencing of the CCL5 and CCR5 genes and investigation of variants for association with diabetic nephropathy," *Journal of Human Genetics*, vol. 55, no. 4, pp. 248–251, 2010.

[34] D.-A. Trégouet, P.-H. Groop, S. McGinn et al., "G/T Substitution in Intron 1 of the UNC13B gene is associated with increased risk of nephropathy in patients with type 1 diabetes," *Diabetes*, vol. 57, no. 10, pp. 2843–2850, 2008.

[35] C. Nobles, E. R. Bertone-Johnson, A. G. Ronnenberg et al., "Correlation of urine and plasma cytokine levels among reproductive-aged women," *European Journal of Clinical Investigation*, vol. 45, no. 5, pp. 460–465, 2015.

[36] K. Shikata and H. Makino, "Microinflammation in the pathogenesis of diabetic nephropathy," *Journal of Diabetes Investigation*, vol. 4, no. 2, pp. 142–149, 2013.

[37] M. G. Pezzolesi and A. S. Krolewski, "The Genetic Risk of Kidney Disease in Type 2 Diabetes," *Medical Clinics of North America*, vol. 97, no. 1, pp. 91–107, 2013.

[38] K. Sulgi, H. E. Abboud, M. V. Pahl et al., "Examination of association with candidate genes for diabetic nephropathy in a Mexican American population," *Clinical Journal of the*

13

Hippocampal Growth Factor and Myokine Cathepsin B Expression following Aerobic and Resistance Training in 3xTg-AD Mice

Gabriel S. Pena, Hector G. Paez, Trevor K. Johnson, Jessica L. Halle, Joseph P. Carzoli, Nishant P. Visavadiya ⓘ, Michael C. Zourdos, Michael A. Whitehurst ⓘ, and Andy V. Khamoui ⓘ

Department of Exercise Science and Health Promotion, Florida Atlantic University, Boca Raton, Florida 33431, USA

Correspondence should be addressed to Michael A. Whitehurst; whitehur@fau.edu and Andy V. Khamoui; akhamoui@fau.edu

Academic Editor: Khoa Nguyen

Aerobic training (AT) can support brain health in Alzheimer's disease (AD); however, the role of resistance training (RT) in AD is not well established. Aside from direct effects on the brain, exercise may also regulate brain function through secretion of muscle-derived myokines. *Aims.* This study examined the effects of AT and RT on hippocampal BDNF and IGF-1 signaling, β-amyloid expression, and myokine cathepsin B in the triple transgenic (3xTg-AD) model of AD. 3xTg-AD mice were assigned to one of the following groups: sedentary (Tg), aerobic trained (Tg+AT, 9 wks treadmill running), or resistance trained (Tg+RT, 9 wks weighted ladder climbing) ($n = 10$/group). Rotarod latency and strength were assessed pre- and posttraining. Hippocampus and skeletal muscle were collected after training and analyzed by high-resolution respirometry, ELISA, and immunoblotting. Tg+RT showed greater grip strength than Tg and Tg+AT at posttraining ($p < 0.01$). Only Tg+AT improved rotarod peak latency ($p < 0.01$). Hippocampal IGF-1 concentration was ~15% greater in Tg+AT and Tg+RT compared to Tg ($p < 0.05$); however, downstream signals of p-IGF-1R, p-Akt, p-MAPK, and p-GSK3β were not altered. Cathepsin B, hippocampal p-CREB and BDNF, and hippocampal mitochondrial respiration were not affected by AT or RT. β-Amyloid was ~30% lower in Tg+RT compared to Tg ($p < 0.05$). This data suggests that regular resistance training reduces β-amyloid in the hippocampus concurrent with increased concentrations of IGF-1. Both types of training offered distinct benefits, either by improving physical function or by modifying signals in the hippocampus. Therefore, inclusion of both training modalities may address central defects, as well as peripheral comorbidities in AD.

1. Introduction

Alzheimer's disease (AD) is the result of genetic susceptibility and environmental influences that present as an incurable progressive brain disorder affecting memory, decision-making, and vital neurobiological systems [1, 2]. AD disproportionately affects the elderly, and in 2016, more than 5 million Americans suffered from AD, with an estimated healthcare cost nearing $236 billion [3].

Neurotrophins derive from a highly conserved family of proteins in mammals essential for maintenance, survival, and neurogenesis [4]. In neurodegenerative diseases such as AD, critically important growth factors including brain-derived neurotrophic factor (BDNF) and insulin-like growth factor 1 (IGF-1) are downregulated, suggesting a pivotal role in the pathophysiology of AD [5–7]. Importantly, neurotrophin expression is upregulated in response to the bioenergetic challenge of voluntary exercise [8, 9]. As such, exercise may offer an alternative or adjuvant therapy to pharmacological interventions aimed at promoting neurotrophin expression [2, 5, 10] and possibly mitigating AD-related neurodegeneration [5, 11–14].

It is well documented that aerobic training (AT) can support brain health by delaying age-related cognitive decline and changing the trajectory of neurodegenerative diseases [5, 11]. For example, murine models of AD show that AT can increase levels of hippocampal BDNF and its high-affinity receptor TrkB concurrent with improved learning behaviors [11]. Similarly, human longitudinal studies have shown that AT helps to maintain and increase grey and white matter, while improving memory and executive function in healthy individuals and older adults with AD [15, 16].

Although studied far less than AT, resistance exercise has been shown to activate anabolic and neurotrophic signals. For instance, acute resistance exercise increased BDNF expression in older adults [17]. However, others reported no change in BDNF expression following either acute loading or chronic resistance training (RT) [18, 19]. Despite the conflicting results, RT may still modulate neuroprotection via IGF-1 [20]. Serum IGF-1 has been shown to increase in response to acute resistance loading and chronic RT, and this may support hippocampal neurogenesis [21, 22], whereas blocking brain uptake of IGF-1 eliminates these effects [23]. Finally, IGF-1 has been linked to AD pathophysiology due to its role in β-amyloid plaque clearance through the upregulation of essential proteins [12, 21, 24]. How RT affects hippocampal expression of BDNF, IGF-1, and β-amyloid in AD is not well defined at present.

In addition to direct effects on the brain, exercise has been suggested to regulate brain function through secretion of skeletal muscle-derived factors termed myokines. Recently, myokine cathepsin B (CatB) has been identified as a peripheral secretory factor that may mediate exercise's effects on brain health [25]. These findings were confirmed in rodents when CatB knockout mice failed to enhance adult hippocampal neurogenesis and spatial memory function in response to voluntary wheel running, suggesting a central role of CatB in aerobic exercise-induced improvements in cognitive function. CatB may mediate improvements in cognitive function by increasing levels of BDNF and degrading Aβ [25–28].

Resistance training (RT), which generates intermittent high muscular tension rather than sustained low muscular tension characteristic of AT, has been shown to increase CatB expression in healthy muscle [29]. To our knowledge, the relationship between CatB, RT, and AD has not been investigated. Therefore, the purpose of this study was to examine the effects of AT and RT on hippocampal BDNF and IGF-1 signaling, expression of β-amyloid, and myokine cathepsin B. *In situ* mitochondrial respiration and motor function were also measured as additional indices to assess the efficacy of exercise training.

2. Methods

2.1. Animals and Design. Three-month-old 3xTg-AD ($N = 30$) females were purchased from The Jackson Laboratory (Bar Harbor, ME). 3xTg-AD mice show AD-related pathology such as intracellular Aβ deposition and reduced performance in behavioral tests as early as 3 months of age [30, 31]. Continued intracellular Aβ accumulation and cognitive deficits occur at 6 months [30, 31], followed by extracellular Aβ deposits at ≥12 months [32]. Therefore, exercise training occurred during anticipated Aβ accumulation, and prior to the onset of Aβ plaque, similar to previous work on exercise and AD mice [33]. Mice were provided a three-day acclimation and not handled during this period. After acclimation, 3xTg-AD mice were randomly assigned to one

of the following groups: sedentary (Tg, $n = 10$), aerobic training (Tg+AT, $n = 10$), or resistance training (Tg+RT, $n = 10$). All mice underwent pretraining assessments to obtain baseline values of physical function. Mice assigned to training groups then underwent a familiarization period for one week where they were introduced to their respective exercises. After familiarization, Tg+AT and Tg+RT performed their respective training for 9 weeks. At posttraining, the same assessments were repeated, followed by euthanasia and tissue collection. Mice were group housed, provided food and water *ad libitum*, and maintained on a 12:12 hr light:dark cycle. All experimental procedures were conducted with prior approval obtained from the Institutional Animal Care and Use Committee at Florida Atlantic University (protocol # A17-08).

2.2. Aerobic Training. Aerobic training was conducted on a 5-lane mouse treadmill (Harvard Apparatus). Mice went through a one-week familiarization period in which they ran at a speed of 15 m/min for 10 minutes daily on three nonconsecutive days, with the duration increased to 15 minutes by the third day of training. After the familiarization period, mice trained at a frequency of 5 days per week on the first week of training, gradually increasing from 30 minutes on day 1 to 60 minutes by day 5. Afterwards, the speed and frequency of training remained constant, but the length of training session was increased to 75 minutes on week 5 and 90 minutes on week 7. Only gentle reinforcement was used in which the researcher lightly touched the hips.

2.3. Resistance Training. Weighted ladder climbing was used to simulate RT. The ladder had a height of 100 cm and 1.5 cm grids and was placed at an 85-degree angle to the ground. A one-week familiarization period was conducted in which mice climbed the ladder unweighted for 4 repetitions with one-minute rest between repetitions. After familiarization, mice underwent 3 training sessions per week on nonconsecutive days for 9 weeks. The initial resistance was 50% of body mass for 16 total repetitions per training session with one minute of rest between repetitions. Load was increased by 12.5% of body mass weekly. After reaching 100% of body mass, total repetitions performed per session were decreased to 10. No positive or negative stimulus was used as incentive for climbing.

2.4. Grip Strength. The mice were allowed to grip the device with their forelimbs while restrained at the base of the tail. The animal was then pulled back by its tail until it released its grip. The force generated while the animal attempted to maintain its grip was quantified in grams by a strain gauge (Harvard Apparatus). The average force of four trials was calculated for each mouse.

2.5. Rotarod. Mice were placed on a rotating tube with an initial speed of 4 rotations per minute (rpm). Once all mice were positioned on the rod (5 mice), the assessment began. The speed of the rotarod increased at a rate of 1 rpm every 8 seconds (up to 40 rpm maximum). When an animal fell off the rotating tube, the timer was deactivated and the time and rpm recorded. After 500 seconds, if the mouse was still active the test was terminated. A total of 4 trials were given with 15 minutes of recovery between trials. The maximum time spent on the rotarod (i.e., peak latency) was used for analysis.

2.6. Tissue Collection. Tissue was collected 48 hours after the final training bout to control for acute effects of exercise. Mice were euthanized by ketamine/xylazine overdose delivered i.p. at 300/30 mg/kg. Skeletal muscle, brain, and vital organs were carefully isolated and removed. The right half of the hippocampus was immediately placed into preservation buffer (BIOPS: 2.77 mM CaK_2EGTA, 7.23 mM K_2EGTA, 5.77 mM Na_2ATP, 6.56 mM $MgCl_2 \cdot 6H_2O$, 20 mM taurine, 15 mM Na_2PCr, 20 mM imidazole, 0.5 mM DTT, and 50 mM MES hydrate) and stored on ice for mitochondrial respiration experiments. The remaining hippocampus was then homogenized, protein extracted, and stored at -80°C. Remaining tissues were snap frozen and stored at -80°C.

2.7. High-Resolution Respirometry. To prepare the hippocampus, duplicate samples ~6 mg each were gently blotted dry on filter paper and weighed before being placed into the respirometer chambers. Chemical permeabilization was performed by addition of saponin directly into the respirometer chambers in accordance with Herbst and Holloway [34]. Oxygen flux per tissue mass ($pmol \cdot s^{-1} \cdot mg^{-1}$) was recorded in real time at 37°C in the oxygen concentration range of 550-350 nmol/ml using high-resolution respirometry (Oxygraph-2 k, Oroboros Instruments, Innsbruck, AT). *In situ* respiration was assessed using a protocol adapted from Burtscher et al. [35].

2.8. Respiration Data Analysis. Oxygen flux for the different respiratory states were corrected by subtracting the residual oxygen consumption. Fluxes from each duplicate measurement were averaged for statistical analysis. To determine flux control ratios, which express respiratory control independent of mitochondrial content, tissue mass-specific oxygen fluxes from the SUIT protocol were divided by maximal electron transfer system capacity as the reference state [36]. The respiratory control ratio (RCR), an index of coupling efficiency of the OXPHOS system, was calculated in the complex I linked state [35].

2.9. ELISA. Hippocampal tissue was homogenized in NP-40 lysis buffer containing protease and phosphatase inhibitors. IGF-1 concentration was measured in the hippocampal homogenate using IGF-1 mouse/rat ELISA kit per manufacturer guidelines (cat# MG100, R&D Systems, Minneapolis, MN).

2.10. Western Blotting. Protein was isolated from the hippocampus using the NP-40 lysis buffer containing a protease/phosphatase inhibitor cocktail (Halt, Thermo Fisher Scientific, cat# 78425 and 78428). For the gastrocnemius muscle, protein was extracted using an ice-cold lysis buffer (150 mM NaCl, 10 mM HEPES, 1 mM EGTA, 0.1 mM $MgCl_2$, and 1% Triton X-100, pH 7.4) containing a freshly made protease/phosphatase inhibitor cocktail (0.5x Sigma-Aldrich P2714, 100 μM PMSF, 0.1 μM okadaic acid, and 1 mM orthovanadate). Protein concentration was determined via Pierce BCA protein assay kit (Thermo Fisher Scientific,

Waltham, MA). Equal amounts of protein (35 μg/lane) were loaded and separated by SDS-PAGE using 4–20% Criterion™ TGX™ Precast Gels (cat# 5671095, Bio-Rad, Hercules, CA) and electrotransferred to PVDF membranes. The membranes were blocked in 6% nonfat dry milk or 5% bovine serum albumin (BSA: in case of phospho-specific antibody) for one hour at room temperature, and then incubated at 4°C overnight with the primary antibody of interest. The primary antibodies used in this study included BDNF (cat# ab108319) and Cathepsin B (Cat# ab58802) from Abcam Inc., Cambridge, MA; IGF-1R (cat# 05-656) and p-IGF-1R (cat# ABE332) from Millipore, Temecula, CA; β-Amyloid (cat# sc-28365), CREB (cat# sc-271), and p-CREB (cat# sc-81486) from Santa Cruz Biotechnology, Santa Cruz, CA; and Akt (cat# 4691), p-Akt, (cat# 4060), GSK3β (cat# 9315), p-GSK3β (cat# 9322), MAPK 42/44 (cat# 9102), p-MAPK 42/44 (cat# 9101), α-tubulin (cat# 3873), and β-actin (cat# 3700) from Cell Signaling Technology, Danvers, MA. For secondary antibodies, we used peroxidase-conjugated horse anti-mouse IgG (cat#7076) and goat anti-rabbit IgG (cat# 7074) from Cell Signaling Technology, Danvers, MA. The immunoreactive protein reaction was revealed using the SuperSignal™ West Pico PLUS Chemiluminescent Substrate (cat# PI34580, Thermo Fisher Scientific). The reactive bands were detected by a ChemiDoc™ XRS+ imaging system (Bio-Rad), and density was measured using the ImageJ software (NIH).

2.11. Statistical Analysis. All data are reported as mean ± SE. A 3 (groups) × 2 (timepoints) factorial ANOVA was used to evaluate differences in physical function (i.e., grip strength and rotarod). Differences in protein expression were determined by one-way ANOVA. Muscle wet mass was analyzed by an unpaired t-test. Follow-up testing was conducted with Tukey's HSD to localize significant interaction or main effects. Statistical significance was set at $p \le 0.05$.

3. Results

3.1. Phenotype of Aerobic- and Resistance-Trained 3xTg-AD Mice. No differences were observed for body weight ($p > 0.05$) (Figure 1(a)). Gastrocnemius mass was greater in Tg+RT compared to Tg ($p < 0.05$) (Figure 1(b)), consistent with resistance training-induced muscle hypertrophy. Gastrocnemius mass related linearly with grip strength ($r = 0.59$, $R^2 = 0.35$, $p < 0.05$) (Figure 1(c)). Peak latency and revolutions were not different between groups at pretraining ($p > 0.05$) (Figures 1(d)–1(e)). Only Tg+AT significantly increased peak latency (+88%) and revolutions (+66%) from pre- to posttraining ($p < 0.01$) (Figures 1(d)–1(e)). Average latency was not different between groups at pretraining ($p < 0.05$) (Figure 1(f)). However, average latency increased ($p < 0.05$) from pre- to posttraining in Tg+AT (+68%, $p < 0.05$) and Tg+RT (+78%, $p < 0.01$) (Figure 1(g)). There were no differences in strength at pretraining ($p > 0.05$) (Figure 1(g)). All groups increased strength from pre- to posttraining; however, Tg+RT had significantly greater strength than Tg and Tg+AT at posttraining (+13%

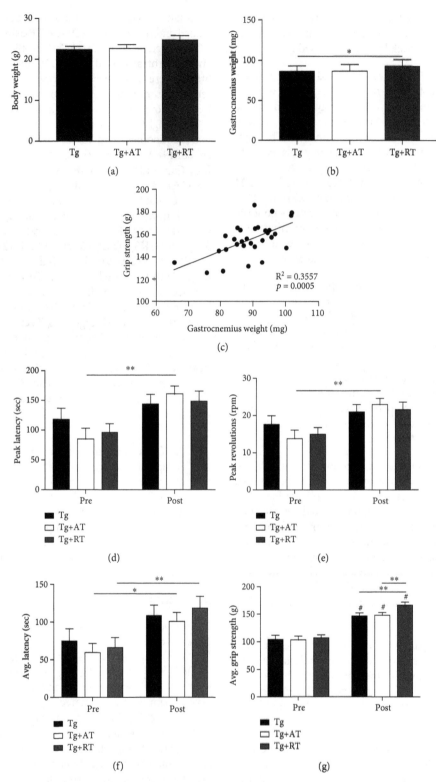

FIGURE 1: Phenotype of aerobic- and resistance-trained 3xTg-AD mice. Three-month-old 3xTg-AD mice were assigned to one of the following groups: nonexercised (Tg), aerobic trained (Tg+AT), or resistance trained (Tg+RT) ($n = 10$/group). Training was performed for 9 weeks, followed by tissue collection. Physical function was evaluated longitudinally, at pre- and posttraining. (a) Final body weight measured at the end of the experiment. (b) Wet weight of the gastrocnemius. (c) Association of gastrocnemius weight with grip strength. (d) Peak latency (time to fall in seconds) on the rotarod test. (e) Peak revolutions per minute (RPM) achieved on the rotarod test. (f) Average latency (time to fall in seconds) averaged across four trials on the rotarod. (g) Average forelimb grip strength across four trials. Data presented as mean ± SE. Differences determined by one-way ANOVA. $^*p < 0.05$ and $^{**}p < 0.01$.

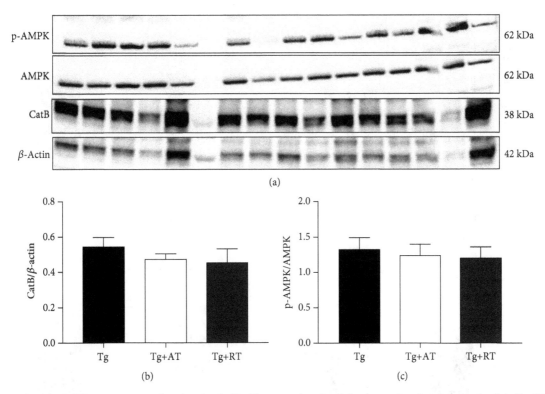

FIGURE 2: Unaltered AMPK activation and cathepsin B (CatB) expression in skeletal muscle of exercise-trained 3xTg-AD mice. (a) Immunoblots for CatB, p-AMPK, and AMPK in skeletal muscle homogenate. (b) CatB expression normalized to β-actin. (c) p-AMPK expression normalized to total AMPK. Data presented as mean ± SE. Tissues assayed from the nonexercised group (Tg), the aerobic-trained group (Tg+AT), or the resistance-trained group (Tg+RT) ($n = 10$/group). Differences determined by one-way ANOVA.

vs. both groups, $p < 0.01$) (Figure 1(g)), indicating greater improvement with resistance training.

3.2. Myokine Cathepsin B Response to Aerobic and Resistance Training in 3xTg-AD Mice. Myokine cathepsin B is a skeletal muscle-secreted factor shown to be important for exercise-induced improvement in cognitive function. Cathepsin B expression in skeletal muscle is regulated in part by the activity of AMPK. No group differences were detected for p-AMPK or mature cathepsin B in skeletal muscle ($p > 0.05$) (Figures 2(a)-2(c)).

3.3. Effect of Aerobic and Resistance Training on Hippocampal Mitochondrial Respiration. Mitochondrial dysfunction is associated with AD, and exercise may alter mitochondrial function. We therefore determined *in situ* mitochondrial respiration in saponin-permeabilized hippocampus by high-resolution respirometry. Tissue mass-specific fluxes were not different between groups ($p > 0.05$) (Figure 3(a)), suggesting no effect of training on hippocampal mitochondrial function per unit of tissue mass. RCR in the complex I-supported state, an index of OXPHOS coupling efficiency, was not different between groups ($p > 0.05$) (Figure 3(b)). Flux control ratios, which express respiratory control independent of mitochondrial mass, were determined as indicators of mitochondrial quality. No differences were observed in any of the flux control ratios calculated ($p > 0.05$) (Figures 3(c)-3(f)), implying no effect of training on hippocampal mitochondrial quality.

3.4. Hippocampal Neurotrophin and β-Amyloid Response to Aerobic and Resistance Training in 3xTg-AD Mice. There were no differences in amyloid precursor protein expression ($p > 0.05$) (Figures 4(a) and 4(c)); however, β-amyloid was 32% lower in Tg+RT vs. Tg ($p < 0.05$) (Figures 4(b) and 4(c)). There were no differences in hippocampal p-CREB or BDNF ($p > 0.05$) (Figures 4(d)-4(f)). IGF-1 concentration in the hippocampus was significantly greater in Tg+AT (+15%) and Tg+RT (+13%) compared to Tg ($p < 0.05$) (Figure 5(b)). No differences were observed in the expression of p-IGF-1R, p-Akt, p-GSK3β, or p-MAPK ($p > 0.05$) (Figures 5(a) and 5(c)-5(g)).

4. Discussion

While the anabolic nature and associated benefits of RT are well established in the general population, very little is known regarding the effects of RT in AD. This study adds to the literature by contributing to a dialogue aimed at describing the role of RT in leveraging an adaptive brain as well as a peripheral response to bioenergetic demands. Moreover, as a clinical exercise modality, RT is unique in that it has the added benefit of being able to promote physical function and combat muscle wasting, comorbidities in AD.

We were somewhat surprised to find that RT significantly improved average latency on the rotarod. Perhaps the inherent instability of the near vertical weighted ladder climb triggered postural control mechanisms (e.g., vestibular and proprioception) as part of an adaptive motor response that

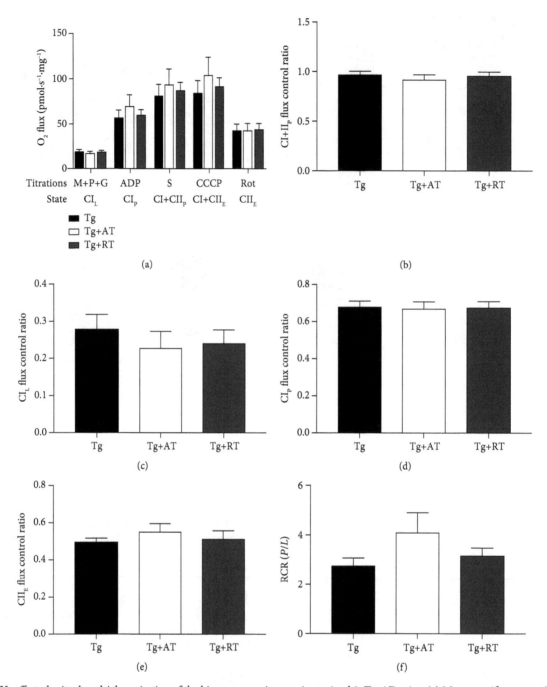

FIGURE 3: Unaffected mitochondrial respiration of the hippocampus in exercise-trained 3xTg-AD mice. (a) Mass-specific oxygen (O_2) flux of the hippocampus determined *in situ* by a substrate-uncoupler-inhibitor titration protocol, including complex I-supported LEAK (CI_L) through addition of malate, pyruvate, and glutamate (M+P+G); complex I-supported oxidative phosphorylation (OXPHOS) (CI_P) by addition of adenosine diphosphate (ADP); complex I+II-supported OXPHOS ($CI+II_P$) by addition of succinate (S); maximal electron transfer system (ETS) capacity ($CI+II_E$) by stepwise titration of carbonyl cyanide m-chlorophenyl hydrazine (CCCP); and complex II ETS (CII_E) by addition of rotenone (Rot). (b) Respiratory control ratio (RCR) determined by dividing CI_P by CI_L. (c–f) Flux control ratios were calculated by normalizing mass-specific fluxes to maximal electron transfer system capacity ($CI+II_E$). Shown are flux control ratios for (c) CI_L, (d) CI_P, (e) $CI+II_P$, and (f) CII_E. Data presented as mean ± SE. Tissues assayed from the nonexercised group (Tg), the aerobic-trained group (Tg+AT), or the resistance-trained group (Tg+RT) (n = 10/group). Differences determined by one-way ANOVA.

included better dynamic balance. In addition, RT was superior to AT in terms of strength and muscle mass. Finally, and consistent with other studies, the low force protracted exercise bouts, hallmarks of AT and our protocol, translated to greater endurance and speed of movement (i.e., peak latency and RPM) when compared to RT.

While the current investigation did not observe a significant increase in the expression of BDNF within the

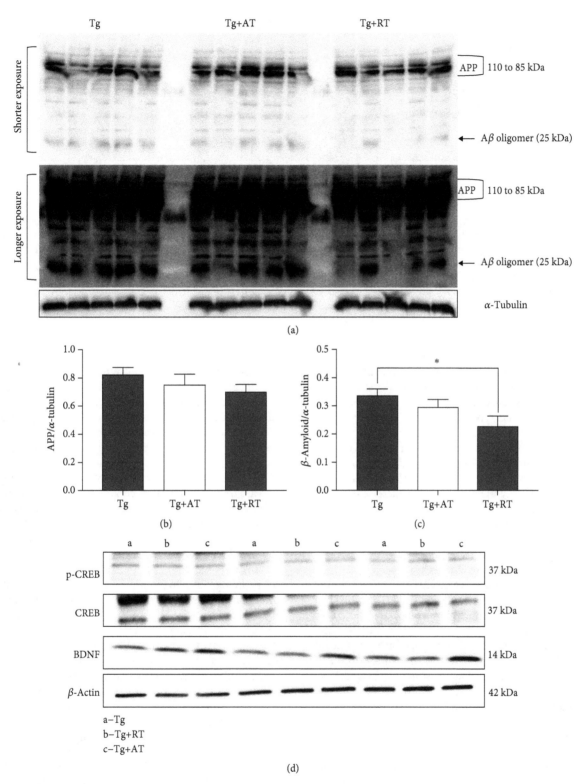

(a)

(b)

(c)

(d)

a–Tg
b–Tg+RT
c–Tg+AT

FIGURE 4: Continued.

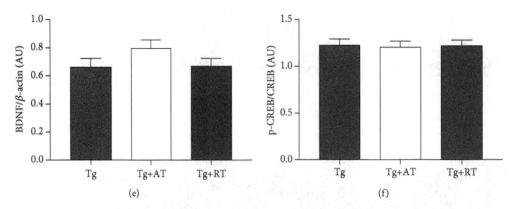

FIGURE 4: Reduced β-amyloid but unaltered CREB and BDNF in resistance-trained 3xTg-AD mice. (a) Representative immunoblots for amyloid precursor protein (APP) and β-amyloid probed in hippocampal homogenate. The shorter and longer exposure clearly revealed APP (110 to 85 kDa) and Aβ oligomer (25 kDa) bands, respectively. (b) Amyloid precursor protein (APP) normalized to tubulin. (c) β-Amyloid expression normalized to tubulin. (d) Representative immunoblots for CREB and BDNF expression. (e) p-CREB normalized to total CREB. (f) BDNF expression normalized to β-actin. Data presented as mean ± SE. Tissues assayed from the nonexercised group (Tg), the aerobic-trained group (Tg+AT), or the resistance-trained group (Tg+RT) ($n = 10$/group). Differences determined by one-way ANOVA. $^{*}p < 0.05$ and $^{**}p < 0.01$.

hippocampus, previous literature suggests that gender differences may aid in the understanding of our results. Following a five-month aerobic exercise intervention, Venezia et al. saw BDNF gene expression to be significantly increased in both female and male wild-type mice, but BDNF protein to be only significantly higher in males and largely unchanged in females [37]. Along these lines, we note that BDNF protein was slightly greater in Tg+AT compared to Tg, and while not as robust as in mixed cohorts, is consistent with existing literature highlighting the use of aerobic exercise to upregulate this neurotrophin.

We note that both exercised groups increased hippocampal IGF-1 without changes in downstream signaling. One possible explanation is that our increased hippocampal IGF-1 is merely reflective of elevated circulating IGF-1. Previous work has shown that the concentration of hippocampal IGF-1 is highly related to circulating levels of IGF-1 [38]. Although we did not measure circulating IGF-1 because we did not collect blood, an increased circulating IGF-1 can be neuroprotective absent direct manipulation of the cellular cascades that regulate neuronal health. Outside of direct modulation of important cellular cascades such as those targeted in the present work, circulating IGF-1 levels have been implicated in the clearance of β-amyloid. In animal models, higher circulating IGF-1 levels have been associated with increased mobilization of clearing proteins—such as albumin and transthyretin—along with lower amyloid deposition and increased release of intracellular amyloid that may ultimately translate to decreased amyloid burden [39, 40]. Thus, exercise modulation of hippocampal and circulating IGF-1 may play other important ancillary roles in preventing accretion of β-amyloid oligomers.

Known to cross the blood-brain barrier from peripheral secretion in muscles during AT in humans, rhesus monkeys, and mice, cathepsin B (CatB) represents a potential therapeutic mechanism to combat AD. Specifically, CatB is a lysosomal cysteine protease that can lower AB levels [25].

However, in the present study, AT did not increase the expression of CatB in skeletal muscle. This may have been due to the use of involuntary treadmill training as our AT exercise. In a quintessential study [25], CatB expression in mouse muscle increased in response to voluntary wheel running, with distance ran reaching an average of over 19,000 meters per week. In the present study, animals ran an average distance of 4,500 meters in the first four weeks of training and 6,750 meters by the last week of training. Attempts to increase training volume on either exercise modality resulted in failure to complete the training session. Thus, it is possible that the total training volume in Tg+AT and Tg+RT may not have been sufficient to induce AMPK activation and CatB peripherally in skeletal muscle.

It is well known that mitochondrial dysfunction triggers AD pathology [39]. In the present study, we carried out mitochondrial function experiments using the hippocampus of 3xTg-AD mice following AT and RT. Our results indicated no significant alternations in any of the bioenergetics parameters. It is possible that the AT and RT protocols were not sufficient to stimulate improvements in hippocampal respiration, and may require greater intensity and/or prolonged training duration to see improvement in mitochondrial function in this mouse model. Alternatively, exercise-dependent mitochondrial adaptations may have been absent due to interference arising from the underlying disease.

A novel finding in our study was a reduction in hippocampal β-amyloid load in RT. Importantly, this finding closely parallels one of only several reports that β-amyloid levels were regulated by RT in AD. For example, Özbeyli et al. found a significant increase in hippocampal IGF-1 expression in conjunction with a decrease in β-amyloid following six weeks of ladder climbing in an AD rodent model [40]. Perhaps the reduction in β-amyloid load in RT represents a complementary adaptive response driven by the high force output and intermittent periods of rest. In support of this explanation, the low force and sustained nature of AT

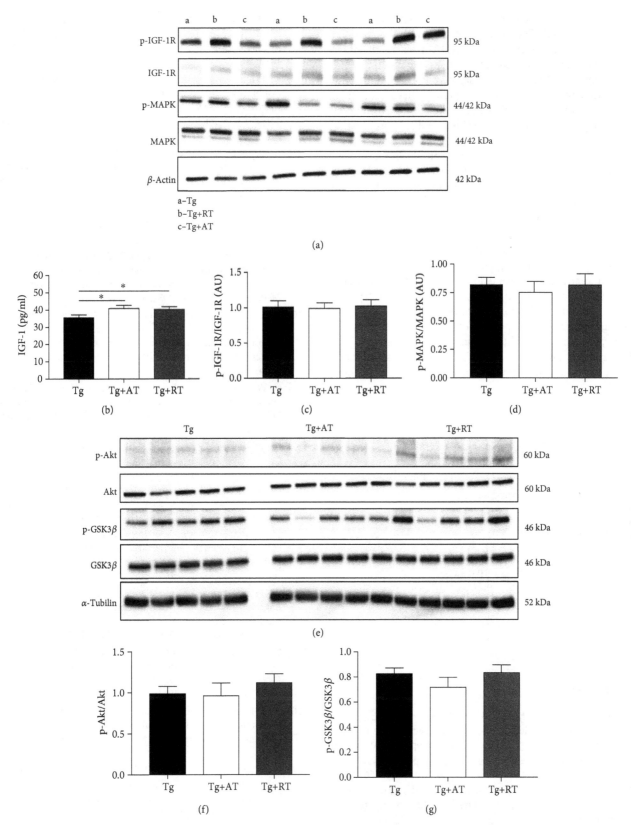

FIGURE 5: IGF-1 expression and signaling in the hippocampus of exercise-trained 3xTg-AD mice. (a) Representative immunoblots for IGF-1R and MAPK. (b) IGF-1 concentration in hippocampal homogenate measured by ELISA. (c) p-IGF-1R normalized to total IGF-1R. (d) p-MAPK normalized to MAPK. (e) Representative immunoblots for Akt and GSK3β. (f) p-Akt normalized to Akt. (g) p-GSK3β normalized to total GSK3β. Data presented as mean ± SE. Tissues assayed from the nonexercised group (Tg), the aerobic-trained group (Tg+AT), or the resistance-trained group (Tg+RT) ($n = 10$/group). Differences determined by one-way ANOVA. $^*p < 0.05$ and $^{**}p < 0.01$.

resulted in an increase in IGF-1 without a significant reduction in β-amyloid. Furthermore, it is conceivable that RT enhanced the expression of proteins, particularly those regulating β-amyloid clearance such as proteolytic degradation enzymes (e.g., α-secretase, neprilysin, and insulindegrading enzyme), molecular chaperones (e.g., heat shock protein 70), and blood-brain barrier efflux proteins; however, these suggestions remain unverified and require further investigation. Thus, this finding suggests that regular RT may promote clearance of β-amyloid from the brain, a major pathological hallmark of AD. Finally, given the lower levels of β-amyloid associated with RT, a more comprehensive therapeutic strategy may be to combine RT and AT in an effort to maximize patient outcomes.

In summary, we found that β-amyloid burden was relieved by RT. This finding suggests that RT may be prophylactic in attenuating unwanted age-related and/or neurodegenerative changes in critical neural tissue/circuitry that underlie learning and memory, and ultimately vital biological systems. Given the propensity of AD to develop in the elderly, RT should be included as part of an exercise intervention prior to and during AD in order to increase strength, muscle mass, and function/independence, all comorbidities of AD.

Authors' Contributions

Gabriel S. Pena and Hector G. Paez contributed equally.

Acknowledgments

We extend our sincere thanks to Ms. Peggy Donnelly and Ms. Denise Merrill for administrative support.

References

[1] A. Kumar, A. Singh, and Ekavali, "A review on Alzheimer's disease pathophysiology and its management: an update," *Pharmacological Reports*, vol. 67, no. 2, pp. 195–203, 2015.

[2] D. J. Selkoe, "Alzheimer's disease: genes, proteins, and therapy," *Physiological Reviews*, vol. 81, no. 2, pp. 741–766, 2001.

[3] Alzheimer's Association, "Alzheimer's & dementia," *Alzheimer's Disease Facts and Figures*, vol. 12, no. 4, pp. 459–509, 2016.

[4] L. Olson and C. Humpel, "Growth factors and cytokines/chemokines as surrogate biomarkers in cerebrospinal fluid and blood for diagnosing Alzheimer's disease and mild cognitive impairment," *Experimental Gerontology*, vol. 45, no. 1, pp. 41–46, 2010.

[5] C. Phillips, M. A. Baktir, D. Das, B. Lin, and A. Salehi, "The link between physical activity and cognitive dysfunction in Alzheimer disease," *Physical Therapy*, vol. 95, no. 7, pp. 1046–1060, 2015.

[6] K. Talbot, H. Y. Wang, H. Kazi et al., "Demonstrated brain insulin resistance in Alzheimer's disease patients is associated with IGF-1 resistance, IRS-1 dysregulation, and cognitive decline," *The Journal of Clinical Investigation*, vol. 122, no. 4, pp. 1316–1338, 2012.

[7] B. Connor, D. Young, Q. Yan, R. L. M. Faull, B. Synek, and M. Dragunow, "Brain-derived neurotrophic factor is reduced in Alzheimer's disease," *Molecular Brain Research*, vol. 49, no. 1-2, pp. 71–81, 1997.

[8] M. P. Mattson, "Evolutionary aspects of human exercise—born to run purposefully," *Ageing Research Reviews*, vol. 11, no. 3, pp. 347–352, 2012.

[9] S. M. Raefsky and M. P. Mattson, "Adaptive responses of neuronal mitochondria to bioenergetic challenges: roles in neuroplasticity and disease resistance," *Free Radical Biology and Medicine*, vol. 102, pp. 203–216, 2017.

[10] H. S. Um, E. B. Kang, Y. H. Leem et al., "Exercise training acts as a therapeutic strategy for reduction of the pathogenic phenotypes for Alzheimer's disease in an NSE/APPsw-transgenic model," *International Journal of Molecular Medicine*, vol. 22, no. 4, pp. 529–539, 2008.

[11] C. W. Cotman, N. C. Berchtold, and L.-A. Christie, "Exercise builds brain health: key roles of growth factor cascades and inflammation," *Trends in Neurosciences*, vol. 30, no. 9, pp. 464–472, 2007.

[12] F. G. de Melo Coelho, S. Gobbi, C. A. A. Andreatto, D. I. Corazza, R. V. Pedroso, and R. F. Santos-Galduróz, "Physical exercise modulates peripheral levels of brain-derived neurotrophic factor (BDNF): a systematic review of experimental studies in the elderly," *Archives of Gerontology and Geriatrics*, vol. 56, no. 1, pp. 10–15, 2013.

[13] M. Garuffi, J. L. Costa, S. S. Hernández et al., "Effects of resistance training on the performance of activities of daily living in patients with Alzheimer's disease," *Geriatrics & Gerontology International*, vol. 13, no. 2, pp. 322–328, 2013.

[14] F. Gómez-Pinilla, Z. Ying, R. R. Roy, R. Molteni, and V. R. Edgerton, "Voluntary exercise induces a BDNF-mediated mechanism that promotes neuroplasticity," *Journal of Neurophysiology*, vol. 88, no. 5, pp. 2187–2195, 2002.

[15] K. I. Erickson, M. W. Voss, R. S. Prakash et al., "Exercise training increases size of hippocampus and improves memory," *Proceedings of the National Academy of Sciences*, vol. 108, no. 7, pp. 3017–3022, 2011.

[16] K. I. Erickson, R. S. Prakash, M. W. Voss et al., "Aerobic fitness is associated with hippocampal volume in elderly humans," *Hippocampus*, vol. 19, no. 10, pp. 1030–1039, 2009.

[17] J. F. Yarrow, L. J. White, S. McCoy, and S. E. Borst, "Training augments resistance exercise induced elevation of circulating brain derived neurotrophic factor (BDNF)," *Neuroscience Letters*, vol. 479, no. 2, pp. 161–165, 2010.

[18] P. R. Correia, A. Pansani, F. Machado et al., "Acute strength exercise and the involvement of small or large muscle mass on plasma brain-derived neurotrophic factor levels," *Clinics*, vol. 65, no. 11, pp. 1123–1126, 2010.

[19] M. Goekint, K. de Pauw, B. Roelands et al., "Strength training does not influence serum brain-derived neurotrophic factor,"

European Journal of Applied Physiology, vol. 110, no. 2, pp. 285–293, 2010.

[20] T. Liu-Ambrose and M. G. Donaldson, "Exercise and cognition in older adults: is there a role for resistance training programmes?," *British Journal of Sports Medicine*, vol. 43, no. 1, pp. 25–27, 2009.

[21] E. Carro, J. L. Trejo, T. Gomez-Isla, D. LeRoith, and I. Torres-Aleman, "Serum insulin-like growth factor I regulates brain amyloid-β levels," *Nature Medicine*, vol. 8, no. 12, pp. 1390–1397, 2002.

[22] R. C. Cassilhas, V. D. Wilson, A. L. Souza et al., "The impact of resistance exercise on the cognitive function of the elderly," *Medicine and Science in Sports and Exercise*, vol. 39, no. 8, pp. 1401–1407, 2007.

[23] R. Cassilhas, K. S. Lee, J. Fernandes et al., "Spatial memory is improved by aerobic and resistance exercise through divergent molecular mechanisms," *Neuroscience*, vol. 202, pp. 309–317, 2012.

[24] A. Angelini, C. Bendini, F. Neviani et al., "Insulin-like growth factor-1 (IGF-1): relation with cognitive functioning and neuroimaging marker of brain damage in a sample of hypertensive elderly subjects," *Archives of Gerontology and Geriatrics*, vol. 49, pp. 5–12, 2009.

[25] H. Y. Moon, A. Becke, D. Berron et al., "Running-induced systemic cathepsin B secretion is associated with memory function," *Cell Metabolism*, vol. 24, no. 2, pp. 332–340, 2016.

[26] W. A. Suzuki, "How body affects brain," *Cell Metabolism*, vol. 24, no. 2, pp. 192-193, 2016.

[27] B. Sun, Y. Zhou, B. Halabisky et al., "Cystatin C-cathepsin B axis regulates amyloid beta levels and associated neuronal deficits in an animal model of Alzheimer's disease," *Neuron*, vol. 60, no. 2, pp. 247–257, 2008.

[28] S. Mueller-Steiner, Y. Zhou, H. Arai et al., "Antiamyloidogenic and neuroprotective functions of cathepsin B: implications for Alzheimer's disease," *Neuron*, vol. 51, no. 6, pp. 703–714, 2006.

[29] F. Norheim, T. Raastad, B. Thiede, A. C. Rustan, C. A. Drevon, and F. Haugen, "Proteomic identification of secreted proteins from human skeletal muscle cells and expression in response to strength training," *American Journal of Physiology Endocrinology and Metabolism*, vol. 301, no. 5, pp. E1013–E1021, 2011.

[30] M. C. Janelsins, M. A. Mastrangelo, S. Oddo, F. M. LaFerla, H. J. Federoff, and W. J. Bowers, "Early correlation of microglial activation with enhanced tumor necrosis factor-alpha and monocyte chemoattractant protein-1 expression specifically within the entorhinal cortex of triple transgenic Alzheimer's disease mice," *Journal of Neuroinflammation*, vol. 2, no. 1, p. 23, 2005.

[31] S. J. Webster, A. D. Bachstetter, P. T. Nelson, F. A. Schmitt, and L. J. Van Eldik, "Using mice to model Alzheimer's dementia: an overview of the clinical disease and the preclinical behavioral changes in 10 mouse models," *Frontiers in Genetics*, vol. 5, p. 88, 2014.

[32] S. Oddo, A. Caccamo, J. D. Shepherd et al., "Triple-transgenic model of Alzheimer's disease with plaques and tangles: intracellular Abeta and synaptic dysfunction," *Neuron*, vol. 39, no. 3, pp. 409–421, 2003.

[33] K. M. Moore, R. E. Girens, S. K. Larson et al., "A spectrum of exercise training reduces soluble Aβ in a dose-dependent manner in a mouse model of Alzheimer's disease," *Neurobiology of Disease*, vol. 85, pp. 218–224, 2016.

[34] E. A. Herbst and G. P. Holloway, "Permeabilization of brain tissue in situ enables multiregion analysis of mitochondrial function in a single mouse brain," *The Journal of Physiology*, vol. 593, no. 4, pp. 787–801, 2015.

[35] J. Burtscher, L. Zangrandi, C. Schwarzer, and E. Gnaiger, "Differences in mitochondrial function in homogenated samples from healthy and epileptic specific brain tissues revealed by high-resolution respirometry," *Mitochondrion*, vol. 25, pp. 104–112, 2015.

[36] D. Pesta and E. Gnaiger, "High-resolution respirometry: OXPHOS protocols for human cells and permeabilized fibers from small biopsies of human muscle," *Methods in Molecular Biology*, vol. 810, pp. 25–58, 2012.

[37] A. C. Venezia, L. M. Guth, R. M. Sapp, E. E. Spangenburg, and S. M. Roth, "Sex-dependent and independent effects of long-term voluntary wheel running on Bdnf mRNA and protein expression," *Physiology & Behavior*, vol. 156, pp. 8–15, 2016.

[38] H. Yan, M. Mitschelen, G. V. Bixler et al., "Circulating IGF1 regulates hippocampal IGF1 levels and brain gene expression during adolescence," *The Journal of Endocrinology*, vol. 211, no. 1, pp. 27–37, 2011.

[39] P. I. Moreira, C. Carvalho, X. Zhu, M. A. Smith, and G. Perryi, "Mitochondrial dysfunction is a trigger of Alzheimer's disease pathophysiology," *Biochimica et Biophysica Acta (BBA)-Molecular Basis of Disease*, vol. 1802, no. 1, pp. 2–10, 2010.

[40] D. Özbeyli, G. Sarı, N. Özkan et al., "Protective effects of different exercise modalities in an Alzheimer's disease-like model," *Behavioural Brain Research*, vol. 328, pp. 159–177, 2017.

14

The Influence of Family History of Type 2 Diabetes Mellitus on Positive Health Behavior Changes among African Americans

Donny Ard,[1] **Naa-Solo Tettey**⊙,[2] **and Shinga Feresu**[3]

[1]*Department of Surgery, Holy Cross Hospital, Silver Spring, MD 20910, USA*
[2]*Department of Public Health, William Paterson University, Wayne 07470, USA*
[3]*Department of Public Health, University of Johannesburg, Auckland Park 2006, South Africa*

Correspondence should be addressed to Naa-Solo Tettey; drntettey@gmail.com

Academic Editor: Khoa Nguyen

Type 2 diabetes mellitus (T2DM) is a disease that affects the body's ability to metabolize glucose effectively. The disease is predicted to be prevalent in over 300 million people by the year 2030. African Americans (AA) have the highest prevalence rates of type 2 diabetes mellitus (T2DM) in the United States. Lifestyle modification and awareness of risk factors, including family history, are important aspects for prevention of developing T2DM. The purpose of this study was to understand if a family history of T2DM played an influential role in individuals making positive health behavior changes for T2DM prevention. The phenomenological study was grounded in the health belief model and also identified barriers associated with inactivity towards positive health behavior changes. Participants selected for this study were at least 18 years of age, self-identified as AA, self-reported a family history of T2DM, and were not diagnosed with the disease themselves. Transcriptions of twenty face-to-face interviews were analyzed via qualitative research software NVivo Version 12 for Mac. Participants demonstrated a strong awareness of T2DM with an accurate definition of T2DM and explanation of signs, symptoms, and prevention. Participants recognized family history as a risk factor in only 55% of the responses. However, family history played a major role in prevention in the lives of the participants. The participants reflected on personal barriers to health behavior changes and were encouraged to incorporate better life choices in their own lives. This research offers communities, healthcare providers, and stakeholders a better understanding of the importance of family history as a risk factor to T2DM as programs are developed to mitigate health disparities in the AA community.

1. Introduction

Diabetes mellitus (DM) is a disease that affects the body's ability to effectively break down sugar for the consumption of energy. There are three types of DM: type 1, type 2, and gestational DM. Type 2 DM (T2DM) deals with the cells of the body not responding to the hormone insulin, the body not producing enough insulin, or both [1]. According to the Centers for Disease Control and Prevention (CDC), diabetes affects approximately 29.1 million individuals each year and is the seventh leading cause of mortality in the United States [2]. The World Health Organization estimates that T2DM will be prevalent among 366 million people by the year 2030, which is a dramatic increase from the 171 million

that was reported globally in 2000 (World Health Organization, 2010 as cited in [3]).

African Americans are twice as likely to be predisposed to develop diabetes as their European American counterparts [4]. This disparity has elevated the issue to a national concern. Healthy People 2020, through the goals and objectives for diabetes, recognizes there is a significant health disparity among African Americans diagnosed with T2DM [5]. As it pertains to race and ethnicity, African Americans are 50%-100% more likely to develop T2DM compared to their European American counterparts [6]. Researchers estimate the rate of T2DM to triple by the year 2050 among African Americans [6]. African Americans are more likely to have disproportionate outcomes as they relate to T2DM and are twice as likely to experience diabetes-related blindness, lower limb amputations, and depression [4, 7].

T2DM remains the leading cause of death for African Americans. The overall goal of Healthy People 2020 in this regard is to reduce the number of newly diagnosed individuals with T2DM and contribute to reducing the economic burden it has on individuals and their families [5]. The keys to this reduction in newly diagnosed individuals are within awareness and prevention. Awareness involves understanding the risk factors associated with the disease. The risk factors related to T2DM include obesity, hypertension, heart disease, family history, and ethnicity. Compared with individuals without a family history of T2DM, persons with a family history in any first-degree relative have a 2- to 3-fold increased risk of developing T2DM [8]. The way a person internalizes the importance of family history varies by disease. Individuals becoming aware of their family history and assessing their personal relationship to a disease may result in a positive change in health behavior [9]. McDowell et al. [9] found that individuals who were aware of a family history of prostate cancer were more likely to undergo screening as compared to those who did not have a family history. In another study, Madlensky et al. [10] showed that women who had a strong family history of breast cancer were more likely to take more of a dramatic approach to the disease as it pertains to surgical management. At the same time, they did not report more preventive measures as compared to breast cancer survivors who did not have a family history.

A shift in thinking within the African American community, healthcare providers, and stakeholders on the role of positive health behavior and family history as it pertains to improving the overall outcome of T2DM is needed. How the family history of T2DM is influential as a positive behavior change agent for African Americans was the area of interest for this study. There are several gaps in the literature specifically in looking at the impact that knowledge of family history has on preventive measures in T2DM. This study provides a perspective of African Americans who have a family history of T2DM and how knowledge of this affects lifestyle choices. This research has the potential to shed light on specific barriers that may hinder individuals in making lifestyle changes. This study adds to the discipline of T2DM, African Americans, and community health promotion and education.

2. Materials and Methods

2.1. Research Design Rationale. To fully understand the influence the knowledge of family history of T2DM has on an individual to engage in positive health behavior changes, a qualitative research method was used. This research method is favored because it allows for interaction with the participants via face-to-face interviews. Focus groups and interviews have been used in prior research that focused on diabetes and some other lived experience. Jagiello and Azulay Chertok [11] illustrated this concept when they looked at women's experiences with early breastfeeding after GDM. Prompting questions were used to initiate conversation in the focus groups and the interviews; detailed accounts from the participants were recorded and analyzed for the research [11].

2.2. Theoretical Foundation. The theoretical framework for this research was the health belief model (HBM). The HBM explores the mindsets of individuals and their willingness to make healthy choices. The HBM provides insight on barriers associated with persons who may refuse to involve themselves in any positive changes towards their health [12]. The HBM for this study assisted in examining African Americans with a family history of diabetes and the influence it has had on positive health behavior changes.

2.3. Conceptual Framework. The conceptual framework for this research was centered on a phenomenological design. Phenomenology is a broad discipline and method of inquiry in philosophy. German philosophers Edmund Husserl and Martin Heidegger were primarily responsible for its conception. Phenomenology is based on the premise that reality consists of objects and events ("phenomena") as they are perceived or understood in the human consciousness and not of anything independent of human consciousness [13]. As described by Mapp [14], phenomenology aspires to construct insight into "lived experience" from the perception of those individuals involved in a particular experience or "phenomenon" [15].

2.4. Research Questions. RQ1-Does knowledge and understanding of a family history of diabetes promote positive health behavior changes in African Americans?

RQ2-For individuals who have not made any changes towards prevention, what are the barriers that have prevented change in their lifestyles?

2.5. Nature of the Study. A qualitative approach with an emphasis on the HBM and phenomenology was the research design for this study. A qualitative study design enables the researcher to gather data and information from participants by allowing them to express their thoughts and concerns through focus groups and interviews (Patton 2002). This study was centered on recruiting African Americans who self-report a known family history of diabetes but themselves are not diagnosed with the disease. The participants composed a convenience sample of interested African American men and women over the age of 18. Participants were recruited from an inclusion questionnaire that was given to various church congregations in Maryland after receiving permission from the church's pastor allowing dialogue and recruitment from these various churches. Data was collected from face-to-face interviews, transcribed, and analyzed through NVivo.

2.6. Participant Selection Logic. African Americans are affected by T2DM more than any other ethnic group [5]. Therefore, individuals who self-identified as African American no matter their place of origin were used in this study. The participants for this research came from the African American population from different churches in the state of Maryland. The counties of interest for the study included Prince George's, Howard, and Montgomery County. Pastors of these churches were approached to discuss the research. The premise of the meetings was to present the information about the research and its importance. Permission was obtained to distribute questionnaires to the churches for their congregations. The pastor in an African American community is held in high regard and is highly respected; hence, building a research partnership with pastors of churches is essential.

2.7. Procedures for Recruitment, Participation, and Data Collection. Sampling in qualitative research has a distinct purpose. The sampling strategies and sizes are meant to mirror the diversity of the population being studied and not be a statistical representation [16]. Therefore, purposive sampling method was used. Sampling sizes are usually dictated based upon methods, research questions, and the type of data that is being collected. Most importantly, the sampling size should be significant enough to gather content that is rooted more in depth than in breadth. This often may produce smaller sampling sizes [16]. Similar studies with qualitative methodology and the HBM used smaller samples sizes. Based on the methodology and the type of data collection utilized, sampling was concluded after the first 20 eligible participants.

An inclusion questionnaire was used during the recruitment process to determine eligibility for the study. The main purpose of the inclusion questionnaire was to help discern individuals who self-identified as African Americans and had a family history of T2DM but they themselves had not been diagnosed with the disease. An informed consent was provided to participants prior to any data collection and interviews. The interviews took place in a mutually agreed upon location that was convenient for both parties. Participants were made aware that the interview would be recorded for later transcription and data collection. Video and audio technology from FaceTime or Skype via the internet were utilized as last resorts to conduct the face-to-face interviews when a location to meet in person was not available. Only the audio portion was recorded from a video conference for later transcription and data collection. The collection of data, including the transcriptions and review of the interviews, took place over a period of 6 to 8 weeks. The analysis of the data from the interviews was completed with the use of NVivo Version 12 for Mac computers.

2.8. Demographics. The study consisted of six men and 14 women. All the participants self-identified as African American; most reported a birthplace within the United States. Only five participants reported having a birthplace outside of the United States. Although these five participants' birthplaces were located outside of the United States, their time of legal residence within the United States was at least 5 years or more. Participants' ages ranged from 25 to 60 years old. All of the participants lived in either Prince George's, Howard, or Montgomery County in Maryland. Participants' highest level of education completed ranged from "some college" to "graduate degree" (see Table 1).

TABLE 1: Frequencies and percentages for participant demographics.

Demographic characteristics	Frequency N = 20	Percentage
Gender		
Male	6	30
Female	14	70
Origin of birthplace		
USA	15	75
Other	5	25
Highest level of education completed		
Some college	3	15
Bachelor's degree	8	40
Master's degree	6	30
Ph.D./PharmD/DPT	3	15

2.9. Data Collection. Data collection began in December 2017 after receiving Institutional Review Board approval (approval number 11-14-17-0165848). Emails were sent to local churches asking to schedule time to speak with the pastor about the study and obtain their permission to recruit participants in their congregation. Four of the seven emails were answered. After speaking in detail with the pastor or the health ministry leader of the church, permission was granted from three churches to make a presentation and distribute inclusion surveys. Participants were required to reside the counties of Prince George's, Howard, or Montgomery. Names of the participants were left out of the recordings and on transcriptions.

2.10. Data Analysis. Each response from the interviews was analyzed for common themes. The open-ended questions allowed for elaborate responses. The questions for the interviews were designed to address the following areas of concern for this research study: (1) knowledge of diabetes and prevention, (2) the participant's family history and events around diabetes, and (3) the participant's health behavior. "Knowledge," "Family History," and "Personal Health Behavior" were the first three themes created. Another theme that was created was "Barriers." This theme was created to analyze the responses given to the overall and personal barriers hindering change in health behaviors. Other themes emerged after reading over the transcriptions and discovering common responses within the original themes. Graphs, tables, and figures assisted in the breakdown of the data. Notes were also taken on participant facial expressions and body positioning details.

3. Results

3.1. Knowledge of Type 2 Diabetes Mellitus. To understand the impact knowledge of a family history of T2DM has on positive health behavior change, it was important to first determine if individuals knew the facts surrounding the disease. Three questions from the interview gauged the overall knowledge of T2DM by assessing its meaning, the signs and symptoms of the disease, and risk factors associated with the disease. Participants had an array of definitions for diabetes, with all of the responses making a connection with T2DM being a disease of the pancreas and the body's inability to process carbohydrates. The most commonly used words or phrases in the definitions included "insulin" or "sugar" in conjunction with the "body's inability to process sugar." Examples of the responses included "diabetes is a disease that affects the pancreas, or your body's ability to produce or secrete insulin" (Participant 201701) and "the failure of the pancreas to produce enough insulin to efficiently metabolize sugars and carbohydrates" (Participant 201703).

Individuals were also asked to identify risk factors that were associated with T2DM. The premise behind this question was to help link the awareness that family history is a known risk factor. The most identified risk factors included poor diet, obesity, a sedentary lifestyle, and heredity. Seventy percent of the responses mentioned poor diet as a risk factor while only 55% of the responses recognized there is a hereditary link to developing T2DM (see Figure 1).

Prevention and awareness are important factors when dealing with chronic diseases and public health. The participants were asked to share their knowledge and thoughts surrounding ways individuals could prevent developing T2DM. Overwhelmingly, all of the participants gave a response that either centered around either changing one's diet, increasing physical activity, weight control, or seeing their doctor regularly (see Figure 2). Diet changes included limiting sugar intake or moving from an animal-based to a plant-based diet. Exercising was defined as being involved in cardio-related activities for at least 30 minutes a day for three to five days a week. Several participants' responses reflected on at least three or all of these prevention modalities.

3.2. Personal Health Behavior. The HBM suggests that health-related decision-making is determined by (a) perceptions about one's susceptibility to and (b) severity of the illness, (c) perceived benefits of treatment, (d) perceived barriers to seeking care, and (e) cues to action [17, 18]. The questions asked during this study that focused on personal health behavior were able to ascertain one or more of the concepts from the HBM. Participants were first asked to describe their feelings surrounding the fact they had a family member who lived or was living with T2DM. The responses varied from "conscious" to "no feelings at all." Others had different responses that expressed "sadness" or "no reaction."

Interestingly, three participants communicated how they felt with describing situational events which occurred in their life with a family member or themselves. Participant 201701 expressed "...there was no concern until their father had a heart attack." Participant 201703 stated the following: "... then I went to the doctor and they told me that my sugar level was high and that if I didn't do something that I was probably going to be diabetic; so that made me feel like OK, I need to get things in check." When Participant 201702 saw their family member having to take insulin injections, this was the turning point for them to say "...that was something that I said I do not ever want to have to do..." (see Figure 3).

Personal health behavior also examined the participant's actions as it pertained to the prevention of T2DM. Participants were asked to give details of their own health-related behavior in reference to their own family history of T2DM. Only one participant stated that their knowledge of the disease and their family contributed little to their overall health behavior: "It has had very little influence. I'm sitting here, and I'm embarrassed to say that; it has had very little influence beyond the fact of me being aware." (Participant 201701). The remaining individuals of the study expressed actions and behavior patterns such as "I purposely watch a lot of what I eat, as far as fat content and sugar content." (Participant 201708); "I try to exercise regularly and limit my sugar intake, and then I go to get my regular checkups like yearly that include blood work." (Participant 201711); and "I have significantly reduced my sugar intake; I think the weight gain and knowing my grandfather's history made me a little nervous because I love sugar. I think that's probably the biggest thing I have modified–my diet overall, but sugar has been the thing I have had to pay more attention to" (Participant 201712). Participants were very interested in the study and how they could better their status. Some individuals saw this study as an opportunity to start their change in health for better. Others even saw this study as a wake-up call to how much really is not known about the T2DM.

3.3. Barriers. The second research question is an intricate part of this study and to the HBM design. The question relates to the participant's self-awareness of negative behavior or the lack of positive behavior. The interview questions linked to the second research question asked participants to explain in their own words "barriers to change in health" from an overall point-of-view. The participants were then asked to identify any barriers within their personal lives they felt were averting them in making positive health behavior changes or altering negative health behaviors. When asked to define "barriers to change in health," all of the participants described the phrase as something that hinders change from happening. Participants gave a variety of reasons for barriers within their life. Some stated "self" was the barrier in their own life. One participant eloquently stated, "The biggest barrier or obstacle, I find personally, in my productivity is me—I am my biggest obstacle" (Participant 201701). Participant 201702 expressed the same by saying "My own laziness–the barrier is me just being lazy. I can definitely do better...."

Others found their professional work life, school, or family responsibilities deprived them of time they needed to incorporate positive changes in their schedules. Participant 201708 shared the following: "My barrier right now is time. Right now, I have an hour commute in the morning, and then I work 9-10 hours a day. Then I have another hour commute home. Just enough time to take my daughter to swimming class or spending a couple of hours with her making dinner and then going to bed. I think my personal schedule is the biggest barrier to anything."

Other participants wanted to invest in their health but realized it would take time, effort, and commitment to maintain things many of the participants did not know how to

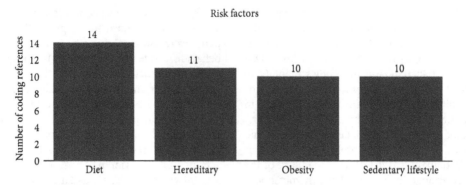

FIGURE 1: Risk factors associated with T2DM according to study participants.

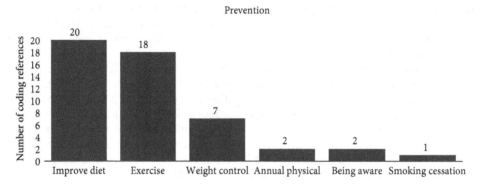

FIGURE 2: Prevention of T2DM according to the responses of the participants.

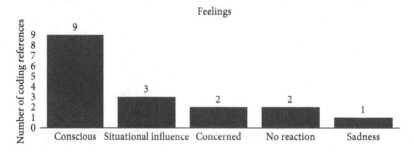

FIGURE 3: Participants' expressed feeling towards family history of T2DM.

include in their compressed schedule—"I think free time is a lot of it. ...it can take anywhere from an hour to two hours one way to get to work. I would definitely go to the gym if I had more time. If I go to the gym, I have to sacrifice something else" (Participant 201710).

4. Discussion

Awareness of a disease's risk factors and preventive measures is paramount for positive health behavior and incorporating lifestyle changes. However, how persons see themselves as being susceptible to developing a disease and how they use the information are the cornerstones of the HBM. This study examined how a family history of T2DM influenced individuals in the African American community in their actions towards positive health behavior change. The study also examined the participant's ideas regarding general and personal barriers to such changes. Whether or not individuals

were involved in preventive activities, the participants discussed how barriers played a role in health behavior changes in the general public and for themselves. Each response provided by the participants alluded to how diabetes was the body's inability to process sugar effectively. Many of the participants were able to identify the pancreas was involved in the process of T2DM as the dysfunctional organ. Every individual in the study was also able to give appropriate signs and symptoms of how someone may present with T2DM, which included having extreme thirst, being obese, consuming a diet rich of foods high in fats, sugar, and salt, or having frequent urination. While participants were able to recognize many risk factors associated with the disease, only 11 of 20 of the responses (55%) recognized a family history as being a risk factor for developing T2DM. Much of the responses acknowledged modifiable risk factors such as obesity and a sedentary lifestyle. The latter correlates with the overwhelming answers given from participants with respect to prevention of the disease. Participants' preventive activities focused more on managing weight with a healthy diet and engaging in cardio-related exercises. These findings are in a horizontal alignment with the current research, which shows healthcare providers stress the importance of awareness through modifiable risk factors, whereas family history is rarely emphasized enough during awareness campaigns on the prevention of diabetes [19].

The second theme of the study was centered around personal health behavior. As mentioned before, participants were asked about prevention activities earlier in the study. This question was followed up with a discussion about the participant's health beliefs and behaviors. According to this study, there was broad acknowledgment that more needed to be done by each participant as it pertained to preventive efforts. The proposed activities involved eating a healthier diet with more fruits and vegetables, doing more cardio-related exercises for at least 30 minutes a day, and seeing a healthcare provider annually for a physical and routine checkup. Interestingly, only one participant did not actively engage in any type of the preventive actions mentioned above, although that participant was aware of the potential complication of T2DM. Furthermore, only three participants actively sought out preventive care with annual health visits to their primary care physicians; these findings show a disconnection to the current literature as it pertains to annual health maintenance. Current recommendations for annual health visits have shown benefits with earlier detection in cancers and preventable diseases, along with proper management of chronic diseases [20].

4.1. Limitations. There are several limitations to this study. The first limitation of the study was the sample size. Although there is a larger than recommended sample size for a qualitative study, this size does not fairly represent a larger community of African Americans. A second limitation to address in this study was the lack of male participants in the research. Considering African Americans are the least represented race and ethnicity in research, this trend has been noted in other research areas for African American males. The third limitation with this study was that it only asked the experiences of African Americans. Allowing the study to engage anyone with a family history of T2DM may have shown different responses with consideration to culture, preventive healthcare beliefs, and barriers.

5. Conclusions

Individuals within the African American community who had a family history of T2DM were the nucleus of this study. The study delved into the communication of health topics within the family and home. Fifty percent of the participants stated health and disease prevention was not a usual topic of discussion in their home growing up. This study could be the catalyst to starting the conversation of disease prevention in the home at an earlier age. Butler and Mead [21] both suggest beginning preventive health messages during the earliest time of developing lifelong habits. The idea of preventive messages within the home at an earlier age feeds into the idea

of changing the mind of generations to come. This study provides a sense of generational awareness of T2DM and the critical impact family history has on disease prevention. The study brings to the forefront the need to address health topics not only in the doctor's office but also more in the home and communities. Health communication strengthens awareness, which in hope encourages action for positive health behavior change at an earlier age.

Awareness, just like communication, is twofold. Awareness campaigns for the community are developed with strategic plans in place with all stakeholders in mind. Policymakers, being a significant contributor to the class of stakeholders, are intricate to the implementation of positive social change. Many African Americans communities are stricken with poverty and less than favorable access to healthcare. Policymakers should be made aware of the challenges such communities face. To fully comprehend the barriers affecting many communities, the difficult conversations between those affected and those who can help with change need to happen more often face-to-face. Just as this study was able to highlight barriers for participants, town hall meetings should occur to have the voices of the communities heard by the policymakers. Change can only take place if people are willing to accept the fact barriers exist and are disproportionate to various communities. Social determinates play a major role in access to healthcare, knowledge and understanding of disease awareness and prevention, and an individual's overall health outcome to chronic disease. More specifically, in communities where socioeconomic disadvantages are the significant barriers, it is proposed that policymakers and public health officials should gather in communities to hear firsthand how healthier eating options are not as available or affordable in some communities. The options to eat healthier are at times far more expensive to families who may be struggling financially versus others who are able to afford a desired meal plan that is organic, plant-based, or vegan [22]. Awareness to every component of this multifaceted problem is the key to proper change.

Social change also pertains to building and maintaining meaningful relationships between the health providers and the communities they serve. This study sheds light on how one can strengthen the healthcare provider and patient relationship, especially among the African American community. African Americans have a deep history of mistrust from health providers dating back to the Tuskegee Experiments [23]. This mistrust of care has planted seeds of doubt for many generations. Specifically, healthcare providers can use the interview questions as a guide to engage their patients to be open about their knowledge of a disease, their family history, their own healthcare practices or beliefs, and personal barriers within their lives which inhibit positive health behavior changes. Furthermore, providers should allow their patients to be more involved in their healthcare decision-making and tailor an action plan to their current lifestyle and recognizable barriers.

According to the CDC, there are more than 29 million people living in America who are diagnosed with T2DM and nearly 60 million individuals who are prediabetic [2]. This puts a financial burden on the healthcare system which paid $245 billion only for T2DM and complications associated with the disease in 2012 [24]. The predicted increase in prevalence, especially among the African American community, has made diabetes a public health concern. The increase has set off a chain reaction of care planning. The main goal for T2DM in the public health realm is geared towards awareness. Awareness focuses on bringing attention to modifiable risk factors. The hope is that awareness will promote preventive actions with lifestyle modification for obesity and a sedentary lifestyle. These modifications include increasing physical activity and eating a healthy diet. Furthermore, awareness campaigns should also shed light on nonmodifiable risk factors, such as a family history of T2DM. Preventative actions can still be put into place while encouraging individuals to visit their healthcare providers routinely to have blood work done which could detect the disease.

This study, with the limitations mentioned, proved to show an individual's family history of T2DM was a strong influence in positive health behavior change for the participants involved. Continuing to focus on awareness and prevention, this study subscribes to the idea of making family history, a nonmodifiable risk factor, just as important as modifiable risk factors. Family history, although it is not a modifiable risk factor, should be added to the awareness campaign. Having providers and patients understand the overall dangers of T2DM with an added focus on family history can be beneficial to all involved. The topic of family history opens the pipe lines of discussion not only for T2DM but also for other healthcare concerns. The provider and patient relationship becomes stronger than ever and flourishes.

Barriers became a topic of discussion as well. Individuals within this study were able to realize the true definition of a barrier and how barriers impacted their desires to do better. Barriers for these participants mainly dealt with time. Fortunately, access to healthy food or a gym membership was not a part of the barriers to change in health for this study. The main goal to overcoming barriers was to set realistic expectations and start small. Setting realistic action plans and expectations aids in an overall better outcome. Furthermore, individuals had a chance to be honest about these goals while taking into considerations their acknowledged barriers. Not all barriers can be modified. However, recognizing that barriers exist and having the difficult conversations between communities and all stakeholders are the beginning many are looking for to start a new healthy lifestyle.

Acknowledgments

This research is based on the dissertation for Donny Ard.

References

[1] S. K. Tanamas, E. Wong, K. Backholer et al., "Age of onset of obesity and risk of type 2 diabetes," *Australian and New Zealand Journal of Public Health*, vol. 40, no. 6, pp. 579–581, 2016.

[2] Centers for Disease Control and Prevention, *National diabetes statistics report: Estimates of diabetes and its burden in the United States, 2014*, U.S. Department of Health and Human Services, Centers for Disease Control and Prevention, Atlanta, GA, USA, 2014.

[3] E. Hansen, B. J. Landstad, O. Hellzén, and S. Svebak, "Motivation for lifestyle changes to improve health in people with impaired glucose tolerance," *Scandinavian Journal of Caring Sciences*, vol. 25, no. 3, pp. 484–490, 2011.

[4] J. McCloskey and D. Flenniken, "Overcoming cultural barriers to diabetes control: a qualitative study of southwestern New Mexico Hispanics," *Journal of Cultural Diversity*, vol. 17, no. 3, pp. 110–115, 2010.

[5] J. Gumbs, "Relationship between diabetes self-management education and self-care behaviors among African American women with type 2 diabetes," *Journal of Cultural Diversity*, vol. 19, no. 1, pp. 18–22, 2012.

[6] L. B. Signorello, D. G. Schlundt, S. S. Cohen et al., "Comparing diabetes prevalence between African Americans and Whites of similar socioeconomic status," *American Journal of Public Health*, vol. 97, no. 12, pp. 2260–2267, 2007.

[7] A. N. Brewer-Lowry, T. A. Arcury, R. A. Bell, and S. A. Quandt, "Differentiating approaches to diabetes self-management of multi-ethnic rural older adults at the extremes of glycemic control," *The Gerontologist*, vol. 50, no. 5, pp. 657–667, 2010.

[8] N. Rautio, J. Jokelainen, H. Oksa et al., "Family history of diabetes and effectiveness of lifestyle counselling on the cardio-metabolic risk profile in individuals at high risk of type 2 diabetes: 1-year follow-up of the FIN-D2D project," *Diabetic Medicine*, vol. 29, no. 2, pp. 207–211, 2012.

[9] M. E. McDowell, S. Occhipinti, and S. K. Chambers, "The influence of family history on cognitive heuristics, risk perceptions, and prostate cancer screening behavior," *Health Psychology*, vol. 32, no. 11, pp. 1158–1169, 2013.

[10] L. Madlensky, S. W. Flatt, W. A. Bardwell, C. L. Rock, J. P. Pierce, and for the WHEL Study group, "Is family history related to preventive health behaviors and medical management in breast cancer patients?," *Breast Cancer Research and Treatment*, vol. 90, no. 1, pp. 47–54, 2005.

[11] K. P. Jagiello and I. R. Azulay Chertok, "Women's experiences with early breastfeeding after gestational diabetes," *Journal of Obstetric, Gynecologic & Neonatal Nursing*, vol. 44, no. 4, pp. 500–509, 2015.

[12] R. M. Huff and M. V. Kline, *Health Promotion in Multicultural Populations: A Handbook for Practitioners and Students*, Sage Publications, Thousand Oaks, CA, USA, 2nd edition, 2008.

"Exploring the lived experience of surviving with both alcoholism and diabetes," *Journal of Addictions Nursing*, vol. 15, no. 2, pp. 65–72, 2004.

[14] T. Mapp, "Understanding phenomenology: the lived experience," *British Journal of Midwifery*, vol. 16, no. 5, pp. 308–311, 2008.

[15] M. Poth and M. Carolan, "Pregnant women's knowledge about the prevention of gestational diabetes mellitus: a qualitative study," *British Journal of Midwifery*, vol. 21, no. 10, pp. 692–700, 2013.

[16] R. Johnson and J. Waterfield, "Making words count: the value of qualitative research," *Physiotherapy Research International*, vol. 9, no. 3, pp. 121–131, 2004.

[17] K. Glanz, B. K. Rimer, and K. Viswanath, Eds., *Health Behavior and Health Education*, Jossey-Bass, San Francisco, CA, USA, 4th edition, 2008.

[18] J. Hayden, *Introduction to Health Behavior Theory*, Jones and Bartlett Learning, Burlington, MA, USA, 2nd edition, 2014.

[19] L. S. Geiss, K. Kirtland, J. Lin et al., "Changes in diagnosed diabetes, obesity, and physical inactivity prevalence in US counties, 2004-2012," *PLoS One*, vol. 12, no. 3, article e0173428, 2017.

[20] D. J. Hain, "The CMS annual wellness visit: bridging the gap," *The Nurse Practitioner*, vol. 39, no. 7, pp. 18–26, 2014.

[21] K. L. Butler and A. S. Mead, "Developing and evaluating a college diabetes prevention and awareness campaign," *American Journal of Health Studies*, vol. 25, no. 4, pp. 196–201, 2010.

[22] D. Kwasnicka, J. Presseau, M. White, and F. F. Sniehotta, "Does planning how to cope with anticipated barriers facilitate health-related behaviour change? A systematic review," *Health Psychology Review*, vol. 7, no. 2, pp. 129–145, 2013.

[23] A. Sharma, "Diseased race, racialized disease: the story of the negro project of American social hygiene association against the backdrop of the Tuskegee syphilis experiment," *Journal of African American Studies*, vol. 14, no. 2, pp. 247–262, 2010.

[24] K. Subramanian, I. Midha, and V. Chellapilla, "Overcoming the challenges in implementing type 2 diabetes mellitus prevention programs can decrease the burden on healthcare costs in the United States," *Journal of Diabetes Research*, vol. 2017, Article ID 2615681, 5 pages, 2017.

15

Comparative Abilities of Fasting Plasma Glucose and Haemoglobin A1c in Predicting Metabolic Syndrome among Apparently Healthy Normoglycemic Ghanaian Adults

Nafiu Amidu,[1] William Kwame Boakye Ansah Owiredu ⓘ,[2] Lawrence Quaye ⓘ,[1] Peter Paul Mwinsanga Dapare ⓘ,[1] and Yussif Adams ⓘ[1]

[1]*Department of Biomedical Laboratory Science, University for Development Studies, Tamale, Ghana*
[2]*Department of Molecular Medicine, Kwame Nkrumah University of Science and Technology, Kumasi, Ghana*

Correspondence should be addressed to Peter Paul Mwinsanga Dapare; pdapare@uds.edu.gh

Academic Editor: Jose Tellez-Zenteno

There are arguments as to whether haemoglobin A1c (HbA1c) better predicts Metabolic syndrome (MetS) than fasting plasma glucose. The aim of the study was to explore the comparative abilities of HbA1c and Fasting plasma glucose (FPG) in predicting cardiometabolic risk among apparently healthy adults in the Tamale metropolis. This study was a cross-sectional study conducted in the Tamale metropolis from September, 2017, to January, 2018, among one hundred and sixty (160) apparently healthy normoglycemic adults. A self-designed questionnaire was administered to gather sociodemographic data. Anthropometric and haemodynamic data were also taken and blood samples collected for haemoglobin A1c (HbA1c), fasting plasma glucose (FPG), and lipid profile. MetS was classified using the harmonised criteria as indicated in the joint interim statement (JIS). Out of the 160 participants, 42.5% were males and 57.5% were females. FPG associated better with MetS and other cardiovascular risk markers, compared to HbA1c. FPG had the largest area under curve for predicting MetS and its components. This study shows a stronger association between FPG and MetS compared with haemoglobin A1c; it also provides evidence of a superior ability of FPG over HbA1c in predicting MetS and other adverse cardiovascular outcomes in apparently heathy normoglycemic individuals.

1. Background

Metabolic syndrome (MetS) is a set of closely associated cardiometabolic risks [1], like obesity, dyslipidemia, hypertension, and hyperglycemia and is seen as a powerful indicator of diabetes and cardiovascular disease (CVD) [2, 3]. The prevalence of metabolic syndrome continues to be on the rise; this is in part as a result of rapid urbanization with the related variations in nutrition and physical activity [4]. Worldwide the prevalence of metabolic syndrome has been reported as being between 10% and 84% [5]. In Africa, prevalence of 2.1% to 34.7% has been reported in several studies from around the continent [6, 7]. In Ghana, a prevalence of metabolic syndrome between 6% and 21.2% has been reported [8] using different criteria.

Haemoglobin A1c (HbA1c), a result of nonenzymatic glycosylation of the β-chain of haemoglobin, is made in proportion to the rise in blood glucose levels. It has been considered a preferable tool since HbA1c assay has superior technical advantages compared to the estimation of plasma glucose; it can be measured in the nonfasted state and has greater reproducibility than fasting glucose [9, 10]. HbA1c is a set-up marker of long haul glycemic control in individuals with diabetes mellitus (DM), and increased HbA1c levels are linked with an increased risk for later microvascular and macrovascular illness [11].

The fasting plasma glucose (FPG) cut-off figure for MetS may differ among various populaces. There are numerous reports recommending that HbA1c is superior to FPG in forecasting cardiometabolic risk even in nondiabetic individuals

[12–14], with many others proposing that HbA1c may be an essential marker for MetS, but it stays a controversy [15–17]. However, HbA1c may be influenced by various haematologic, genetic, and disease-related factors [18]. The most important factors globally affecting HbA1c levels are some anaemias, haemoglobinopathies, and disorders linked with increased red blood cell turnover like malaria [9, 19].

A 1% rise in HbA1c raises the risk of CVD by 18% and positive relation between CVD and HbA1c has been shown in nondiabetic individuals even within normal values of HbA1c [20]. Many population-based studies from Western nations have investigated the link between HbA1c and the risk of CVDs (MetS) among nondiabetics [14, 21, 22], while only a few studies were from Africa and for that matter Ghana has examined this issue. Moreover, there is scarce evidence about whether or not adding HbA1c to other possible risk factors improves the ability to predict the Metabolic syndrome.

Previous studies have related HbA1c to glucose and weighed the option of replacing glucose with HbA1c for the criterion or adding HbA1c as an extra criterion for diabetes [17, 23–26]. However, data on the use of HbA1c as an indicator of MetS particularly in nondiabetic people are scanty and inconclusive, with some studies supporting the possible use of HbA1c as a marker for MetS, while other studies show divergence [15, 24, 27, 28]. While some studies have observed the importance of haemoglobin A1c in MetS, few have studied it in individuals with normal glucose levels. The aim of the study was to explore the comparative abilities of HbA1c and FPG in predicting metabolic syndrome in apparently healthy normoglycemic adults within the Tamale metropolis of Ghana.

2. Methods

2.1. Subjects.
This study was a cross-sectional study conducted among apparently healthy adults (18 years and above) with no history of diabetes within the Tamale metropolis from September, 2017, to January, 2018.

2.1.1. Exclusion Criteria.
Diabetics, hypertensives, persons treating diabetes or hypertension, persons with a fasting blood glucose >7.0 mmol/l or HbA1c ≥6.5% at the time of the study, pregnant women, persons showing signs of any acute illnesses, and persons with other chronic diseases were excluded from this study.

2.1.2. Sample Size.
The minimum sample size for the study was calculated to be 105 adults, based on the assumption that 7.4% of the normal adult populations have metabolic syndrome [29], with an expected difference of 5% between the sample and the general population and a type I error (α) of 0.05.

This study was limited to only apparently healthy adults who answered at least 75% of the questions in the questionnaire and did not have an FPG of >7.0 mmol/l or an HbA1c of >6.5; hence, the sample size was recalculated to adjust for any possible loss of respondents. Assuming a response rate of 90%, the sample size was recalculated to be approximately

117. One hundred and twenty (120) participants were therefore targeted for this study.

2.2. Data Collection

2.2.1. Sociodemographic and Anthropometric Data.
A self-designed semistructured questionnaire was administered to consented study participants for sociodemographic data. Weight to the nearest 0.1 kg was measured using a digital flat floor weighing scale (with weighing capacity of 250 kg) manufactured by SECA (Hamburg, Germany) and height to the nearest 1 cm was measured using a portable microtoise (measuring range: 0 cm to 220 cm) manufactured by SECA. Waist circumference (to the nearest centimetre) was measured with a Gulick II spring-loaded measuring tape (Gay Mill, WI) midway between the inferior angle of the ribs and the suprailiac crest. Hip circumference was measured as the maximal circumference over the buttocks in centimetre.

2.2.2. Blood Pressure.
Blood pressure was measured in sitting position, with a sphygmomanometer cuff and a stethoscope. Measurements were taken from the left brachial artery after subjects had been sitting for at least five (5) minutes in accordance with the recommendation of the American Heart Association [30]. Triplicate measurements were taken with a five (5) minute rest interval between measurements and the mean value was recorded to the nearest 2.0 mmHg.

2.2.3. Sample Collection, Preparation, and Analysis.
Ten milliliters (10 ml) of venous blood sample was collected under strict aseptic conditions from each participant in the morning between 07.00 and 09.00 GMT into fluoride oxalate tube, Serum Separator Tubes (SST), and ethylenediaminetetraacetic acid (EDTA) anticoagulated tube (Becton Dickinson, Rutherford, NJ), after an overnight (8-12 hours) fast. Samples in the fluoride oxalate tubes were centrifuged and plasma was used for glucose measurement (within 2 hours after sample collection) using the Glucose oxidase peroxidase (GOD-POD) method whilst samples in the SST were centrifuged at 3000 g for 5 minutes and the serum was aliquoted and stored in cryovials at a temperature of -80°C until time for biochemical assays. Lipid profile and fasting blood glucose levels were determined using the Mindray BS-240 Chemistry Analyser (Mindray, China); MedSource Diagnostics reagents were used in all of these assays. The anticoagulated (EDTA) blood was used for the HbA1c Assay using the MedSource Diagnostics reagents for Glycosylated Haemoglobin (A1-fast fraction) test kit which uses the Cation Exchange Method. For the within run (intra-assay) precision, a % CV was 2.7 in normal HbA1c samples and 1.7 in elevated HbA1c samples was quoted while for the run to run (Inter run) precision a % CV was 4.1 for normal samples and 4.6 for elevated samples were quoted by manufacturers. Samples from subjects with haemoglobinopathies or decreased erythrocytes survival times may show incorrect results. This method is not listed in the 2019 National Glycohemoglobin Standardization Program (NSGP) method traceability list.

2.3. Definitions of Metabolic Syndrome

2.3.1. Metabolic Syndrome: Harmonised Criteria by the Joint Interim Statement (JIS). Metabolic syndrome was defined to include individuals with any three or more of the following five components: (1) abdominal obesity (waist circumference, Male ≥94, Female ≥80), (2) high triglyceride ≥ 1.7 mmol/L (150 mg/dl), (3) low HDL-C: Male< 1.0, Female <1.3 mmol/L, (4) High BP (systolic BP ≥ 130 mm Hg or diastolic BP ≥ 85 mm Hg or treatment of hypertension), and (5) high fasting glucose ≥ 5.6 mmol/l [31].

2.4. Statistical Analysis. All analyses were performed using MedCalc® version 10.2.0.0 (www.medcalc.be) for windows and GraphPad version 6.0, San Diego, California, USA. Unpaired T-test was used to compare continuous variables. Association between variables was assessed with linear regression analysis. Receiver Operator Characteristics (ROC) was used to compare the relative abilities of various parameters to predict MetS and other cardiovascular risk factors. In all statistical analyses, a p value of <0.05 was considered significant.

3. Results

3.1. General Characteristics of Studied Population. A total of 160 complete questionnaires were analysed, of which 68 (42.5%) were males and 92 (57.5%) females. Subjects with metabolic syndrome were significantly older than subjects without the metabolic syndrome. The average HbA1c and FPG of the study population were 4.8±1.2% and 4.95±0.92 mmol/L, respectively. These parameters were higher in respondents with MetS; however, only the difference in FPG was statistically (p<0.001) significant as shown in Table 1

3.2. Biochemical Parameters of Studied Population Stratified by Gender. Table 2 summarises the biochemical parameters of the studied population stratified by gender. Female respondents were older (43.8±14.3 years) than the male (41.4±14.8 years) but this was not statistically significant. Female respondents with MetS however were significantly older than those without MetS. In females only, FPG was significantly higher in MetS as shown in Table 2.

3.3. Biochemical Characteristics according to MetS Score. Table 3 shows the anthropometric and biochemical variations in MetS scores. Generally, FPG significantly showed an increasing trend while moving from a score of 0 to a score of 3 or more.

3.4. Association between HbA1c, FPG, Lipid Parameters, and MetS Score. A linear regression between HbA1c, FPG, and selected cardiometabolic risk is shown in Table 4. HbA1c had significant positive association with triglyceride and VLDL-c. A percentage increase in HbA1c results in a 0.12 mmol (r^2=0.03, p<0.05) increase in Triglyceride and 0.05 mmol (r^2=0.03, p<0.05) increase in VLDL-c. FPG however showed significant positive association with SBP, DBP, total

cholesterol, triglyceride, and VLDL-c. A 1 mmol/L increase in FPG is associated with an increase in 0.33 mmol/L (r^2=0.05, p<0.01) of total cholesterol, 0.21 mmol/L (r^2=0.05, p<0.01) of triglyceride, and a 0.10 mmol/L (r^2=0.05, p<0.01) increase in VLDL-c.

3.5. Receiver Operator Characteristics (ROC) for HbA1c and FPG in the Studied Population. The ROC curves and the Area under Curve (AUC) between HbA1c and FPG against MetS and its individual components are shown in Figure 1 and Table 5. FPG had the largest AUC for all variables assessed, that is, MetS, 2 or more nonglycemic components, abdominal obesity, elevated BP, elevated triglyceride, and reduced HDL-c (Table 5).

4. Discussion

The role of impaired glucose metabolism in the pathogenesis of MetS and its adverse effects on CVDs and diabetes outcomes has been well documented [32, 33]. Hyperglycemia is known to compound the problem in MetS through the formation of advanced glycation end products [34].

Fasting plasma glucose and haemoglobin A1c measurements have been used over the years in the diagnosis of impaired glucose metabolism. However, proper consensus has not been reached about which there is a better diagnostic tool, associates better with cardiometabolic risk, and can be used as a predictive tool for MetS, especially among normoglycemic individuals. Some studies have shown that haemoglobin A1c associates better with cardiometabolic risk [16, 24, 35].

This study however found that haemoglobin A1c does not associate better with cardiometabolic risk and has no superior ability in predicting the presence of MetS among a normoglycemic northern Ghanaian population. Succurro and Marini [23] pointed out that the classification of MetS using a HbA1c criterion instead of glucose performed worse in detecting some subjects who still had an unfavourable cardiometabolic risk profile. Several other studies have reported similar findings, especially among a normoglycemic population [36].

The adverse effects of impaired glucose metabolism and diabetes are as a result of the elevated glucose levels and not elevated levels of haemoglobin A1c which is only reflective of a chronic exposure to high plasma glucose concentration [37]. There is evidence that each of the glycemic measures used to identify prediabetes represents a different domain of glucose metabolism. While FPG reflects basal dysglycemia, HbA1c reflects chronic exposure to basal and postprandial hyperglycemia [37]. A nonlinear relationship between glycemia and the haemoglobin A1c in normoglycemic populations has been observed in a number of studies which have shown that glycemia may be a less important determinant of hemoglobin glycation and that other factors operate to produce consistent changes in HbA1c. Potential explanations for this variation in hemoglobin glycation at or near normal glucose levels have focused on interindividual variation in red cell turnover [38], differences between the

TABLE 1: Biochemical parameters of studied population stratified by MetS.

Variables	Total (n=160)	No MetS (n=132)	MetS (n=28)	P value
Age (years)	42.8±14.5	41.6±14.6	48.2±12.9	0.030
HbA1c (%)	4.8±1.2	4.8±1.2	5.2±1.3	0.080
FPG (mmol/L)	5.0±0.9	4.8±0.9	5.8±0.7	<0.001

HbA1c: Haemoglobin A1c and FPG: Fasting Blood Glucose. Data are presented as mean ± SD and compared using T-test.

TABLE 2: Biochemical parameters of studied population stratified by gender.

| Variables | Male | | | Female | | |
	Total (n=68)	No MetS (n=60)	MetS (n=8)	Total (n=92)	No MetS (n=72)	MetS (n=20)
Age (years)	41.4±14.8	41.8±15.2	38.6±10.9	43.8±14.3	41.5±14.2‡‡	52.0±11.8
HbA1c (%)	4.8±1.3	4.8±1.3	5.1±1.1	4.9±1.2	4.7±1.1	5.3±1.3
FPG (mmol/L)	5.0±0.9	5.0±0.9	5.6±0.7	4.9±1.0	4.6±0.9‡‡‡	5.8±0.7

HbA1c: Haemoglobin A1c and FPG: Fasting Blood Glucose. Data are presented as mean ± SD and compared using T-test. ‡Comparing females with MetS with females without MetS. ‡Comparison is significant at the 0.05 level, ‡‡Comparison is significant at the 0.01 level, and ‡‡‡Comparison is significant at the 0.001 level.

TABLE 3: Biochemical characteristics stratified by MetS component score.

| Variable | MetS score | | | | F Value | P Value |
	0 (n=42)	1 (n=52)	2(n=38)	≥3(n=28)		
Age (years)	34.6±11.8	42.4±14.2	48.3±15.0	48.2±12.9	8.66	<0.001
HbA1c (%)	4.8±1.1	4.8±1.3	4.6±1.2	5.2±1.3	1.24	0.297
FPG (mmol/L)	4.43±0.78	4.9±0.9	5.0±0.9	5.8±0.7	14.46	<0.001

HbA1c: Haemoglobin A1c and FPG: Fasting Blood Glucose. Data are presented as mean ± SD and compared using One-way ANOVA.

TABLE 4: Linear regression analysis between HbA1c, FPG, and selected indicators of cardiometabolic risk factors.

| Variable | HbA1c | | FPG | |
	β	r^2	β	r^2
SBP (mmHg)	0.58	0.00	4.10**	0.06
DBP (mmHg)	-0.26	0.00	2.17*	0.03
HbA1dc-Dcct (%)	-	-	0.12	0.01
FPG (mmol/L)	0.07	0.01	-	-
Total cholesterol (mmol/L)	0.07	0.00	0.33**	0.05
Triglyceride (mmol/L)	0.12*	0.03	0.21**	0.05
HDL-c (mmol/L)	0.00	0.00	0.22	0.04
LDL-c (mmol/L)	0.02	0.00	0.01	0.00
VLDL-c (mmol/L)	0.05*	0.03	0.10**	0.05
MetS score	0.06	0.00	0.56***	0.20

*Regression is significant at the 0.05 level, **regression is significant at the 0.01 level, and ***regression is significant at the 0.001 level.

TABLE 5: AUC for HbA1c and FPG in predicting MetS and its components.

Variable	HbA1c	FPG
MetS	0.62(0.54-0.69)	0.84(0.78- 0.89)
2 or more nonglycemic criteria	0.53(0.45- 0.61)	0.62(0.54- 0.69)
Abdominal obesity	0.53(0.45-0.61)	0.61(0.53- 0.69)
Elevated BP	0.54(0.46- 0.62)	0.64(0.56- 0.71)
Elevated triglyceride	0.62(0.54- 0.69)	0.66(0.58- 0.73)
Reduced HDL-c	0.58(0.50- 0.66)	0.73(0.65- 0.80)

Results are expressed as Area under Curve (confidence interval).

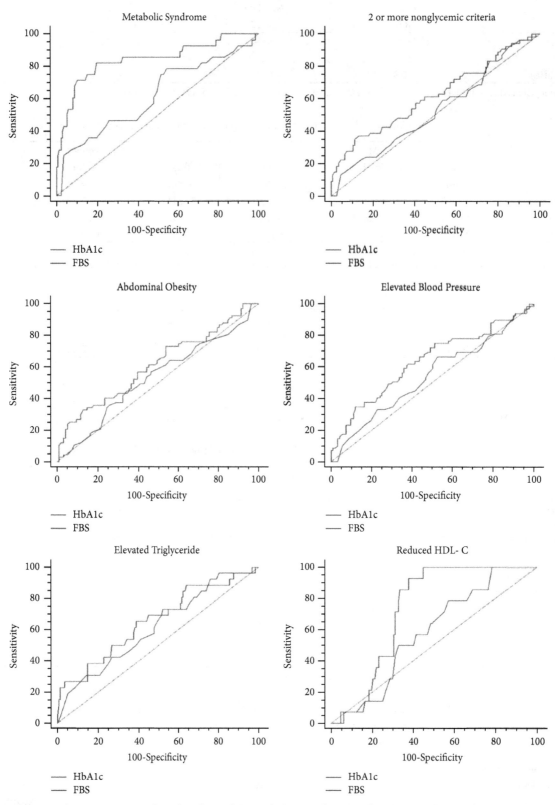

FIGURE 1: ROC curves for MetS. Compared are the relative abilities of HbA1c and FPG to identify respondents with MetS and its components.

intraerythrocyte and extraerythrocyte environment [39], and genetic variation in hemoglobin glycation [40]. This means that, in a normoglycemic population, estimation of glucose levels will correlate better with adverse cardiometabolic outcomes than haemoglobin A1c as shown in the present study.

In this study, though there was no estimation of haemoglobin glycation index (HGI) and data on HGI among African populations that remain sparse, some studies in developed countries have revealed a lower glycation index among African Americans and Caucasians compared with Hispanics [41]. This means that, even at elevated glucose levels, formation of haemoglobin A1c among the population in the present study may have been slow and hence haemoglobin A1c did not reflect the glycemia. Hence, the subsequent absence of association between glycation and the cardiometabolic risk factors and its inability to properly predict MetS and its components compared to Fasting Blood Glucose.

Various combinations of haemoglobin variants C and S have been reported to falsely lower the values of HbA1c. The reported higher frequencies of these variants especially haemoglobin C among sub-Saharan Africans [42, 43] could be linked to the nonperformance of HbA1c in this study, and therefore the impact of haemoglobinopathies in this current study cannot be underestimated especially among a study population of predominantly Northern descent where the prevalence of the haemoglobin C has been shown to be appreciable [44].

5. Conclusion

This study demonstrates that, in a normoglycemic population, FPG associates better with Metabolic syndrome and other cardiometabolic risks than HbA1c and that fasting blood glucose estimation is shown to be the best predictor of MetS and its components among an apparently normoglycemic population.

5.1. Limitations. The estimation of haemoglobin A1c in this study was limited to only one method (Medsource Ozone Biomedicals Pvt., Ltd.) which is not listed on the 2019 NSGP certified methods list.

Abbreviations

MetS: Metabolic syndrome
HbA1c: Haemoglobin A1c
FPG: Fasting blood glucose
CVD: Cardiovascular disease
DM: Diabetes mellitus
SST: Serum separator tube
EDTA: Ethylene diamine tetraacetic acid
HDL-c: High density lipoprotein cholesterol
LDL-c: Low density lipoprotein cholesterol
VLDL-c: Very low-density lipoprotein cholesterol
HGI: Haemoglobin glycation index.

Consent

A consent was sought from each participant before being included in the study. Subjects who did not give their consent were excluded from the study. Subject confidentiality was ensured and hence consent to publish findings from data was obtained.

Authors' Contributions

This work was carried out in collaboration with all authors. Nafiu Amidu, William Kwame Boakye Ansah Owiredu, Lawrence Quaye, Peter Paul Mwinsanga Dapare, and Yussif Adams designed the study, performed the statistical analysis, wrote the protocol, and wrote the first draft of the manuscript. Nafiu Amidu, Peter Paul Mwinsanga Dapare, and Yussif Adams managed the analyses of the study. William Kwame Boakye Ansah Owiredu and Lawrence Quaye managed the literature searches. All authors read and approved the final manuscript.

Acknowledgments

Authors acknowledge the contribution of all research assistants who helped in the collection of data. The authors express their profound gratitude to all participants in the study.

References

[1] R. H. Eckel, S. M. Grundy, and P. Z. Zimmet, "The metabolic syndrome," *The Lancet*, vol. 365, no. 9468, pp. 1415–1428, 2005.

[2] R. A. DeFronzo and E. Ferrannini, "Insulin resistance: a multifaceted syndrome responsible for NIDDM, obesity, hypertension, dyslipidemia, and atherosclerotic cardiovascular disease," *Diabetes Care*, vol. 14, no. 3, pp. 173–194, 1991.

[3] M. P. Stern, "Diabetes and cardiovascular disease: the "common soil" hypothesis," *Diabetes*, vol. 44, no. 4, pp. 369–374, 1995.

[4] C. E. Mbada, R. A. Adedoyin, and O. Ayanniyi, "Socioeconomic status and obesity among semi-urban nigerians," *Obesity Facts*, vol. 2, no. 6, pp. 356–361, 2009.

[5] J. Kaur, "A comprehensive review on metabolic syndrome," *Cardiology Research and Practice*, vol. 2014, Article ID 943162, 21 pages, 2014.

[6] I. I. Ulasi, C. K. Ijoma, and O. D. Onodugo, "A community-based study of hypertension and cardio-metabolic syndrome in semi-urban and rural communities in Nigeria," *BMC Health Services Research*, vol. 10, article no. 71, 2010.

[7] O. O. Oladapo, L. Salako, O. Sodiq, K. Shoyinka, K. Adedapo, and A. O. Falase, "A prevalence of cardiometabolic risk factors among a rural Yoruba south-western Nigerian population: a population-based survey," *Cardiovascular Journal of Africa*, vol. 21, 2010.

[8] R. Ofori-Asenso, A. A. Agyeman, and A. Laar, "Metabolic syndrome in apparently "healthy" ghanaian adults: a systematic review and meta-analysis," *International Journal of Chronic Diseases*, vol. 2017, Article ID 2562374, 9 pages, 2017.

[9] American Diabetes Association, "Standards of medical care in diabetes—2009," *Diabetes Care*, vol. 32, Suppl 1, p. S13, 2009.

[10] M. Mitka, "Hemoglobin A1c poised to become preferred test for diagnosing diabetes," *Journal of the American Medical Association*, vol. 301, no. 15, pp. 1528-1528, 2009.

[11] K. Malmberg, L. Rydén, and H. Wedel, "Intense metabolic control by means of insulin in patients with diabetes mellitus and acute myocardial infarction (DIGAMI 2): effects on mortality and morbidity," *European Heart Journal*, vol. 26, no. 7, pp. 650–661, 2005.

[12] S. Park, E. Barrett-Connor, D. L. Wingard, J. Shan, and S. Edelstein, "GHb is a better predictor of cardiovascular disease than fasting or postchallenge plasma glucose in women without diabetes: the rancho bernardo study," *Diabetes Care*, vol. 19, no. 5, pp. 450–456, 1996.

[13] F. De Vegt, J. M. Dekker, H. G. Ruhé et al., "Hyperglycaemia is associated with all-cause and cardiovascular mortality in the Hoorn population: The Hoorn Study," *Diabetologia*, vol. 42, no. 8, pp. 926–931, 1999.

[14] E. Selvin, M. W. Steffes, H. Zhu et al., "Glycated hemoglobin, diabetes, and cardiovascular risk in nondiabetic adults," *The New England Journal of Medicine*, vol. 362, no. 9, pp. 800–811, 2010.

[15] K. Osei, S. Rhinesmith, T. Gaillard, and D. Schuster, "Is glycosylated hemoglobin a1c a surrogate for metabolic syndrome in nondiabetic, first-degree relatives of african-american patients with type 2 diabetes?" *The Journal of Clinical Endocrinology & Metabolism*, vol. 88, no. 10, pp. 4596–4601, 2003.

[16] C. Lorenzo, L. E. Wagenknecht, A. J. Hanley, M. J. Rewers, A. J. Karter, and S. M. Haffner, "A1C between 5.7 and 6.4% as a marker for identifying pre-diabetes, insulin sensitivity and secretion, and cardiovascular risk factors: the insulin resistance atherosclerosis study (IRAS)," *Diabetes Care*, vol. 33, no. 9, pp. 2104–2109, 2010.

[17] K. L. Ong, A. W. Tso, K. S. Lam, S. S. Cherny, P. C. Sham, and B. M. Cheung, "Using glycosylated hemoglobin to define the metabolic syndrome in united states adults," *Diabetes Care*, vol. 33, no. 8, pp. 1856–1858, 2010.

[18] E. J. Gallagher, D. Le Roith, and Z. Bloomgarden, "Review of hemoglobin A(1c) in the management of diabetes.," *Journal of Diabetes*, vol. 1, no. 1, pp. 9–17, 2009.

[19] W. L. Roberts, B. K. De, D. Brown et al., "Effects of hemoglobin C and S traits on eight glycohemoglobin methods," *Clinical Chemistry*, vol. 48, no. 2, pp. 383–385, 2002.

[20] E. P. Joslin and C. R. Kahn, *Joslin's Diabetes Mellitus*, C. Ronald Kahn, G. Weir, G. King, A. Jacobson, R. Smith, and A. Moses, Eds., Lippincott Williams & Wilkins, 2005.

[21] K. Khaw, N. Wareham, S. Bingham, R. Luben, A. Welch, and N. Day, "Association of hemoglobin A1c with cardiovascular disease and mortality in adults: the European prospective investigation into cancer in Norfolk," *Annals of Internal Medicine*, vol. 141, no. 6, pp. 413–420, 2004.

[22] H. C. Gerstein, J. Pogue, J. F. Mann et al., "The relationship between dysglycaemia and cardiovascular and renal risk in diabetic and non-diabetic participants in the HOPE study: a prospective epidemiological analysis," *Diabetologia*, vol. 48, no. 9, pp. 1749–1755, 2005.

[23] E. Succurro, M. A. Marini, F. Arturi et al., "Usefulness of hemoglobin A1c as a criterion to define the metabolic syndrome in a cohort of italian nondiabetic white subjects," *American Journal of Cardiology*, vol. 107, no. 11, pp. 1650–1655, 2011.

[24] K. C. Sung and E. J. Rhee, "Glycated haemoglobin as a predictor for metabolic syndrome in non-diabetic Korean adults," *Diabetic Medicine*, vol. 24, no. 8, pp. 848–854, 2007.

[25] H. Kim, C. Kim, E. Kim, S. Bae, and J. Park, "Usefulness of hemoglobin A1c as a criterion of dysglycemia in the definition of metabolic syndrome in Koreans," *Diabetes Research and Clinical Practice*, vol. 95, no. 3, pp. 333–339, 2012.

[26] M. Janghorbani and M. Amini, "Comparison of glycated hemoglobin with fasting plasma glucose in definition of glycemic component of the metabolic syndrome in an Iranian population," *Diabetes & Metabolic Syndrome: Clinical Research & Reviews*, vol. 6, no. 3, pp. 136–139, 2012.

[27] J. Dilley, A. Ganesan, R. Deepa et al., "Association of A1C with cardiovascular disease and metabolic syndrome in asian indians with normal glucose tolerance," *Diabetes Care*, vol. 30, no. 6, pp. 1527–1532, 2007.

[28] Q. M. Nguyen, S. R. Srinivasan, J. Xu, W. Chen, and G. S. Berenson, "Distribution and cardiovascular risk correlates of hemoglobin A1c in nondiabetic younger adults: the Bogalusa Heart Study," *Metabolism*, vol. 57, no. 11, pp. 1487–1492, 2008.

[29] W. Owiredu, N. Amidu, E. Gockah-Adapoe, and R. Ephraim, "The prevalence of metabolic syndrome among active sportsmen/sportswomen and sedentary workers in the Kumasi metropolis," *Journal of Science and Technology (Ghana)*, vol. 31, no. 1, 2011.

[30] A. M. Kirkendall, W. E. Connor, F. Abboud, S. P. Rastogi, T. A. Anderson, and M. Fry, "The effect of dietary sodium chloride on blood pressure, body fluids, electrolytes, renal function, and serum lipids of normotensive man," *Translational Research*, vol. 87, no. 3, pp. 418–434, 1976.

[31] K. G. Alberti, R. H. Eckel, S. M. Grundy et al., "Harmonizing the metabolic syndrome: a joint interim statement of the international diabetes federation task force on epidemiology and prevention; National heart, lung, and blood institute; American heart association; World heart federation; International atherosclerosis society; and international association for the study of obesity," *Circulation*, vol. 120, no. 16, pp. 1640–1645, 2009.

[32] E. Ferrannini, "Is insulin resistance the cause of the metabolic syndrome?" *Annals of Medicine*, vol. 38, no. 1, pp. 42–51, 2009.

[33] S. R. Kashyap and R. A. Defronzo, "The insulin resistance syndrome: physiological considerations," *Diabetes and Vascular Disease Research*, vol. 4, no. 1, pp. 13–19, 2016.

[34] M. Brownlee, "Biochemistry and molecular cell biology of diabetic complications," *Nature*, vol. 414, no. 6865, pp. 813–820, 2001.

[35] S. H. Park, J. S. Yoon, K. C. Won, and H. W. Lee, "Usefulness of glycated hemoglobin as diagnostic criteria for metabolic syndrome," *Journal of Korean Medical Science*, vol. 27, no. 9, pp. 1057–1061, 2012.

[36] X. Zhou, Z. Pang, W. Gao et al., "Performance of an A1C and fasting capillary blood glucose test for screening newly diagnosed diabetes and pre-diabetes defined by an oral glucose tolerance test in Qingdao, China," *Diabetes Care*, vol. 33, no. 3, pp. 545–550, 2010.

[37] L. Monnier, H. Lapinski, and C. Colette, "Contributions of fasting and postprandial plasma glucose increments to the overall diurnal hyperglycemia of type 2 diabetic patients: variations with increasing levels of HbA1c," *Diabetes Care*, vol. 26, no. 3, pp. 881–885, 2003.

[38] R. M. Cohen, R. S. Franco, P. K. Khera et al., "Red cell life span heterogeneity in hematologically normal people is sufficient to alter HbA1c," *Blood*, vol. 112, no. 10, pp. 4284–4291, 2008.

[39] P. K. Khera, C. H. Joiner, A. Carruthers et al., "Evidence for Interindividual Heterogeneity in the Glucose Gradient Across the Human Red Blood Cell Membrane and Its Relationship to Hemoglobin Glycation," *Diabetes*, vol. 57, no. 9, pp. 2445–2452, 2008.

[40] R. M. Cohen, H. Snieder, C. J. Lindsell et al., "Evidence for independent heritability of the glycation gap (glycosylation gap) fraction of HbA1c in nondiabetic twins," *Diabetes Care*, vol. 29, no. 8, pp. 1739–1743, 2006.

[41] J. M. Boltri, I. S. Okosun, M. Davis-Smith, and R. L. Vogel, "Hemoglobin A1C levels in diagnosed and undiagnosed Black, Hispanic, and White persons with diabetes: Results from NHANES 1999-2000," *Ethnicity & Disease*, vol. 15, no. 4, pp. 562–567, 2005.

[42] F. B. Piel, A. P. Patil, R. E. Howes et al., "Global epidemiology of Sickle haemoglobin in neonates: a contemporary geostatistical model-based map and population estimates," *The Lancet*, vol. 381, no. 9861, pp. 142–151, 2013.

[43] B. Modell and M. Darlison, "Global epidemiology of haemoglobin disorders and derived service indicators," *Bulletin of the World Health Organization*, vol. 86, no. 6, pp. 480–487, 2008.

[44] F. Mockenhaupt, S. Ehrhardt, J. Cramer et al., "Hemoglobin C and resistance to severe malaria in ghanaian children," *The Journal of Infectious Diseases*, vol. 190, no. 5, pp. 1006–1009, 2004.

16

Sustaining, Forming and Letting Go of Friendships for Young People with Inflammatory Bowel Disease (IBD): A Qualitative Interview-Based Study

Alison Rouncefield-Swales,[1] Bernie Carter [ID],[1] Lucy Bray,[1] Lucy Blake,[1] Stephen Allen,[2] Chris Probert,[3] Kay Crook,[4] and Pamela Qualter[5]

[1]Faculty of Health, Social Care & Medicine, Edge Hill University, Ormskirk, UK
[2]Liverpool School of Tropical Medicine, Liverpool, UK
[3]Institute of Translational Medicine, University of Liverpool, Liverpool, UK
[4]St. Mark's & Northwick Park, London North West University Healthcare NHS Trust, London, UK
[5]Manchester Institute of Education, University of Manchester, Manchester, UK

Correspondence should be addressed to Bernie Carter; bernie.carter@edgehill.ac.uk

Academic Editor: Katarzyna Zorena

Inflammatory bowel disease (IBD) is an incurable, chronic, gastrointestinal condition that can constrain young people's social relationships. Few studies have specifically explored friendships of people with IBD. This qualitative, participatory study used interviews, photographs, and friendship maps to explore friendships and friendship networks of young people with IBD. An online Young Person's Advisory Group was actively engaged throughout the study. Thirty-one young people participated ($n = 16$ males, $n = 15$ female; $n = 24$ Crohn's disease, $n = 6$ ulcerative colitis, $n = 1$ IBD-unclassified; the mean age at study was 18.7 years; range 14-25 years). Findings present a metatheme "The importance and meaning of friendships" and three interwoven subthemes of "Sustaining friendships," "Forming new friendships," and "Letting go of friendships." Friendship was important to the young people with IBD, providing support, but associated with challenges such as disclosure. Such challenges could be mitigated by clearer conversations with clinicians about friendships and more extensive conversations about friendships and long-term conditions in education settings.

1. Introduction

Inflammatory bowel disease (IBD) is an incurable, chronic, relapsing, and debilitating gastrointestinal condition [1], which includes Crohn's disease and ulcerative colitis and IBD-unclassified. It is characterised by uncertainty, unpredictability, and the intrusiveness of symptoms [2, 3]. Research on IBD and young people has been primarily biomedical, with scant attention paid to the psychosocial aspects of living with IBD [4], such that we know little about the challenges of IBD on peer relationships and friendships.

1.1. Challenges of IBD. IBD is challenging for young people [5]; common symptoms are diarrhoea, abdominal pain, weight loss, blood in the stools, and fatigue [6, 7]. Treatments for IBD, such as high-dose steroids, can have adverse effects on mood and behaviour. Young people with IBD can experience psychological morbidity [8] and have a reduced Health Related Quality of Life (HRQoL) compared to their peers [9, 10]. Living with IBD increases anxiety and stress among young people and their families, although the reported levels and prevalence of anxiety and depressive symptoms vary across studies [2, 11–16].

The unpredictability of the course of IBD and the embarrassing nature of the symptoms can result in uncomfortable social experiences and constrained social relationships. Young people may conceal their disease [17] from other people in an effort to reduce stigma and people's negative perceptions [18] and avoid rejection by their peers [4]. Having to take time away from their peer group due to symptoms and hospitalisation can heighten loneliness [19, 20] and the feeling of missing out on life [2].

1.2. Friendships and Peer Relationships. Friendship is defined as "a relationship between two individuals characterised by support, time, intimacy, trust, affection, and the ability to manage conflict" [21] ^{p330}. Young people's friendships are complex, dynamic, and fragile with "deep intrapersonal and interpersonal implications" [22] ^{p2}. As they grow up, young people increasingly seek companionship, intimacy, romantic relationships and emotional support, and a sense of identity and belonging from their friends rather than their family [23–25]. Friendships play an increasingly central role in young people's lives as they move into adolescence [26]. Friendships provide a context for the development of values, definition of roles, and refinement of the social skills which are necessary to maintain future relationships [27]. While instability and change are typical during childhood, friendships [28] by adolescence friendships often become more stable with young people seeking intimacy and emotional support from their friends [28, 29].

Friendships and positive peer relationships can provide benefits, supporting young people's social-emotional development [30, 31], mental health [32, 33], self-esteem, and well-being [34] and buffering them from social disconnection and disappointment [35]. However, peer relationships entail costs [36, 37]. While care, concern, trust, loyalty, emotional support, understanding, and intimacy are salient qualities in friendships [38, 39], friendships can also lead to vulnerability, rejection, and unmet expectations [36]. Persistent peer relationship problems can be a source of conflict [36], negatively impacting engagement with education [40] and resulting in higher self-reported levels of depression, anxiety, and loneliness [41, 42]. These issues contribute to poor health well into adulthood [43], with long-term impacts on future friendship quality [44].

Theories of friendship development suggest they are developed and maintained through interconnected factors such as proximity, mutual appeal and positive outcomes [45], shared values, interests, activities, and the level of affection the relationship provides [37]. Changes to those factors can affect their stability [45] as changes can to social networks and health status of members of the dyad [46]. The path of friendship varies; friendships may remain, dissolve, or transform [47].

Few studies have specifically explored friendship quality of people with IBD [48, 49]. Our study is aimed at addressing this deficit by exploring the impact of IBD on the social relationships and psychological functioning of young people (14-25 years) with the condition. We chose to do this by adopting a methodological approach that offered young people with IBD the opportunity to narrate and contextualise their friendship experiences.

2. Method

This paper reports qualitative findings from a sequential two-phase study that explored the social lives of young people with IBD. Phase 1 (quantitative) findings are reported elsewhere. The in-depth qualitative study (Phase 2) used an Interpretive Description [50] approach and participatory interview methods.

2.1. Aim. The specific aim of the qualitative study was to explore young people's friendships and their friendship networks. The research question underpinning this study was "What experiences of friendship do young people with IBD have and what sort of friendship networks do they have?"

2.2. Settings. The settings were clinical areas (outpatient clinics and day case wards) within two university hospitals serving a major city situated in the North West of England; one provides children's services, the other adult services. Using convenience sampling, young people were recruited to participate in the Phase 1 survey via invitation letters sent out from hospital clinics.

2.3. Recruitment. Young people aged 14-25 years, diagnosed with IBD, at any point in their disease trajectory beyond the first three months post-diagnosis and who participated in the Phase 1 survey, could express interest in participating in Phase 2. If interested in Phase 2, they were asked to complete an "expression of interest" form which included their preferred means of being contacted (text, phone, or email). We then contacted the young person 2-3 weeks before their scheduled clinic/hospital visit (usually this was 2-3 months following survey completion). If they were still interested in participating, we posted or emailed information sheets that provided more details about the interview and the creative methods (maps, photographs). Young people had the opportunity to discuss whether they wanted to use creative methods, with additional guidance, if needed, being provided. In the week before their appointment, we made arrangements to meet them at their clinic/hospital visit. Consent/assent or a decision to not participate was finalised at the visit and the interview undertaken, if appropriate. Of those who participated in Phase 1, 59 young people provided contact details and expressed an interest in participating in Phase 2. Of these, 28 were unable to participate due to not having a scheduled clinic appointment within the timescale of the study, not attending their clinic appointment or researcher unavailability.

2.4. Methods. Our use of multiple qualitative methods (interviews, friendship maps, and photographs) was aimed at promoting conversation and exploration; the young people could choose which method(s) to engage with. All three methods were underpinned by the values of person-centredness and aimed at positioning the young people as experts of their own experience and facilitating their control over what they shared during their interaction with the researcher. Person-centeredness emphasises the importance of building relationships based on mutual respect and understanding [51]. In research practice, the values of person-centredness are expressed through reciprocity, mutuality, and being present in the research relationships [52].

2.4.1. Interviews. The interview was conversational in nature, creating opportunities for the young people to talk about the things that mattered to them; an interview guide was available (see Supplementary File). The interviews, including the dialogue about the maps and photos, were audio-recorded with the young person's permission and later transcribed. All interviews were conducted in a quiet and private setting at a routine clinic or hospital visit (October 2018-April 2019). Researchers had no clinical relationship with the young people, though on some occasions, the interviewer had met the young person in Phase 1.

2.4.2. Friendship Maps. Our approach to friendship maps was based on a participatory mapping technique [53]. Participatory mapping is an interactive approach which uses accessible and straightforward visualisations (e.g., spider diagrams) to enable participants to describe, depict, and theorise how they have represented features on their map through drawing and talking [53]. The visual mapping of friendships enabled the young people to reflect on the evolution of their friendships (e.g., how friendships had started and how long they had lasted) and exploring changing dynamics, the complexities and nuances of friendship practices, and how the young people experienced different forms of friendship (e.g., what made them good friends, what activities they enjoyed doing together, and what difficulties were encountered). The researchers provided the young people who wanted to create a map with the relevant materials (paper, pencils, and coloured pens), and the young people created their map at the start of their interview. Most maps were simple "spider diagrams" (see Supplementary File, Figures 1 and 2) but were creative in using colours as a way of describing friends "I did her in blue because she's often very depressed, unfortunately" (ID29, F25, CD). Young people used line thickness and length to represent the closeness of relationships with less strong lines representing more tenuous friendships such as "I think with this one [line], it's like friends of a friend" (ID17, F15, CD).

2.4.3. Photographs. The use of photographs drew on photo-elicitation technique [54, 55] as a means of enabling young people to use visual images of their friends and friendships to prompt conversation. The use of photographs to trigger discussion enables a repositioning of power [56], and we hoped that this would help the young people feel more in control of what they wanted to talk about. We anticipated that the photographs would evoke emotions, memories, and ideas and unfold different layers of meaning [55]. We asked the young people to take new or use existing photographs as a trigger for our interviews with them. Some young people came prepared with printed photographs and allowed us to retain copies. However, others shared images on phones and tablets; we did not obtain copies of those. Within the interviews, the young people selected which photographs they wanted to talk about and then we used prompts such as "why did you choose this photograph?," "what is happening?," and "who is in this photograph?" to elicit their experi-

ences and perceptions. Most photographs were of the young person's friends, taken at memorable gatherings or activities, and enabled them to talk about their lives, in particular to describe different connections and friendships.

2.5. Ethical Issues. The study was approved by the North West-Liverpool East Research Ethics Committee (18/NW/0178) and research ethics committees at Edge Hill University and the University of Manchester. Conversations about participation and consent (or assent) were undertaken with the young people (and parents, as appropriate). Specific written consent/assent was gained for the use of photographs and friendship maps.

2.6. Young Person's Advisory Group. Key to our commitment to participatory values, an online Advisory Group of ten young people (15-26 years) with IBD contributed to writing the proposal, was influential in determining methods (e.g., suggesting creative methods to use in the interviews) and advising on dissemination. The benefits to the researchers and the study were that research materials and our dissemination were age-relevant. Benefits reported by the young people were that they could see the impact that their suggestions had made to the progress and quality of the study.

2.7. Analysis. Interview data were subjected to an iterative, interpretive approach in line with Interpretive Description [50], with analysis being supported through the use of field notes and synopses of each young person's data. Analysis initially focused on each young person's data (interview, friendship map or photographs). Each interviewer (AR-S, BC, LBr, and LBl) who had personally undertaken the interview read and reread the transcription to refamiliarise themselves with the data and created a synopsis for each young person. Each interviewer identified preliminary themes and meanings and proposed tentative theoretical connections to reflect the social relationships and psychological functioning of young people. Then, working collaboratively, we shared these themes and ideas with each other and started to group the data in different ways (e.g., age, gender, and disease severity) looking for new patterns, resonances, and differences and a deeper understanding. Some ideas were dropped, but others were strengthened. The highly reflexive process we followed is aimed at enhancing the rigour of the study by ensuring that we challenged any preconceptions, looked deeper for stronger interpretations, and were able to fully justify any claims made [57]. Part of this process involved two researchers (AR-S and BC) working across all interviews to ensure an overall perspective was achieved. This iterative, collaborative process allowed us to reach consensus and create the metatheme "The importance and meaning of friendships" and three interwoven subthemes of "Sustaining friendships," "Forming new friendships," and "Letting go of friendships."

3. Findings

Thirty-one young people participated; of these, five created friendship maps and six utilised photographs within their interviews. Interviews ranged in length from approximately 20 to 60 minutes. In seven of the interviews, at the request

TABLE 1: Key demographics of participants.

ID	Gender	Age years (age diagnosed)	Diagnosis	Surgery (stoma)	Disease activity[(1-4)]
2	Female	14 (11)	Crohn's	No	Mild[4]
4	Male	14 (13)	Crohn's	No	Remission[4]
7	Male	14 (12)	Crohn's	No	Mild[4]
3	Male	15 (9)	Crohn's	Yes (stoma)	Remission[4]
5	Male	15 (9)	Crohn's	Yes	Mild[4]
16	Male	15 (11)	Crohn's	No	Remission[4]
17	Female	15 (12)	Crohn's	No	Moderate[4]
27	Female	15 (11)	Crohn's	No	Remission[4]
1	Female	16 (11)	Crohn's	No	Mild[4]
6	Female	16 (13)	Crohn's	No	Remission[4]
14	Female	16 (10)	Crohn's	Yes	Remission[4]
15	Male	16 (15)	Crohn's	No	Remission[4]
28	Female	19 (8)	Crohn's	Yes	Remission[3]
21	Female	20 (19)	Crohn's	No	Remission[3]
24	Male	20 (12)	Crohn's	No	Mild[3]
31	Female	20 (12)	Crohn's	Yes	Moderate[3]
23	Male	21 (14)	Crohn's	No	Remission[3]
25	Male	21 (20)	Crohn's	Yes (stoma)	Remission[3]
19	Male	22 (21)	Crohn's	Yes	Remission[3]
12	Female	23 (15)	Crohn's	Yes	Mild[3]
22	Male	24 (16)	Crohn's	No	Moderate[3]
30	Male	24 (19)	Crohn's	No	Remission[3]
18	Female	25 (23)	Crohn's	Yes	Mild[3]
29	Female	25 (23)	Crohn's	Yes	Mild[3]
13	Female	16 (15)	Ulcerative colitis	No	Remission[1]
26	Male	16 (12)	Ulcerative colitis	No	Mild[1]
9	Female	21 (8)	Ulcerative colitis	No	Remission[2]
11	Female	21 (16)	Ulcerative colitis	No	Moderate[2]
10	Male	23 (20)	Ulcerative colitis	No	Moderate[2]
20	Male	24 (22)	Ulcerative colitis	No	Remission[2]
8	Male	14 (12)	IBD unclassified	No	Remission[1]

[1]Paediatric Ulcerative Colitis Activity Index (PUCAI); [2]Simple Clinical Colitis Activity Index (SSCAI); [3]Harvey-Bradshaw Index (HB Index); [4]weighted Paediatric Crohn's Disease Activity Index (wPCDAI).

of the young person, a parent was present, often informally contributing by clarifying the researcher's questions, supplementing the young person's response, or reminding the young person of activities or events.

Sixteen participants were male, and 15 were female; on average, the age at study was 18.7 years (range 14-25 years); the mean age at diagnosis was 14.4 years (range 8-23 years). Most were White. Most ($n = 21$) had been diagnosed five years or fewer. Twenty-four young people had Crohn's disease (two had stomas), and seven had colitis (six with ulcerative colitis and one with IBD-unclassified). Seventeen were classified as being in remission (a decrease or disappearance of the symptoms), nine had mild disease severity, and five had moderate disease severity (Table 1).

The findings presented in this paper focus on the metatheme "The importance and meaning of friendships" and three interwoven subthemes of "Sustaining friendships," "Forming new friendships," and "Letting go of friendships."

Another paper (Authors, in press) explores young people's decisions about disclosing their diagnosis to friends.

Anonymous quotations are linked to interview number (e.g., ID2), gender, age (F12), and conditions: CD (Crohn's disease), UC (ulcerative colitis), or UnC (IBD-unclassified).

3.1. *The Importance of and Meaning of Friendship to Young People with IBD.* Friends and friendship groups that provided companionship, closeness, connection, acceptance, and fun were important to the young people in this study. Friends provided the young people with opportunities to escape and put their IBD into the background, particularly when they encountered tough times associated with flare-ups, hospitalisation, treatments, surgery, and the ongoing symptoms of IBD. One young person explained:

> *My friends are great... if you've been off a couple of weeks or even if you've got a tube sticking out*

of your nose…. it's just, 'oh what's that?' and I explain quite quick and they're like 'oh, sure, fine '.. back to normal, so that's great (ID3, M15, CD).

Having "people that I can have fun with" (ID17, F15, CD) was important. Equally important was that those friends were "honest with each other" (ID19, M22, CD). Having friends who would be there for them, "to talk to like if I'm not well or something" (ID26, M16, UC) and whom they could trust was essential:

I can talk to them and I trust them a lot, I trust them all, I can tell them anything and they tell me anything (ID17, F15, CD)

Friends who understood and accepted the disruptions associated with IBD and did not blame the young person for those disruptions were important:

My best friend …. Like, I'll be at her house and I'll be like 'oh my tummy hurts. I'm going to the toilet'. She's like, 'don't worry I know you're going to be an hour. I'll be waiting' (ID28, F19, CD).

Some young people mentioned stigma and rejection as issues, reflecting that some people mistakenly believed that IBD was a transmittable disease, noting that "the word disease scares them" (ID6, F16, CD):

… some people don't like it or just because you are different they don't want to see you or speak to you because you've got a disease. (ID1, F16, CD)

Acceptance and "having friends who are very open" (ID11, F21, UC) were core to meaningful friendships and the "sort of people" (ID11, F21, UC) that were valued within the young people's lives. Such friends "grew" with the young person and came to "understand" and accept the stranger aspects of IBD, such as tube-feeding, and could act "normal" even if they had little experience of such things and shared responsibility for sitting with their friend "they would swap each day" (ID27, F15, CD).

Although IBD did not necessarily dominate their lives, young people felt that their IBD was always present, "it's [Crohn's] always there. I think that's the main thing that needs to be said. It's never gone" (ID12, F23, CD).

3.2. Sustaining Friendships. Sustaining existing friendships was important. Having friends meant a lot to the young people; close and trusted friends were key to feelings of connection. Some talked about how some friends who had known them before they got sick "kind of went through that kind of journey with me" (ID22, M24, CD).

Good friendships were reciprocal. Young people acknowledged that when their friends faced difficulties, they were "there" for them: "[I] allowed her to complain like a lot, I tried to be supportive and then the next day I will dump all my load on her and she will help" (ID29, F25, CD). Many friendships were strengthened as a result of IBD

with young people describing their friends becoming "protective" and closer. This closeness did not necessarily require friends to fully understand what the young person was going through:

… they are understanding although they don't understand… they appreciate that I have difficulties sometimes with food or change of bags or whatever… (ID25, M21, CD).

However, some young people found it difficult to sustain friendships; one explained she had "gone into a shell, making it difficult to maintain friendships" (ID21, F20, CD) whereas others found that "It's a lot harder to keep in contact with people" (ID29, F25, CD) or found "it difficult to make plans because… I hate letting them down (ID10, M23, UC). This extra effort to sustain friendships was reflected in the stories they shared:

I was really thankful to them for still being friends with me, I'd been off for quite a while, whilst it didn't become stronger, I knew I could rely on them to remain friends whatever, I'd do the same for them obviously, because that's what friends do (ID3, M15, CD).

IBD created physical and emotional limitations that impacted on young people's ability to maintain friendships. The disruption to the taken-for-granted social aspect of eating was a limitation that many of the young people talked about. This disruption ranged from the apparently modest disruption of sitting in the cinema and "just smelling the popcorn" (ID1, F16, CD) to the challenge of trying to fit special diets in around family routine and time with friends, for example "they say 'Oh let's go get something to eat' and I can't, I've got to have a shake in half an hour" (ID7, M14, CD).

Being able to join in activities they enjoyed with their friends meant working around IBD-related restrictions. Sometimes, that involved self-limiting behaviour to ensure they fit in, such as at university, where going out and drinking were part of social activities:

I won't drink as much as they do… I want to be in a good state in case my bag does come off, which has happened because I dance quite mad…to change it if I need to (ID25, M21, CD).

Some young people talked of being onlookers "just watching them all like having fun" (ID6, F16, CD) with fatigue limiting their ability to participate in normal social activities:

I used to get extremely fatigued so a day at school 9-3:30pm would just exhaust me. So then maybe to think that everyone would go out and do an activity, I'm too tired, I can't go and join in on that. (ID9, F21, UC)

Many went out less often than their friendship group "… If I go out like four or five times a week, week after week, it does put toll on me. So I see them once a week" (ID30, M24, CD). Instead, they often sustained connections with their friends through social media or by phone as "just a phone call. It just completely changes your whole, the whole, feeling your whole surroundings" (ID30, M24, CD).

Good friends were described as those who understood and accommodated young peoples' particular needs, acknowledged their fatigue, and chose activities they could engage in. Tricky conversations with friends, such as those about types of social activities or toilets, often resulted in good friends being accommodating in their plans, "we'll go to this place' cause the toilet's actually quite nice there, you can use it" (ID22, M24, CD). Despite friends being accommodating, some young people felt anxious about worst-case scenarios and "what if" situations when they were out with friends, "It's the sort of fear of what if suddenly I don't feel very well – what if I suddenly have to run to the toilet..." (ID24, M20, CD).

3.3. Forming New Friendships. Forming new friendships was important to the young people. Some talked of feeling confident about making new friends and did not think that their IBD made much difference, and it was a case of "finding the time" (ID11, F21, UC). However, others expressed concerns about how their IBD may influence the perception of them by potential friends. While many talked of the importance of preserving a sense of being "normal" in relationships that were developing, they also expressed a desire to establish friendships with those people who would be understanding about the difficulties that may accompany their IBD:

> I think I'll naturally be more drawn to be closer with people that take it seriously.... Obviously, I wouldn't want to stay friends with someone who just forgets the differences between me and them... in general....my illness isn't really at the forefront of my mind when making friends (ID20, M24, UC).

Situations and transitions such as moving schools, starting college or university, starting work, or becoming involved with new social or group activities were not only opportunities to form new friendships, but also situations where IBD might constrain their chances of making new friends. Worries often reflected the degree to which the young people's identity was linked to their IBD. Many young people wanted to project an identity in which they would be seen as being the "same as" peers:

> Like everyone I want to be perceived as normal, not average but you know the same as everyone else. I don't want it to be that I come with a list of exceptions (ID9, F21, UC).

Projecting "normal" meant that some young people kept their diagnosis to themselves because of fears that it would change their interactions with friends, noting that "I don't think [talking about] bowel movements is the way to go" (ID29, F25, CD) and explaining "I don't want people to start

feeling sorry for me or change the way they treat me because of it" (ID21, F20, CD). The reactions of people where a friendship was in an early stage of development were a real concern, especially in relation to the potential reaction to knowledge about their disease:

> The few times I have brought up my colostomy and Crohn's in Uni... it just turns people feeling sorry for me and which then puts me off talking about it more because I don't want them to feel sorry for me (ID25, M21, CD).

This led to concerns that their identity would be framed by their condition and that potential friendships may stem from people "feel[ing] sorry for me – a sympathy friendship" rather than a true friendship. The young people wanted to make sure they were "not being defined by it [their condition]" (ID10, M23, UC) and wanted friends who knew they were "more than Crohn's" (ID21, F20, CD).

3.4. Letting Go of Friendships. Although IBD had not resulted in the loss of friendships for some young people, "I don't think I've ever lost a friend because of the effects of Crohn's disease" (ID24, M20, CD), others recalled friendships broken by their IBD or times when they felt let down by friends who had failed to understand the magnitude, variety, and impact of symptoms. Some young people talked of how people they had considered to be friends "couldn't be bothered" with them anymore. This often led to questioning the value of those particular friendships:

> I've lost a few friends... because they haven't understood or they'll try and push the matter... They don't realise it's quite hard at times. (ID30, M24, CD).

Some young people talked of how a response to their IBD could negatively affect a friendship:

> I remember her being like....cringey I don't want that [IBD]... you just know who your friends are when you get diagnosed and stuff like that happens (ID21, F20, CD).

Friends "making fun" or making negative or insensitive comments regarding their IBD were difficult to deal with, as was a perception that the young people were somehow using their illness as an excuse to gain benefits such as "sympathy" or the opportunity to "miss exams," even when these supposed benefits "made no sense when you think about it" (ID12, F23, CD).

Negativity from people they had hoped to rely on for support and comfort, feeling abandoned, and rejected by friends were distressing for young people who were already dealing with the physical and emotional consequences of IBD. Some talked of this as a tipping point, a point at which managing their IBD became really difficult. However, the passage of time allowed most of the young people to see the loss of friends in context despite the pain and distress they experienced at the time:

> ... I kind of feel like I'm better off and like I know who is there for me and who's not. So I'm not really bothered. At the time, you know, it was the worst thing in the world (ID28, F19, CD).

4. Discussion

This qualitative, participatory study facilitated young people with IBD to share their experiences of friendship. They recounted the importance of friendships and the personal and emotional challenges of sustaining, forming, and letting go of friendships, adding depth to earlier reports of how IBD may impact on a young person's friendships and social relationships [48, 49]. Although all young people face challenges associated with friendships, the awareness of the importance of friendships was heightened for these young people with IBD by the stress, unpredictability, uncertainty, and stigma associated with the condition, its trajectory, and treatment. Our findings add depth and insight about the nuances of adolescent and young adult friendships which is missing in a previous work [4, 13, 18].

Young people with IBD in the current study talked of the importance of having good friends, friends who were understanding and accepting, friends they could trust and talk to and who made them laugh, and friends who helped them feel socially connected even during illness flares. Those qualities are ones that any young person may view as positive characteristics of a friend [58]. But as with other studies of young people with IBD or other long-term conditions, such qualities were particularly important [59, 60], unsurprisingly considering the challenges they reported about life with IBD.

Interconnection is necessary to develop and maintain friendships [45], and this is often established through being together and shared activities. However, for the young people in the study, establishing and sustaining interconnection were sometimes difficult and, as with other studies, opportunities to make new friends were sometimes diminished [6]. Absence from school, college, or work or symptoms restricting social activities meant that some young people with IBD experienced a sense of isolation. This is at a time when friendships are particularly important, as young people are learning how to navigate, create, and sustain peer group relationships [61]. Other studies addressing the impact of long-term conditions reveal the importance of friends in mitigating the social difficulties, restrictions of the condition, and sense of isolation [62, 63]. We found that while maintaining a sense of being "normal" and keeping pace with peers were important for many young people, they developed tactics and adaptions to work around the physical and emotional limitations imposed by their IBD, as found in other studies of young people with a long-term health condition [62, 64, 65].

Whether through choice or not, the young people tended to concentrate on relationships with their closest, most supportive, and understanding friends who could accommodate the strain and difficulties associated with their IBD. The

breakdown of a friendship might be potentially problematic for young people with IBD who may be perceived as, and indeed may perceive themselves as, different and not conforming with social norms or expectations, as seen with other studies of long-term conditions [66]. As was found in previous studies, young people acknowledged the fragility of friendships and the costs of rejection and unmet expectations [36] but acknowledged the benefits of robust relationships. The loss of some friendships resulted in some young people reporting smaller friendship networks; other studies have also reported ill health impacting on friendships and resulting in smaller friendship networks [13]. Falci and McNeely [67] note that smaller networks can be associated with low perceptions of friend support and belonging but this did not seem to be the case in our study, as the smaller networks were often cohesive and supportive. Our findings align with the research on social networks which emphasise the dynamic landscape of friendships [68]; our young people acknowledged this fluidity in friendships but found conflict perceived as being connected to their IBD difficult to contend with.

Social support after being diagnosed with a long-term condition is important [66], especially for those with stigmatised identity [69]. Some young people in the current study concealed their IBD from friends, while others downplayed the seriousness of their condition. Limiting disclosure and explanations about the "gory detail" are aimed at both protecting their friends and minimising the risk of rejection [17], although a consequence of this could be limiting access to the support that close friends can offer. Friends with a better understanding of IBD and its implications could help sustain social support and potentially mitigate some of the impact of living with IBD. As seen with adults with IBD, young people who were more open about their IBD to a close and trusted network of friends often experienced positive responses: friends developed an understanding of the condition and accommodated restrictions [69] and often became conduits to broader peer relationships [66]. This connects to the work of Flynn et al. [44] who found young people with a supportive network are better able to form reliable and compassionate friendships. Young people in our study described certain friendships as being closer and more meaningful since disclosure [17], possibly reflecting a type of post-traumatic growth, sometimes experienced by young people after trauma exposure [70].

Recommendations arising from our study include the need for better support for young people in terms of managing their concerns and experiences of sustaining, forming, and letting go of friendships. Opportunities exist for conversations to occur that ensure that young people, their friends, and wider peer group can explore friendship, IBD and other long-term conditions. As a result of our findings and in collaboration with our online Advisory Group, we developed a resource to support such conversations (see "Telling My Friends" https://ehu.ac.uk/CrohnsorColitis).

4.1. Limitations. Our findings need to be considered in the context of some limitations. The recruitment of the sample for this phase of the study was from two hospitals within the same city; most participants identified as White, affecting the representativeness of our findings for a broader population. Although only about 20% of the young people created maps and/or shared photographs, we do not perceive this as a limitation. Giving young people choice over which aspects to participate in was fundamental to our person-centred approach, and it generated a supportive context for the interviews. Although parental presence may have shaped what was shared by some young people [71], parental presence was always at the request of the young people, and it always appeared supportive and nondirective. Fewer young people with colitis were interviewed than those with Crohn's, and no young people with severe disease activity chose to participate. Further research exploring the experiences of this population is needed.

Acknowledgments

This work was supported by funding awarded by Crohn's and Colitis UK.

References

[1] A. S. Day, O. Ledder, S. T. Leach, and D. A. Lemberg, "Crohn's and colitis in children and adolescents," *World Journal of Gastroenterology*, vol. 18, no. 41, pp. 5862–5869, 2012.

[2] D. B. Nicholas, A. Otley, C. Smith, J. Avolio, M. Munk, and A. M. Griffiths, "Challenges and strategies of children and adolescents with inflammatory bowel disease: a qualitative examination," *Health and Quality of Life Outcomes*, vol. 5, no. 1, p. 28, 2007.

[3] C. M. Roberts, K. L. Gamwell, M. N. Baudino et al., "Youth and parent illness appraisals and adjustment in pediatric inflammatory bowel disease," *Journal of Developmental and Physical Disabilities*, vol. 31, no. 6, pp. 777–790, 2019.

[4] C. Barned, A. Stinzi, D. Mack, and K. C. O'Doherty, "To tell or not to tell: a qualitative interview study on disclosure decisions among children with inflammatory bowel disease," *Social Science & Medicine*, vol. 162, pp. 115–123, 2016.

[5] L. M. Mackner, R. N. Greenley, E. Szigethy, M. Herzer, K. Deer, and K. A. Hommel, "Psychosocial issues in pediatric inflammatory bowel disease: report of the North American Society for Pediatric Gastroenterology, Hepatology, and Nutrition," *Journal of Pediatric Gastroenterology and Nutrition*, vol. 56, no. 4, pp. 449–458, 2013.

[6] J. J. Ashton, M. Cullen, N. A. Afzal, T. Coelho, A. Batra, and R. M. Beattie, "Is the incidence of paediatric inflammatory bowel disease still increasing?," *Archives of Disease in Childhood*, vol. 103, no. 11, 2018.

[7] J. J. Ashton, A. Harden, and R. M. Beattie, "Paediatric inflammatory bowel disease: improving early diagnosis," *Archives of Disease in Childhood*, vol. 103, no. 4, pp. 307-308, 2018.

[8] A. J. Brooks, G. Rowse, A. Ryder, E. J. Peach, B. M. Corfe, and A. J. Lobo, "Systematic review: psychological morbidity in young people with inflammatory bowel disease – risk factors and impacts," *Alimentary Pharmacology & Therapeutics*, vol. 44, no. 1, pp. 3–15, 2016.

[9] G. Engelmann, D. Erhard, M. Petersen et al., "Health-related quality of life in adolescents with inflammatory bowel disease depends on disease activity and psychiatric comorbidity," *Child Psychiatry and Human Development*, vol. 46, no. 2, pp. 300–307, 2015.

[10] R. N. Greenley, K. A. Hommel, J. Nebel et al., "A meta-analytic review of the psychosocial adjustment of youth with inflammatory bowel disease," *Journal of Pediatric Psychology*, vol. 35, no. 8, pp. 857–869, 2010.

[11] D. Jelenova, J. Prasko, M. Ociskova et al., "Quality of life and parental styles assessed by adolescents suffering from inflammatory bowel diseases and their parents," *Neuropsychiatric Disease and Treatment*, vol. 12, 2016.

[12] E. V. Loftus Jr., A. Guérin, P. Y. Andrew et al., "Increased risks of developing anxiety and depression in young patients with Crohn's disease," *The American Journal of Gastroenterology*, vol. 106, no. 9, pp. 1670–1677, 2011.

[13] J. Haapamäki, R. P. Roine, H. Sintonen, and K. L. Kolho, "Health-related quality of life in paediatric patients with inflammatory bowel disease related to disease activity," *Journal of Paediatrics and Child Health*, vol. 47, no. 11, pp. 832–837, 2011.

[14] K. L. Loreaux, W. N. Gray, L. A. Denson, and K. A. Hommel, "Health-related quality of life in adolescents with inflammatory bowel disease: the relation of parent and adolescent depressive symptoms," *Children's Health Care*, vol. 44, no. 2, pp. 119–135, 2014.

[15] L. Stapersma, G. van den Brink, J. van der Ende et al., "Illness perceptions and depression are associated with health-related quality of life in youth with inflammatory bowel disease," *International Journal of Behavioral Medicine*, vol. 26, no. 4, pp. 415–426, 2019.

[16] G. van den Brink, L. Stapersma, L. E. Vlug et al., "Clinical disease activity is associated with anxiety and depressive symptoms in adolescents and young adults with inflammatory bowel disease," *Alimentary Pharmacology & Therapeutics*, vol. 48, no. 3, pp. 358–369, 2018.

[17] B. Carter, A. Rouncefield-Swales, L. Bray et al., ""I don't like to make a big thing out of it": A qualitative interview-based study exploring factors affecting whether young people tell or do not tell their friends about their IBD," *International Journal of Chronic Diseases*, vol. 2020, Article ID 1059025, p. 11, 2020.

[18] B. Saunders, "Stigma, deviance and morality in young adults' accounts of inflammatory bowel disease," *Sociology of Health & Illness*, vol. 36, no. 7, pp. 1020–1036, 2014.

[19] S. Fourie, D. Jackson, and H. Aveyard, "Living with inflammatory bowel disease: a review of qualitative research studies," *International Journal of Nursing Studies*, vol. 87, pp. 149–156, 2018.

[20] K. L. Gamwell, M. N. Baudino, D. M. Bakula et al., "Perceived illness stigma, thwarted belongingness, and depressive symptoms in youth with inflammatory bowel disease (IBD)," *Inflammatory Bowel Diseases*, vol. 24, no. 5, pp. 960–965, 2018.

[21] A. Roach, "A concept analysis of adolescent friendship," *Nursing Forum*, vol. 54, no. 3, pp. 328–335, 2019.

[22] J. A. Evered, "Friendship in adolescents and young adults with experience of Cancer," *Cancer Nursing*, vol. 43, no. 2, pp. E61–E70, 2020.

[23] W. Furman and A. J. Rose, *Friendships romantic relationships and other dyadic peer relationships in childhood and adolescence: a unified relational perspective*, Wiley, 2015.

[24] A. K. Reitz, J. Zimmermann, R. Hutteman, J. Specht, and F. J. Neyer, "How peers make a difference: the role of peer groups and peer relationships in personality development," *European Journal of Personality*, vol. 28, no. 3, pp. 279–288, 2014.

[25] B. M. Newman, B. J. Lohman, and P. R. Newman, "Peer group membership and a sense of belonging: their relationship to adolescent behavior problems," *Adolescence*, vol. 42, no. 166, pp. 241–263, 2007.

[26] C. L. Bagwell and M. E. Schmidt, *Friendships in Childhood and Adolescence*, The Guilford Press, New York, NY, 2011.

[27] K. H. Rubin, W. M. Bukowski, and B. Laursen, *Handbook of Peer Interactions, Relationships, and Groups*, Guilford Press, 2011.

[28] F. Poulin and A. Chan, "Friendship stability and change in childhood and adolescence," *Developmental Review*, vol. 30, no. 3, pp. 257–272, 2010.

[29] T. J. Berndt, *Obtaining support from friends during childhood and adolescence*, Children's social networks and social supports, 1989.

[30] D. L. Rubin, J. Parmer, V. Freimuth, T. Kaley, and M. Okundaye, "Associations between older adults' spoken interactive health literacy and selected health care and health communication outcomes," *Journal of Health Communication*, vol. 16, Supplement 3, pp. 191–204, 2011.

[31] B. H. Schneider, *Childhood Friendships and Peer Relations: Friends and Enemies*, Routledge, London, Second edition, 2016.

[32] A. Roach, "Supportive peer relationships and mental health in adolescence: an integrative review," *Issues in Mental Health Nursing*, vol. 39, no. 9, pp. 723–737, 2018.

[33] K. Ueno, "The effects of friendship networks on adolescent depressive symptoms," *Social Science Research*, vol. 34, no. 3, pp. 484–510, 2005.

[34] B. Lee, H. J. Park, M. J. Kwon, and J. H. Lee, "A sound mind in a sound body?: the association of adolescents' chronic illness with intrinsic life goals and the mediating role of self-esteem and peer relationship," *Vulnerable Children and Youth Studies*, vol. 14, no. 4, pp. 338–350, 2019.

[35] R. D. Stanton-Salazar and S. U. Spina, "Adolescent peer networks as a context for social and emotional support," *Youth & Society*, vol. 36, no. 4, pp. 379–417, 2016.

[36] D. M. Casper and N. A. Card, ""We were best friends, but . . . ": two studies of antipathetic relationships emerging from broken friendships," *Journal of Adolescent Research*, vol. 25, no. 4, pp. 499–526, 2010.

[37] W. W. Hartup, "The company they keep: friendships and their developmental significance," *Child Development*, vol. 67, no. 1, pp. 1–13, 1996.

[38] M. Azmitia, A. Ittel, and K. Radmacher, "Narratives of friendship and self in adolescence," *New Directions for Child and Adolescent Development*, vol. 2005, no. 107, pp. 23–39, 2005.

[39] W. M. Bukowski, A. F. Newcomb, and W. W. Hartup, *The company they keep: friendships in childhood and adolescence*. *Cambridge*, Cambridge University Press, New York, NY, USA, 1996.

[40] C. Furrer, E. Skinner, and J. Pitzer, "The influence of teacher and peer relationships on students' classroom engagement and everyday resilience," in *NSSE Yearbook: Engaging Youth in Schools: Evidence-Based Models to Guide Future Innovations*, D. Shernoff and J. Bempechat, Eds., Teachers College Records, 2014.

[41] R. A. Harris, P. Qualter, and S. J. Robinson, "Loneliness trajectories from middle childhood to pre-adolescence: impact on perceived health and sleep disturbance," *Journal of Adolescence*, vol. 36, no. 6, pp. 1295–1304, 2013.

[42] P. Qualter, S. L. Brown, K. J. Rotenberg et al., "Trajectories of loneliness during childhood and adolescence: predictors and health outcomes," *Journal of Adolescence*, vol. 36, no. 6, pp. 1283–1293, 2013.

[43] E. Landstedt, A. Hammarström, and H. Winefield, "How well do parental and peer relationships in adolescence predict health in adulthood?," *Scandinavian Journal of Public Health*, vol. 43, no. 5, pp. 460–468, 2015.

[44] H. K. Flynn, D. H. Felmlee, and R. D. Conger, "The social context of adolescent friendships: parents, peers, and romantic partners," *Youth & Society*, vol. 49, no. 5, pp. 679–705, 2014.

[45] G. A. Fine, "The natural history of preadolescent male friendship groups," in *Friendship and social relation in children*, H. C. Foot, A. J. Chapman, and J. R. Smith, Eds., pp. 293–320, Transaction Publishers, Piscataway, NJ, USA, 1980.

[46] S. A. Haas, D. R. Schaefer, and O. Kornienko, "Health and the structure of adolescent social networks," *Journal of Health and Social Behavior*, vol. 51, no. 4, pp. 424–439, 2010.

[47] J. G. Parker and J. Seal, "Forming, losing, renewing, and replacing friendships: applying temporal parameters to the assessment of children's friendship experiences," *Child Development*, vol. 67, no. 5, pp. 2248–2268, 1996.

[48] L. M. Mackner and W. V. Crandall, "Brief report: psychosocial adjustment in adolescents with inflammatory bowel disease," *Journal of Pediatric Psychology*, vol. 31, no. 3, pp. 281–285, 2006.

[49] R. Purc-Stephenson, D. Bowlby, and S. T. Qaqish, ""A gift wrapped in barbed wire" positive and negative life changes after being diagnosed with inflammatory bowel disease," *Quality of Life Research*, vol. 24, no. 5, pp. 1197–1205, 2015.

[50] S. E. Thorne, *Interpretive Description: Qualitative Research for Applied Practice*, Routledge, London, United Kingdom, 2016.

[51] B. McCormack and T. McCance, *Person-Centred Practice in Nursing and Health Care: Theory and Practice*, John Wiley & Sons, 2016.

[52] A. Titchen, S. Cardiff, and S. BiongK. Skovdahl and T. Eide, "The knowing and being of person-centred research practice across worldviews: an epistemological and ontological framework," in *Person-centred Healthcare Research*, B. McCormack, S. Dulmen, and H. Eide, Eds., pp. 31–50, Wiley Blackwell, Chichester, UK, 2017.

[53] N. Emmel, *Participatory mapping: an innovative sociological method*, Real Life Methods, 2008.

[54] K. Ford, L. Bray, T. Water, A. Dickinson, J. Arnott, and B. Carter, "Auto-driven photo elicitation interviews in research with children: ethical and practical considerations," *Comprehensive Child and Adolescent Nursing*, vol. 40, no. 2, pp. 111–125, 2017.

[55] D. Harper, "Talking about pictures: a case for photo elicitation," *Visual Studies*, vol. 17, no. 1, pp. 13–26, 2002.

[56] E. A. Bates, J. J. McCann, L. K. Kaye, and J. C. Taylor, ""Beyond words": a researcher's guide to using photo elicitation in psychology," *Qualitative Research in Psychology*, vol. 14, no. 4, pp. 459–481, 2017.

[57] H. Rettke, M. Pretto, E. Spichiger, I. A. Frei, and R. Spirig, "Using reflexive thinking to establish rigor in qualitative research," *Nursing Research*, vol. 67, no. 6, pp. 490–497, 2018.

[58] L. Wagner, "Good character is what we look for in a friend: character strengths are positively related to peer acceptance and friendship quality in early adolescents," *The Journal of Early Adolescence*, vol. 39, no. 6, pp. 864–903, 2018.

[59] P. A. Forgeron, C. T. Chambers, J. Cohen, B. D. Dick, G. A. Finley, and C. Lamontagne, "Dyadic differences in friendships of adolescents with chronic pain compared with pain-free peers," *Pain*, vol. 159, no. 6, pp. 1103–1111, 2018.

[60] E. Long, T. Barrett, and G. Lockhart, "Chronic health conditions and adolescent friendship: perspectives from social network analysis," *International Journal of Adolescent Medicine and Health*, 2019.

[61] A. Lum, C. E. Wakefield, B. Donnan, M. A. Burns, J. E. Fardell, and G. M. Marshall, "Understanding the school experiences of children and adolescents with serious chronic illness: a systematic meta-review," *Child: Care, Health and Development*, vol. 43, no. 5, pp. 645–662, 2017.

[62] D. J. Tunnicliffe, D. Singh-Grewal, J. Chaitow et al., "Lupus means sacrifices: perspectives of adolescents and young adults with systemic lupus erythematosus," *Arthritis Care & Research*, vol. 68, no. 6, pp. 828–837, 2016.

[63] C. D. Adams, R. M. Streisand, T. Zawacki, and K. E. Joseph, "Living with a chronic illness: a measure of social functioning for children and adolescents," *Journal of Pediatric Psychology*, vol. 27, no. 7, pp. 593–605, 2002.

[64] A. J. Brooks, G. Rowse, A. Ryder et al., "PTU-059 "i can cope right now, because i know where i have come from"; a qualitative exploration of the lived experience of young adults with inflammatory bowel disease," *Gut*, vol. 64, Supplement 1, pp. A85.2–A8A86, 2015.

[65] K. Polidano, C. A. Chew-Graham, B. Bartlam, A. D. Farmer, and B. Saunders, "Embracing a 'new normal': the construction of biographical renewal in young adults' narratives of living with a stoma," *Sociology of Health & Illness*, vol. 42, no. 2, pp. 342–358, 2019.

[66] S. Kirk and D. Hinton, ""I'm not what I used to be": a qualitative study exploring how young people experience being diagnosed with a chronic illness," *Child: Care, Health and Development*, vol. 45, no. 2, pp. 216–226, 2019.

[67] C. Falci and C. McNeely, "Too many friends: social integration, network cohesion and adolescent depressive symptoms," *Social Forces*, vol. 87, no. 4, pp. 2031–2061, 2009.

[68] S. Heath, A. Fuller, and B. Johnston, "Chasing shadows: defining network boundaries in qualitative social network analysis," *Qualitative Research*, vol. 9, no. 5, pp. 645–661, 2009.

[69] N. L. Defenbaugh, "Revealing and concealing ill identity: a performance narrative of IBD disclosure," *Health Communication*, vol. 28, no. 2, pp. 159–169, 2013.

[70] T. E. A. Waters, J. F. Shallcross, and R. Fivush, "The many facets of meaning making: comparing multiple measures of meaning making and their relations to psychological distress," *Memory*, vol. 21, no. 1, pp. 111–124, 2013.

[71] H. Gardner and D. Randall, "The effects of the presence or absence of parents on interviews with children," *Nurse Researcher*, vol. 19, no. 2, pp. 6–10, 2012.

17

Health Conditions, Access to Care, Mental Health and Wellness Behaviors in Lesbian, Gay, Bisexual and Transgender Adults

Richard S. Henry, Paul B. Perrin ⓘ, Ashlee Sawyer, and Mickeal Pugh Jr.

Department of Psychology, Virginia Commonwealth University, Richmond, Virginia, USA

Correspondence should be addressed to Paul B. Perrin; pperrin@vcu.edu

Academic Editor: Karen Hirschman

This study examined relationships among wellness behaviors, physical health conditions, mental health, health insurance, and access to care among a sample of 317 lesbian, gay, bisexual, and transgender (LGBT) adults. Participants completed a web-administered survey from May 2013 to April 2014. Of the sample, 41.6% of the participants reported having one or more health conditions. Most participants (92.1%) reported access to a health care facility and current health insurance coverage (84.9%), though 24.9% of those with health insurance reported being incapable of paying the copayments. Physical health conditions, age, and self-esteem explained 24% of the variance in engagement in wellness behaviors; older age, a greater number of health conditions, higher self-esteem, possession of health insurance, and ability to access to care were associated with increased wellness behaviors. Providing affordable insurance coverage, improving access to care, and properly treating mental health in LGBT individuals could improve wellness behaviors.

1. Introduction

On Oct. 6, 2016, the director of the U.S. National Institute on Minority Health and Health Disparities (NIMHD) announced sexual and gender minority (SGM) individuals as a designated population for health disparity research under the National Institute of Health [1]. This formal designation came about because of the increasing evidence that SGM individuals have higher burdens of certain diseases (e.g., depression, HIV/AIDs, and cancer) and less access to health care [1]. Lesbian, gay, bisexual, and transgender (LGBT) individuals were also included in the *2020 Healthy People* objectives for the first time [2]. *Healthy People* reports are 10-year U.S. national objectives for setting benchmarks and monitoring progress for improving the health of individuals and society [3]. The *2020 Healthy People* report suggests that LGBT individuals face health disparities related to discrimination, social stigma, and denial of civil and human rights [4]. This discrimination has been linked to higher rates of substance use, psychiatric disorders, and suicide [4]. These inclusions have brought greater attention to documenting and understanding the health disparities that exist in the LGBT community.

The LGBT community houses an extremely diverse set of communities, as both gender and sexual minorities are lumped under the same umbrella. These communities face many intersecting issues, including race/ethnicity, ability status, and socioeconomic issues [5]. Different segments of these communities face individual health needs and risks related to their differing social statuses. Despite these individual differences, there are common challenges to their health status [5]. Many of these challenges center on discrimination (both from providers and society), social stigma, and negative stereotypes [6]. LGBT individuals are often grouped together within the research context, despite the existence of unique subgroups; however, some group differences have been documented.

Research into sexual minorities is often limited to those with lesbian, gay, and sometimes bisexual identities. However, this work shows that sexual minorities (lesbian, gay, and bisexual individuals) as a group share increased risk for health disparities compared to heterosexual peers. LGB individuals are more likely to self-identify as having poorer health overall [5]. LBG individuals are also at higher risk for poor mental health, psychological distress, suicidal ideation, mental health disorders (e.g., depression and anxiety), disability, asthma, and physical limitations [2], as well as self-harm, and risky sexual behaviors [7]. Additionally, LGB individuals have higher rates of tobacco, alcohol, and drug use [6, 7] and experience higher rates of homelessness than heterosexual adults [7].

Lesbian and bisexual women report worse global ratings of physical health than heterosexual women [8]. They are less likely to have routine care and cancer screenings including mammography or cervical screenings [5–7]. Lesbian and bisexual women are also more likely to be overweight or obese [5, 8] and experience higher rates of asthma [2, 8] and arthritis [8]. Lesbian and bisexual women are also more likely to become disabled younger [5] and, as they age, experience higher risk of cardiovascular disease [9].

Gay and bisexual men are at increased risk for certain sexually transmitted infections (STIs) and also represent more than half of all HIV cases in the U.S. [2, 5–7]. Evidence is mixed regarding whether they experience higher risk of prostate, anal, testicular, and colon cancer [7]. Gay and bisexual men, similar to lesbian and bisexual women, are more likely to become disabled at a younger age [5]. As they age, they are also more likely to experience poor general health and to live alone [9].

There has been very limited research that has focused specifically on the health status of transgender/gender nonconforming (TGNC) individuals [2]. Trans women experience higher rates of HIV than the general population [2, 6]. Compared to the general population, TGNC individuals also experience higher rates of disability, stress, and poor mental and physical health [9]. The TGNC population experiences higher rates of suicide [7], depression, anxiety, and overall psychological distress [2]. Additionally, TGNC individuals report higher rates of military service [2], incarceration [2], victimization and sexual violence [2, 9], poor general health [2], being uninsured or underinsured [6], poverty, unemployment [7], and violent crime victimization [7].

Poor mental health has been linked to risky/negative health behaviors [10]. In one U.S.-based study examining 28 health risks, 18 were found to differ across genders and 23 were found to differ across sexual orientation [11]. Groups in this study at higher risk were transgender men and pansexual participants (self-harm), bisexual participants (substance use), and transgender women (diet and exercise behaviors) [11]. Subgroups, particularly transgender individuals and queer-identified sexual minority individuals, have limited access to care, are less likely to utilize care, and are more likely to report experience with discrimination in health care [12].

It has been well-documented that LGBT individuals have certain poorer health behaviors compared to heterosexual/-cisgender peers (e.g., lesbian and bisexual women are more likely to smoke) and worse access to care [13–15]. Research into men who have sex with men likewise has documented risky health behaviors (e.g., smoking and not being HIV-tested) and having more restricted access to care [16, 17]. TGNC individuals also face challenges accessing medically necessary and culturally sensitive care, and some rely on two sets of providers, one to assist with general health care and the other to address gender-related concerns [18, 19]. This can be a financial burden, may lead to duplication in medical

tests, getting differing advice on treatment, and could lead to medical errors. However, these studies have primarily documented health behaviors and access to care based on LGBT identity, without examining the relationships existing between access to care and engagement in wellness behaviors.

Broadly defined, health behaviors are those actions taken to improve or maintain health [20, 21]. Wellness behaviors, more specifically, are those behaviors which are designed not merely to prevent illness but to improve overall health and wellness [21, 22]. Wellness behaviors include things such as exercising, having regular doctor and dental visits, and gathering information about one's health [21, 22]. Being diagnosed with a chronic health condition [23] and having high self-esteem [24] are both linked with higher engagement in wellness behaviors.

The purpose of the current study was to document rates of common, potentially serious, and/or chronic health conditions, of health care insurance, and of access to care among a sample of LGBT adults. The study also sought to examine the relationships among common, potentially serious, and/or chronic health conditions, mental health, insurance status, access to care, and wellness behaviors.

2. Methods

2.1. Procedure. This study was conducted using a web-administered survey with data collection occurring from May 2013 to April 2014. Participants were recruited via online groups and forums hosted in the United States. If groups and forums were open, study information and recruitment details were posted directly to community message boards. For closed groups, moderators were contacted to post study information. Both regional and national LGBT organizations were also emailed information about the study and details about recruitment. A research coordinator screened those interested in the study to determine eligibility. Those who met the study criteria were emailed a study survey link using Research Electronic Data Capture (REDCap) a secure web-based database [25, 26] and code. Additionally, in the survey, participants were asked demographic questions including their age and to self-identify (through selecting among a list of options) an identity. Only those who selected sexual and/or gender minority options and were aged 18 or older were included in the current study.

For the study, participant inclusion criteria were to be at least 18 years old and self-identify as a sexual or gender minority. A $15 electronic http://Amazon.com gift card was provided as compensation to participants for completing the survey. An informed consent was obtained from participants, and the study was approved by the host university Institutional Review Board.

2.2. Participants. The sample included 317 individuals who identified as a gender or sexual minority (or both) and were at least 18 years of age. The mean age of participants was 31.0 (SD = 11.16), and the range was 18-66. Participant sexual orientation, gender identity, relationship status, employment status, and family socioeconomic status (SES) can be found in Table 1.

TABLE 1: Participant demographics.

Variable	Total sample n	%
Age M (SD); range	31.0 (11.16); 18-66	—
Gender		
Man	89	28.1
Woman	150	47.3
Transman	26	8.2
Transwoman	29	9.1
Other	23	7.3
Sexual orientation		
Heterosexual	12	3.8
Bisexual	84	26.5
Gay/lesbian	122	38.5
Queer	80	25.2
Other	19	6
†Race/ethnicity		
Asian/Asian-American/Pacific islander	57	18
Black/African-American (non-Latino)	66	20.8
Latino/Hispanic	26	8.2
American-Indian/Native-American	9	2.8
White/European-American (non-Latino)	117	36.9
Multiracial/multiethnic	38	12
Other	4	1.3
Relationship status		
Long term (>12 months) with 1 person	126	39.7
New relationship (<12 months) with 1 person	39	12.3
Dating/in a relationship 1+ person	43	13.6
Not currently dating or in a relationship	109	34.4
Employment status		
Full-time	141	44.5
Part-time	47	14.8
Full-time student	41	12.9
Student and employed	53	16.7
Unemployed	35	11
Family income		
$7,000-14,999	38	12
$15,000-29,999	45	14.2
$30,000-59,999	113	35.6
$60,000-199,999	114	36
$200,000+	7	2.2
Health insurance (yes)	269	84.9
Access to a health care facility (yes)	292	92.1
Insurance, but incapable of paying copayment (yes)	79	24.9

Note. N = 317. †Participants responded to the question "Which racial/ethnic label best describes you?" and were able to select the single best answer choice.

2.3. Measures

2.3.1. Demographics. Survey respondents were asked to report their age (in years), gender, sexual orientation, race/ethnicity, relationship status, education, employment status, and family income level (ranges of USD).

2.3.2. Health-Protective Behavior Scale (HPBS). Health behaviors were measured using the HPBS [21, 27]. There are three subscales of the HPBS: one focused on preventative behaviors, a second on risk-taking behaviors, and a third assessing traffic risk [21]. Only the preventative behavior subscale was used in the current study, which contains 10 items answered on a five-point self-report scale ranging from 1 (*Not at all like me*) to 5 (*Very much like me*). Scores are totaled and range from 10 to 50, with higher scores indicating stronger engagement in wellness behaviors. In the current study, the internal validity was acceptable ($\alpha = .79$).

2.3.3. Hopkins Symptom Checklist 25 (HSCL-25). Anxiety and depressive symptomology was assessed using the HSCL-25 [28]. The HSCL-25 contains a 15-item self-report measure for depression and a 10-item self-report measure for anxiety to evaluate how much over the previous week an individual was bothered or distressed by their symptoms. A mean score is calculated from participants' responses using a four-point Likert-type scale ranging from 1 (*Not at all*) to 4 (*Extremely*), with more severe symptoms indicated by higher scores. Established clinically significant cutoffs of 1.75 are used for each subscale [29, 30]. In the current study, internal validity for the anxiety items was good ($\alpha = .89$) and excellent for the depression items ($\alpha = .93$).

2.3.4. Rosenberg Self-Esteem Scale (RSES). Self-esteem was measured using the RSES [31]. It is a 10-item scale in which statements are rated on a four-point Likert-type scale from 0 (*Strongly disagree*) to 3 (*Strongly agree*). Scores can range from 0 to 30, and a sum score is calculated such that higher scores indicate higher self-esteem [31]. In the current study, internal validity was excellent ($\alpha = .91$).

2.3.5. Satisfaction with Life Scale (SWLS). The SWLS is a measure of global subjective well-being without specific time parameters. There are five self-report items answered on a six-point Likert-type scale ranging from 1 (*Strongly disagree*) to 5 (*Strongly agree*). The five items each examine a different domain to create an overall satisfaction score, with higher scores indicating higher levels of satisfaction [32]. In the current study, internal validity was good ($\alpha = .88$).

2.3.6. Insurance and Access. Three researcher-generated questions were used to assess whether participants were insured ("Do you currently have health insurance"), if they otherwise had access to care ("If not, do you have access to a health care facility if you needed care"), or were able to utilize the health insurance ("Do you have health insurance, but find yourself incapable of paying your copayment for care").

2.3.7. Health Conditions. A researcher-generated questionnaire of common, potentially serious, and/or chronic health conditions regularly assessed for in primary care clinic intake forms was used to assess self-reported health conditions.

2.4. Data Analysis Plan. Skewness and kurtosis coefficients were calculated for the primary variables under scrutiny

TABLE 2: Health conditions.

Condition	n	%
AIDS/HIV	4	1.3
Arthritis/gout	16	5
Asthma	52	16.4
Blood disease	2	.6
Cancer	9	2.8
Diabetes	9	2.8
Epilepsy/seizures	5	1.6
Hepatitis A	1	.3
Hepatitis B or C	4	1.3
Leukemia	1	.3
Sickle cell disease	1	.3
Thyroid disease	13	4.1

Note. $N = 317$.

(anxiety, depression, self-esteem, satisfaction with life, and number of self-reported health conditions). In terms of the main analyses, first, the rates of health care access and health conditions in the sample were calculated. Second, descriptive statistics for the mental health variables, as well as health insurance and access, were calculated and presented. Third, a bivariate correlation table showing the relationships between all primary variables and demographics in the study was calculated. Fourth, the data were analyzed using a hierarchical multiple regression. In the first step, all demographic variables significantly associated with the outcome were entered. In the second step, access to care and health insurance were entered. In the third step, the number of health conditions was added. In the fourth step, mental health variables (anxiety, depression, satisfaction with life, and self-esteem) were added. All statistical analyses were performed using IBM SPSS 26 statistics software.

3. Results

3.1. Assumption Checks. All skewness coefficients were below a magnitude of .80, and all kurtosis coefficients were below a magnitude of .77, with the exception of self-reported health conditions, which had a skewness coefficient of 1.83 and kurtosis coefficient of 3.44, as would be expected given that over half of the sample did not report a health condition.

3.2. Mental and Physical Health Rates. Of the current survey respondents, 132 individuals (41.6%) reported having one or more health conditions. Of the 132 individuals, 76 reported just one condition (24.0%), 32 reported two conditions (10.1%), 15 reported three conditions (4.7%), 4 reported four conditions (1.3%), and 5 reported five conditions (1.6%). Thus, of the 132 individuals with health conditions, approximately 24 (7.6%) reported three or more health conditions. The most common health conditions reported were asthma (16.4%, $n = 52$), arthritis/gout (5%, $n = 16$), and thyroid disease (4.1%, $n = 13$). See Table 2 for the rates of health conditions.

For mental health, 13% ($n = 42$) of the survey respondents scored above the 1.75 cutoff for clinically significant

depression and 9% ($n = 29$) for clinically significant anxiety (for mean scores, see Table 3). For satisfaction with life, the mean score was 19.36 (SD = 7.38). This score falls in the boundaries between slightly below average and average. For self-esteem, the mean score was 18.01 (SD = 6.17). Among the respondents, 32.50% ($n = 103$) scored below 15—which represents low self-esteem—while only 14.60% ($n = 46$) of respondents' scores fell in the high self-esteem range (25 or above). The mean score for engagement in preventive health behaviors was 32.32 (SD = 6.98), indicating an average endorsement of two-thirds of the preventative health behaviors.

In addition to health rates, participants were asked about health insurance status (i.e., whether they possessed health insurance), ability to pay their copay, and access to care (Table 3). The majority of participants (92.1%, $n = 292$) reported access to a health care facility if they needed once. Most of the respondents (84.9%, $n = 269$) also reported current health insurance coverage. However, of the 269 participants who stated they currently had health insurance, 24.9% ($n = 67$) stated that they found themselves incapable of paying the copayments.

3.3. Correlation Matrix. A correlation table was calculated showing the bivariate relationships among variables in the current study (Table 3). Wellness behaviors were correlated with all the four mental health indicators (depression, anxiety, self-esteem, and satisfaction with life) and number of health conditions. Wellness behaviors were also correlated with having health insurance and access to a health care facility but not with the ability to pay one's copay. Age was positively correlated with wellness behaviors, satisfaction with life, and number of health conditions and was negatively correlated with anxiety, depression, and having insurance but being unable to pay the copay. Family income was positively correlated with wellness behaviors, self-esteem, satisfaction with life, having health insurance, and access to health care and negatively with anxiety and depression. Education level was positively correlated with wellness behaviors, self-esteem, satisfaction with life, number of health conditions, and age and negatively with anxiety, depression, and having insurance but not being able to pay the copay.

3.4. Hierarchical Multiple Regression. In the hierarchical multiple regression predicting health behaviors (Table 4), demographic variables significantly related to wellness behaviors from the correlation matrix (age, family income, and education) were entered into the first step, health insurance status and access to health care into the second step, number of health conditions into the third step, and depression, anxiety, satisfaction with life, and self-esteem into the fourth step. The overall model was significant $F(10, 306) = 9.85$, $p < .001$. After controlling for demographic factors, insurance status, access to care, and number of physical health conditions, age ($\beta = .21$, $p = .001$), having health insurance ($\beta = .12$, $p = .039$), access to health care ($\beta = .15$, $p = .007$), and self-esteem ($\beta = .18$, $p = .010$) were unique predictors of engagement in wellness behaviors.

TABLE 3: Correlations and means.

Variable	1	2	3	4	5	6	7	8	9	10	11	Mean	SD
1. Wellness behaviors												32.32	6.98
2. Anxiety	-.16**											.84	.63
3. Depression	-.25**	.76**										.97	.7
4. Self-esteem	.27**	-.40**	-.58**									18.01	6.17
5. Satisfaction with life	.34**	-.45**	-.60**	.62**								19.36	7.38
6. Health insurance? (yes)	.23**	.02	.04	.06	.10							—	—
7. Access to a health care facility? (yes)	.23**	-.08	-.04	.13*	.05	—						—	—
8. Insurance but incapable of paying copayment? (yes)	-.02	.23**	.18**	-.06	-.08	—	—					—	—
9. Health condition (number)	.04	.08	-.01	-.10	.02	.09	.03	-.11				—	—
10. Age	.27**	-.19**	-.14*	.03	.19**	.07	.11	-.13*	.38**			—	—
11. Family income	.19**	-.18**	-.16**	.24**	.18**	.15**	.32**	-.07	.00	-.01		—	—
12. Education	.25**	-.21**	-.19**	.22**	.24**	-.01	.11*	-.13*	.16**	.37**	-.23**	—	—

Note. $N = 317$; *$p < .05$; **$p < .01$. Correlations between two dichotomous variables were calculated as a Pearson correlation and between a dichotomous and continuous variable as a point-biserial correlation. Correlations between two dichotomous variables are not reported.

4. Discussion

This study examined relationships among physical health conditions, mental health, health insurance, and access to care among a sample of LGBT adults, with a specific focus on engagement in wellness behaviors. As noted in previous literature, the most influential method for reducing chronic illness is through altering individual health behaviors [33]. In the current study, LGBT adults engaged in wellness behaviors at average rates compared to the general population. A hierarchical multiple regression showed that after controlling for demographic factors, health insurance and access to care, and the number of health conditions, anxiety, depression, satisfaction with life, and self-esteem explained an additional 7% of the variance in engagement in wellness behaviors, with 24% explained overall. Within these models, older age, having a higher number of health conditions, greater self-esteem, and having health insurance and access to care were associated with greater wellness behavior engagement.

Over 40% of LGBT adults in this study reported having one or more health conditions, with asthma, arthritis/gout, and thyroid disease being the most commonly reported. These findings are similar to the rates of health conditions documented among LGBT individuals in other research which note higher rates of physical health issues among LGBT individuals [2]. A notable proportion of participants scored within the clinically significant ranges for depression and anxiety (13% and 9%, respectively). These findings are also in line with previous work noting elevated rates of mental health issues among LGBT individuals [2, 7].

The finding that number of health conditions was positively associated with engagement in wellness behaviors in both the correlation matrix and multiple regression supports existing literature showing that diagnosis of chronic health conditions can serve as a "teachable moment" for individuals and can result in increased engagement in wellness behaviors [23]. Individuals with health conditions may become moti-

vated to make changes in their health behaviors to limit their experience of symptoms and slow the progression of the illness [23]. Having chronic health conditions has also been related to more frequent visits with medical providers [23], which can create more opportunities for providers to educate the individual about health behaviors and encourage them to engage in wellness behaviors [34].

Self-esteem was positively associated with engagement in wellness behaviors and—aside from age—represented the strongest relationship among all predictors, which supports previous work showing that higher self-esteem is related to positive health behaviors [24], psychosocial health [31], and well-being in health [35]. Recent work by Taylor and colleagues [36] has also investigated self-esteem as it relates to self-injury (including self-mutilation, attempted suicide, and substance abuse behaviors) among LGBT individuals and found that self-esteem negatively predicted this relationship above and beyond anxiety and depressive symptoms. The present study, in conjunction with previous work, suggests that feelings of self-worth among LGBT individuals may be a crucial factor in determining engagement in wellness and health promoting behaviors.

Health insurance and access to care were positively associated with wellness behaviors. This finding illustrates a connection between access to care and health behaviors. Although most participants reported having insurance and access to a health care facility (85% and 92%, respectively), approximately one out of every four of those with insurance indicated that they were unable to pay their copayment to receive care. This may indicate that although LGBT people in this study reportedly having access to health care facilities and insurance, a substantial proportion still experienced barriers in being able to utilize health services. This is an especially important issue when considering wellness, given that higher rates of health care visits have been associated with positive health outcomes [37, 38]. Health care visits serve as a good opportunity for providers to encourage engagement

TABLE 4: Hierarchical multiple regression analysis: wellness behaviors.

Independent variable	ΔR^2	β
Step 1	.12***	
Age		.22***
Family income		.16**
Education		.13*
Step 2	.05***	
Age		.19**
Family income		.10
Education		.15*
Access to care		.11
Health insurance		.16**
Step 3	.01	
Age		.22***
Family income		.10
Education		.15**
Access to care		.10
Health insurance		.17**
Health conditions		−.08
Step 4	.07***	
Age		.21**
Family income		.06
Education		.11
Access to care		.12*
Health insurance		.15**
Health conditions		−.08
Anxiety		.15
Depression		−.17
Satisfaction with life		.05
Self-esteem		.18*
Total R^2	.24***	

Note. $N = 317$; *$p < .05$, **$p < .01$, ***$p < .001$, two-tailed.

in health behaviors [34]. If LGBT individuals cannot afford to access health services, they may miss out on important opportunities for wellness behavior intervention.

Results from this study provide implications for clinical care and public policy. From a public health perspective, affordability of health care may be a common barrier to services among LGBT individuals. Study results also suggest that health behaviors may be malleable given that health insurance status, access to a health care facility, health conditions, and self-esteem uniquely predicted health behaviors. Increasing affordable insurance coverage, improving access to care, and properly treating mental health in LGBT individuals could have the effect of improving health behaviors.

For providers, because 41.6% of the sample endorsed one or more health conditions, there is a high necessity for established health care access and utilization for LGBT individuals. Factors related to mental health were found to correlate with wellness behaviors, which suggest that

poorer mental health status may curtail proactive health care behaviors. This trend may result in the proliferation of comorbid health conditions which can lead to an exacerbation of health disparities observed in LGBT populations. Due to the elevated rates of mental health concerns among both the current study sample and previous literature, routine screeners by health care providers that sensitively assess mental health functioning and feelings about oneself (including self-esteem) as a part of treatment planning may be beneficial in identifying individuals who may need additional support in maintaining their wellness behaviors.

4.1. Limitations. The current study has several limitations and, as a result, directions for future research. Researchers recruited participants using web-based convenience sampling, which may not have generated a representative sample of the LGBT community. Although the sample was quite diverse in terms of gender and sexual minority identities, as well as race/ethnicity, these results can only be applied to individuals with access to the online forums similar to where the study recruited. The relationship among insurance status, access to health care services, and wellness behaviors may operate differently among populations with limited access to online forums and internet-based social networking. Thus, future research should recruit participants through both online and in-person domains in order to obtain a more inclusive sample. Another limitation of this study is that some of the data were collected before most of the Affordable Care Act (ACA) went into effect which occurred on January 1, 2014. Thus, the difference in insurance coverage status may have differentially affected health care behaviors for a part of the sample. Because the location of participants is unknown, the rollout of ACA-mandated health coverage may or may not have occurred in their state during the time of data collection. Finally, during data collection, gay and lesbian identities were collected in one category ("gay/lesbian"), and these differences cannot be distinguished, particularly for the TGNC subsample. As a result, differences in the primary variables could not be broken down by sexual orientation, and future research should consider doing so.

5. Conclusion

This is the first study to assess the relationships among health condition status, insurance coverage, access to care, mental health, and health behaviors in LGBT individuals. These findings underscore the moderate to high rates of physical and mental health conditions in this population and emphasize the necessity of accessible, affordable, and culturally sensitive care.

Acknowledgments

The survey software for this study was funded by the National Center for Research Resources (award number UL1TR002649).

References

[1] National Institute for Health, *Director's Message*, 2016, https://www.nimhd.nih.gov/about/directors-corner/message.html.

[2] K. I. Fredriksen-Goldsen, J. M. Simoni, H.-J. Kim et al., "The health equity promotion model: reconceptualization of lesbian, gay, bisexual, and transgender (LGBT) health disparities," *American Journal of Orthopsychiatry*, vol. 84, no. 6, pp. 653–663, 2014.

[3] US Department of Health and Human Services, *About healthy people*https://www.healthypeople.gov/2020/About-Healthy-People.

[4] US Department of Health and Human Services, *Lesbian, gay, bisexual, and transgender health*https://www.healthypeople.gov/2020/topics-objectives/topic/lesbian-gay-bisexual-and-transgender-health.

[5] H. Daniel, R. Butkus, and Health and Public Policy Committee of American College of Physicians, "Lesbian, gay, bisexual, and transgender health disparities: executive summary of a policy position paper from the American College of Physicians," *Annals of Internal Medicine*, vol. 163, no. 2, pp. 135–137, 2015.

[6] L. Mollon, "The forgotten minorities: health disparities of the lesbian, gay, bisexual, and transgendered communities," *Journal of Health Care for the Poor and Underserved*, vol. 23, no. 1, pp. 1–6, 2012.

[7] B. McKay, "Lesbian, gay, bisexual, and transgender health issues, disparities, and information resources," *Medical Reference Services Quarterly*, vol. 30, no. 4, pp. 393–401, 2011.

[8] J. M. Simoni, L. Smith, K. M. Oost, K. Lehavot, and K. Fredriksen-Goldsen, "Disparities in physical health conditions among lesbian and bisexual women: a systematic review of population-based studies," *Journal of Homosexuality*, vol. 64, no. 1, pp. 32–44, 2017.

[9] K. I. Fredriksen-Goldsen, C. P. Hoy-Ellis, J. Goldsen, C. A. Emlet, and N. R. Hooyman, "Creating a vision for the future: key competencies and strategies for culturally competent practice with lesbian, gay, bisexual, and transgender (LGBT) older adults in the health and human services," *Journal of Gerontological Social Work*, vol. 57, no. 2–4, pp. 80–107, 2014.

[10] S. Cohen, J. E. Schwartz, E. J. Bromet, and D. K. Parkinson, "Mental health, stress, and poor health behaviors in two community samples," *Preventive Medicine*, vol. 20, no. 2, pp. 306–315, 1991.

[11] K. B. Smalley, J. C. Warren, and K. N. Barefoot, "Differences in health risk behaviors across understudied LGBT subgroups," *Health Psychology*, vol. 35, no. 2, pp. 103–114, 2016.

[12] K. Macapagal, R. Bhatia, and G. J. Greene, "Differences in healthcare access, use, and experiences within a community sample of racially diverse lesbian, gay, bisexual, transgender, and questioning emerging adults," *LGBT Health*, vol. 3, no. 6, pp. 434–442, 2016.

[13] A. L. Diamant, C. Wold, K. Spritzer, and L. Gelberg, "Health behaviors, health status, and access to and use of health care: a population-based study of lesbian, bisexual, and heterosexual women," *Archives of Family Medicine*, vol. 9, no. 10, pp. 1043–1051, 2000.

[14] B. D. Kerker, F. Mostashari, and L. Thorpe, "Health care access and utilization among women who have sex with women: sexual behavior and identity," *Journal of Urban Health*, vol. 83, no. 5, pp. 970–979, 2006.

[15] J. C. White and V. T. Dull, "Health risk factors and health-seeking behavior in lesbians," *Journal of Women's Health*, vol. 6, no. 1, pp. 103–112, 1997.

[16] M. D. Kipke, K. Kubicek, G. Weiss et al., "The health and health behaviors of young men who have sex with men," *The Journal of Adolescent Health*, vol. 40, no. 4, pp. 342–350, 2007.

[17] D. J. McKirnan, S. N. Du Bois, L. M. Alvy, and K. Jones, "Health care access and health behaviors among men who have sex with men: the cost of health disparities," *Health Education & Behavior*, vol. 40, no. 1, pp. 32–41, 2013.

[18] E. Lombardi, "Enhancing transgender health care," *American Journal of Public Health*, vol. 91, no. 6, pp. 869–872, 2001.

[19] J. Xavier, J. Bradford, M. Hendricks et al., "Transgender health care access in Virginia: a qualitative study," *International Journal of Transgenderism*, vol. 14, no. 1, pp. 3–17, 2013.

[20] M. Bąk-Sosnowska and V. Skrzypulec-Plinta, "Health behaviors, health definitions, sense of coherence, and general practitioners' attitudes towards obesity and diagnosing obesity in patients," *Archives of Medical Science*, vol. 13, no. 2, pp. 433–440, 2017.

[21] R. R. Vickers Jr., T. L. Conway, and L. K. Hervig, "Demonstration of replicable dimensions of health behaviors," *Preventive Medicine*, vol. 19, no. 4, pp. 377–401, 1990.

[22] P. Lebensohn, S. Dodds, R. Benn et al., "Resident wellness behaviors: relationship to stress, depression, and burnout," *Family Medicine*, vol. 45, no. 8, pp. 541–549, 2013.

[23] X. Xiang, "Chronic disease diagnosis as a teachable moment for health behavior changes among middle-aged and older adults," *Journal of Aging and Health*, vol. 28, no. 6, pp. 995–1015, 2016.

[24] C. L. Holt, D. L. Roth, E. M. Clark, and K. Debnam, "Positive self-perceptions as a mediator of religious involvement and health behaviors in a national sample of African Americans," *Journal of Behavioral Medicine*, vol. 37, no. 1, pp. 102–112, 2014.

[25] P. A. Harris, R. Taylor, B. L. Minor et al., "The REDCap consortium: building an international community of software platform partners," *Journal of Biomedical Informatics*, vol. 95, article 103208, 2019.

[26] P. A. Harris, R. Taylor, R. Thielke, J. Payne, N. Gonzalez, and J. G. Conde, "Research electronic data capture (REDCap)—a metadata-driven methodology and workflow process for providing translational research informatics support," *Journal of Biomedical Informatics*, vol. 42, no. 2, pp. 377–381, 2009.

[27] D. M. Harris and S. Guten, "Health-protective behavior: an exploratory study," *Journal of Health and Social Behavior*, vol. 20, no. 1, pp. 17–29, 1979.

[28] L. R. Derogatis, R. S. Lipman, K. Rickels, E. H. Uhlenhuth, and L. Covi, "The Hopkins Symptom Checklist (HSCL): a self-report symptom inventory," *Behavioral Science*, vol. 19, no. 1, pp. 1–15, 1974.

[29] P. T. Hesbacher, K. Rickels, R. J. Morris, H. Newman, and H. Rosenfeld, "Psychiatric illness in family practice," *The Journal of Clinical Psychiatry*, vol. 41, no. 1, pp. 6–10, 1980.

[30] I. Sandanger, T. Moum, G. Ingebrigtsen, T. Sørensen, O. S. Dalgard, and D. Bruusgaard, "The meaning and significance of caseness: the Hopkins Symptom Checklist-25 and the Composite International Diagnostic Interview II," *Social Psychiatry and Psychiatric Epidemiology*, vol. 34, no. 1, pp. 53 59, 1999.

[31] M. Rosenberg, *Society and the Adolescent Self-Image*, Princeton University Press, 1965.

[32] E. Diener, R. A. Emmons, R. J. Larsen, and S. Griffin, "The satisfaction with life scale," *Journal of Personality Assessment*, vol. 49, no. 1, pp. 71–75, 1985.

[33] D. R. Smith, "Reducing healthcare costs through co-op care," *Nursing Management*, vol. 25, no. 6, pp. 44–47, 1994.

[34] V. Kemppainen, K. Tossavainen, and H. Turunen, "Nurses' roles in health promotion practice: an integrative review," *Health Promotion International*, vol. 28, no. 4, pp. 490–501, 2013.

[35] U. Orth and R. W. Robins, "The development of self-esteem," *Current Directions in Psychological Science*, vol. 23, no. 5, pp. 381–387, 2014.

[36] P. J. Taylor, K. Dhingra, J. M. Dickson, and E. McDermott, "Psychological correlates of self-harm within gay, lesbian and bisexual UK university students," *Archives of Suicide Research*, pp. 1–16, 2018.

[37] K. Baicker, S. L. Taubman, H. L. Allen et al., "The Oregon experiment—effects of Medicaid on clinical outcomes," *The New England Journal of Medicine*, vol. 368, no. 18, pp. 1713–1722, 2013.

[38] B. D. Sommers, S. K. Long, and K. Baicker, "Changes in mortality after Massachusetts health care reform: a quasi-experimental study," *Annals of Internal Medicine*, vol. 160, no. 9, pp. 585–593, 2014.

18

The Prevalence and Associated Factors of Hypertension among Adults in Southern Ethiopia

Belachew Kebede,[1] Gistane Ayele,[2] Desta Haftu,[2] and Gebrekiros Gebremichael ⓘ[3]

[1]Public Health, John Snow Inc., Ethiopia
[2]School of Public Health, Arba Minch University, Ethiopia
[3]School of Public Health, Mekelle University, Ethiopia

Correspondence should be addressed to Gebrekiros Gebremichael; gebrekiros.meles@mu.edu.et

Academic Editor: Ivor J. Katz

Background. Hypertension is a growing public health problem in many developing countries including Ethiopia. Determining the prevalence of hypertension and identifying the associated factors is crucial. *Objective.* To assess the prevalence of hypertension and associated factors, among adult population of Arba Minch town, Gamo Zone, Southern Nations, Nationalities and Peoples Region, Ethiopia. *Methods.* A cross-sectional study design was conducted from December 1 to 30, 2017 among adults. Study participants were selected using a multistage systematic sampling method. Data were collected by face-to-face interview after getting written informed consent by using a structured questionnaire. Additionally, weight, height, and blood pressure of participants were measured following standard procedures. Data were entered into a computer using EPI INFO 7 and exported into SPSS version 20 for analysis. Bivariate and multivariable analyses were performed to explore the association between hypertension and associated factors. Multivariable logistic regressions were fitted to control the effect of confounders. *Results.* A total of 784 study participants were included in this study. The overall prevalence of hypertension in Arba Minch Town was 35.2%, (95% CI: 32.4%, 38.4%). Nearly 90% of hypertensive patients were screened for the first time. Age ≥55 years [AOR = 7.74; 95% CI: 2.19, 27.23], income level which is greater than 2501 Ethiopian Birr [AOR = 9.5; 95% CI: 4.5, 20.20], working hour less than seven hours per day [AOR = 12.5; 95% CI: 4.3, 36.1], and chewing "khat" [AOR = 11.06: 95% CI: 4.3, 27.7] were the independently associated factors with hypertension. *Conclusion.* The prevalence of hypertension is found to be high. Increasing awareness on control use of "khat," increasing physical activity, and strengthening community-based periodic screening programs of high-risk populations are recommended.

1. Introduction

Noncommunicable diseases (NCDs) are a major cause of morbidity and mortality globally accounting for about three-fourths of all deaths worldwide [1]. Hypertension is one of the main public health challenges because of its high frequency and associated risks of cardiovascular and kidney diseases such as myocardial infarctions, strokes, and renal failures [2, 3]. Hypertension is the top leading cause of the global burden of disease [4]. The African region did not differ from the global epidemic of NCDs, and, in fact, suffered from the double burden of diseases (communicable and noncom-

municable diseases) [5]. The World Health Organization (WHO) predicted deaths from NCDs would increase globally by 17% over the next ten years where the greatest increase will be in the African region (by 27% or 28 million deaths from NCDs) [6].

Little is known about the magnitude and factors of hypertension in Ethiopia; although, recent evidences indicate that hypertension and raised blood pressure are increasing partly because of the increase in risk factors including smoking, obesity, use of alcohol, and lack of exercise [7].

A systematic meta-analysis from Ethiopia showed about 19.6% prevalence of hypertension with a higher proportion in urban than rural [8]. Similarly, a 15.8% prevalence of raised blood pressure was reported from the national NCDs STEPS survey in 2015 [9].

An up-to-date and comprehensive assessment of the evidence concerning hypertension in Ethiopia is lacking. On the other hand, urbanization is expanding, lifestyles are changing, the literacy rate is low, and people are still living in poverty. Thus, this study assessed the prevalence and associated factors of hypertension among the adult population of Arba Minch town.

2. Methods

2.1. Study Settings. A community-based cross-sectional study was conducted among adult population living in Arba Minch town from December 1 to 30, 2017. The study was done at Arba Minch Town, which is zonal capital city, and it is 505 km from Addis Ababa and 273 km south of the regional capital Hawassa. Based on figures obtained from 2007 National Population and Housing Census of Ethiopia, the adjusted population projection of the total population of the Arba Minch town was 110,104, of whom 54,833 (49.8%) were males and 55,271 (50.2%) were females. Arba Minch town is administratively divided into four subcities, namely, Secha, Sikela, Nechsar, and Abaya. The town had two health centers, 11 kebeles, and 38 urban health extension workers. The town has a total of 57,397 (53.13%) adult population, which means ages 15 years and above [10].

2.2. Population. The source population were all adult persons living in Arba Minch town, and the study population were all selected adult populations who live in the town during the study period. All adult persons whose age is 18-70 years and lived at least 6 months in the town were included. Those who were disabled individuals, pregnant women, known hypertensive patients (self-declared), and persons who were severely diseased were excluded from the study.

2.3. Sample Size and Sampling Procedures. The required sample size for this particular study was determined by the Epi Info version 7 software using a single-population proportion formula $n = (z2^{*} P (1 - P)/d2)$, where "$n$" is the sample size, "$z$" is the standard normal score set at 1.96, "d" is the desired degree of accuracy, and "p" is the estimated proportion of the target population. By taking, $p = 25.1\%$ [11], $z = 1.96$ and $d = 4.5\%$. Based on these assumptions, the final sample size with the design effect of 2 and 10% for nonresponse rate was 784.

Arba Minch town has 11 administrative units or kebeles. Multistage systematic sampling was used, and at first stage, five of the eleven kebeles (45.5%) were selected by lottery method to get representative samples of the population. The second stage was used to select study households by using systematic sampling method, and the sample was proportionally distributed to each selected kebeles. Total number of households was obtained from the town administrative office.

Then, after determining the number of individuals to be studied in each kebele, the sample size in each kebele was divided by the number of households in the kebele to determine the proportion of individuals to be studied in each selected kebele. After getting the sampling fraction in the selected kebeles or administrative units, systematic sampling was used to select the households and a lottery method was used to select the first household. Then, every 3rd unit of households were visited to get the required number of study participants in all selected kebeles of the city. If more than one eligible adult was present in the selected household, one household member was selected randomly using lottery method.

2.4. Variables of the Study

2.4.1. Dependent Variables. Presence or absence of hypertension.

(1) Independent Variables.

  (i) **Socio-demographic variables**: Age, gender, marital status, family history of hypertension, height, weight, body mass index, feeding practice, and sedentary lifestyle (physical inactivity).

  (ii) **Socio-economic variables**: Occupation, monthly income, highest education attained, history of smoking, and alcohol consumption.

(2) Definition of Terms. **Hypertension**: the average of casual systolic Blood Pressure readings ≥140 mmHg and/or diastolic pressure readings ≥90 mmHg [7, 12].

Sedentary lifestyle (physical inactivity): is measured as a response of being always or usually engaged in light/leisure activities for most days of the week or a response of sometimes/never engagement in moderate to intense physical activity outside work for most days of the week that would add up to at least three hours per week of moderate to intense (vigorous) physical activity [13].

Sufficient Fruit and Vegetable Intake: Intake of seven-day history was use and 4-7 days use of fruit and vegetables in a day was regarded as sufficient [12].

Khat: stimulant leaves of a shrub that have a stimulating and euphoric effect when chewed [14, 15].

2.5. Data Collection Procedures. The data were collected using a structured questionnaire through interview and physical measurements. The questionnaire was adapted from the "WHO STEP wise approach to chronic disease risk factor surveillance (STEPS)" [16].

A digital measuring instrument was used to measure the weight of adult individuals to the nearest 100 grams. Weight measuring scales were checked and adjusted to zero levels between each measurement. Height was measured with stadiometer following the standard steps. Blood pressure was measured twice in a sitting position (using a standard sphygmomanometer blood pressure cuff with an appropriate size to cover two-thirds of the upper arm) after the participant rested for at least 5 minutes, with no smoking or caffeine allowed for 30 minutes before measurement. The second measurement was taken 5 minutes after the first measurement. Finally, the mean of the two measurements was taken to determine hypertension. Eight clinical nurses were selected as data collectors, and two experienced health professionals were recruited as supervisors for the fieldwork.

2.6. Data Quality Management. Quality of data were assured by using a structured questionnaire which was translated into Amharic language, back-translated into English, and pretested before the actual survey. A pretest was done among 5% of the sample size among individuals in kebeles that were not included in the study. Data collectors and supervisors were trained for three days on procedures of measuring blood pressure, heart rate, weight, and height of the participants and were also made familiar with the questionnaire.

2.7. Data Processing and Analysis. After the questionnaires were checked for errors and coded, data were entered and cleaned using EPI info version 7 software. Then, it was exported into SPSS version 20 software package for further cleaning and analysis. Data were cleaned by doing simple frequency and cross-tabulation between each independent and dependent variable. Body mass index (BMI) was calculated dividing the weight in kilograms of the participants by the squares of their height in meters. Then, it was categorized as underweight (less than 18.5), normal (18.5-24.9), overweight (25-29.9), and obese (30 and above). Cross-tabulation and bivariate logistic regression were used to explore the relation between hypertension and the different independent variables using crude odds ratio (COR) with 95% CI. Finally, to determine the independent factors associated with hypertension, multivariable logistic regression model was done. Model fitness was checked using Hosmer-Lemeshow test which was 0.23. Variables with $p < 0.05$ in the multivariable analysis were considered significant and presented by adjusted odds ratio (AOR) with 95% CI.

3. Results

3.1. Socio-Demographic Characteristics. A total of 784 participants of ages 18 and above years participated in the study yielding in 100% response rate. Of the total respondents, 344 (43.9%) were males and 440 (56.1%) were females. Nearly half of the study participants (41.5%) were in the age group of 45-54 years followed by 35-44 years (30.1%). Majority of the participants can read and write (89%), were married (74.4%), and had a family history of chronic health diseases (71%). The median monthly income of the respondents was 4500ETB (Table 1).

3.2. Prevalence of Hypertension. The prevalence of adult hypertension was 35.2% (95% CI: 32.4%, 38.4%). The prevalence of hypertension was 54.7% among females and 44.9% among males. Among the hypertensive cases, around ninety percent 251 (90.9%) were newly screened for the first time but the twenty-five participants (9%) had been screened for hypertension before.

3.3. Behavioral Characteristics of Study Participants. Overall, 201 (25.6%) respondents reported that they have ever smoked cigarettes in their lifetime. Eighty-three (10.6%) respondents have ever chewed "khat." Among the study participants, 510 (65.1%) reported that they ever took alcoholic drinks in their lifetime. Daily drinkers were, however, found in only 22 (8.0%) of all ever drinkers who constitute 34.9% of the total study participants. Out of the total study respondents, 208 (26.5%) reported that they regularly have moderate to intense physical activities some times in a week, but the rest 576 (73.5%) did not.

3.4. Biological Characteristics of Study Participants. The body mass index (BMI) of the respondents ranged from 14.6 to 33.8 kg/m^2, with a mean of $24.5 \pm 2.9 \text{ kg m}^2$. Overall, 330 (42.0%) of participants had BMI $< 25.0 \text{ kg/m}^2$, and 454 (57.9%) of respondents had BMI $\geq 25.0 \text{ kg/m}^2$. Three hundred sixteen (40.3%) participants were overweight and 14 (1.8%) were obese. The mean $\pm$ SD systolic blood pressure of the study population was $137.9 \pm 16.5 \text{ mmHg}$, while the diastolic mean $\pm$ SD was $86.2 \pm 10.9 \text{ mmHg}$.

3.5. Factors Associated with Hypertension. In the bivariate analysis of the socio-demographic variables with hypertension, age was found to have a statistically significant association with the more odds of hypertension among the age group 45-54, (COR = 4.9; 95% CI: 2.1, 11.2), and those $\geq$55 years, (COR = 8.95; 95% CI: 3.6, 22.6), compared to the younger age group (18-24 years).

An increase in the odds of hypertension with increasing income level was noted in the bivariate analysis, and it was statistically significant. Those who earned between 1,001 and 2,500 ETB, (COR = 3.8; 95% CI: 2.09, 6.83), and >2501ETB, (COR = 5.9; 95% CI: 3.6, 9.7), were more likely having hypertension compared to those earning less than one thousand ETB. Sex and marital status did not show any statistically significant association with hypertension in the study population.

Among the behavioral characteristics, being obese was found to be positively associated with the odds of hypertension. Those who had body mass index greater or equal to 30 kg/m2 more likely to have hypertension (COR = 10.0; 95% CI: 2.3, 43.2) than those with a BMI lower than 30 kg/m^2.

Similarly, a positive association was found for "khat" chewers. Using "khat" regularly had more chance to develop hypertension than nonchewers, (COR = 23.0; 95% CI: 11.0, 49.2), and also working hour also has an association; those working less than seven hours daily are less likely to develop hypertension (COR = 22.9; 95% CI: 9.2, 57.1).

In the same way using fruits and vegetables have an association with hypertension, those peoples using fruits and vegetables 4-7 days per week were less likely to develop hypertension when compared to not consuming totally (COR = 0.024; 95% CI: 0.003, 0.22). Similarly, using salt always in food is associated with more likelihood to develop hypertension when compared to not using salt all (COR = 11.5; 95% CI: 4.1, 31.8). Other behavioral variables such as smoking, alcohol drinking, and transportation

TABLE 1: Sociodemographic characteristics of the study participants at Arbaminch town, Gamo, Ethiopia, 2018.

Variables		Number ($n = 784$)	Percent (%)
Sex	Male	344	43.9
	Female	440	56.1
Age group	18-24	54	6.9
	25-34	98	12.5
	35-44	236	30.1
	45-54	326	41.6
	≥55	70	8.9
Educational status	Can read and write	698	89
	Cannot read and write	86	11
Marital status	Married	583	74.4
	Single	111	14.2
	Divorced/widowed	67	8.5
Income (ETB)	≤1,000 ETB	171	21.8
	1,001-2,500 ETB	129	16.5
	≥2,501 ETB	484	61.7
Family history of chronic heart diseases	No	226	29
	Yes	558	71.1

method used did not show any significant associations with hypertension in the study participants (Table 2).

In the multivariable logistic regression analysis, age group 45-54 and ≥55 years, proved to have an independently significant association with hypertension among the study participants. Persons in the age group 45-54 and ≥55 years were found to be 6 and 7.7 times at more odds of having hypertension than 18-24 years of age (AOR = 6.5; 95% CI: 2.1,20.7 and AOR = 7.74, 95% CI: 2.19, 27.23), respectively.

Income level of participants also showed an independent association with hypertension. Respondents with income level 1,001-2,500 ETB and ≥2,501 ETB were found to be almost five and nine times at more likelihood of having hypertension than those families whose income level was ≤1,000ETB (AOR = 5.1; 95% CI: 2.19, 12.14 and AOR = 9.5 ; 95% CI: 4.5, 20.2).

Respondents who work less than seven hours per day were 10.29 times more likely to develop hypertension when compared to respondents working more than eleven hours per day (AOR = 10.29; 95% CI: 3.29, 32.14).

Respondents who had ever chew "khat" were found to be more likely of having hypertension (AOR = 11; 95% CI: 4.3, 27.7) than those who do not chew "khat." Although usage of salt in food, body mass index, and use of fruit and vegetables showed significant association with hypertension in the bivariate analysis, the variables were not statistically significant in the final logistic regression analysis.

4. Discussion

The prevalence of hypertension in this study was 35.2%. The finding is slightly comparable to a community-based study among police officers in Bengal, India 32% [17]. The prevalence of hypertension in this study is higher than the studies in Gonder with the prevalence of 28.3% (26), Addis Ababa 31.5% [7], among a ministry of civil servants 27.3% [18], Durame 22.4%, Bahir Dar city 25.1% and 27.3% [2, 19, 20], Ethiopia and Hawwasa 19.6% [8, 21], Jigjiga 28.3%, and Tigray 16% [22, 23]. This discrepancy may be explained by the study methodology and setting difference. Secondly, the time of study may make such a difference since the prevalence of hypertension is increasing.

The prevalence of hypertension in this study was lower than that reported in Ghana ranged from 19 to 48% between studies [12], and those reported from population-based studies is 55.9% [24, 25]. This discrepancy may be due to age difference as 18-70 years were used in this study and others use 30 years and above. On top of this, genetic difference may probably affect the prevalence of hypertension.

In this study age group, 45-54 and ≥55 years were found to have a significantly associated with hypertension even after adjusting for confounders, which has been confirmed in previous studies [23, 25]. This may be because of the biological effect of increased arterial resistance due to arterial thickening as one gets older. High-income level of families, less working hour per day, and regular "khat" chewing were significantly associated with hypertension [19]. This study further strengthens the previous reports in this country.

On the other hand, being literate, cigarette smoking, regular use of alcohol, gender, and positive family history of hypertension were not significantly associated with hypertension in this study.

No significant statistical associations were found in this study between hypertension and using salty foods, sedentary lifestyles, use of fruits and vegetables, and religion. This was not in line with other studies which presented paradoxical results [14, 25]. Such differences maybe due to disparities in methodologies and due to the fact that majority of the

TABLE 2: Factors associated with hypertension of the study participants in Arba Minch town, Gamo, Ethiopia, 2018.

Variables		Hypertension Yes	No	COR (95% CI)	AOR (95% CI)
Age	18-24	7	47	1	1
	25-34	15	83	1.21 (0.5, 3.2)	1.5 (0.5, 5.4)
	35-44	76	160	3.19 (1.4, 7.2)	4.49 (1.4, 14.5)
	45-54	138	188	4.92 (2.2, 11.2)*	6.5 (2.1, 20.7)*
	≥55	40	30	8.95 (3.6, 22.6)*	7.74 (2.2, 27.2)*
Income	≤1,000 ETB	20	151	1	1
	1,001-2,500 ETB	43	86	3.8 (2.1, 6.8)*	5.16 (2.2, 12.1)*
	≥2,501	213	271	5.9 (3.6, 9.8)*	9.5 (4.5, 20.2)*
"Khat" users	No	201	500	1	1
	Yes	75	8	23.(11, 49.2)*	11.06 (4.3, 27.7)*
Working hour	≤7 hours per day	70	7	22.9 (9.2, 57.1)*	12.5 (4.3, 36.1)*
	8-10 hours per day	182	405	0.94 (0.6, 1.6)	0.5 (0.3, 0.9)
	≥11 hours per day	24	96	1	1
Use of fruits and vegetables	Not at all	6	1	1	1
	1-3 days per week	261	444	0.1 (0.012, 0.8)	34 (1.9, 585.3)
	4-7 days per week	9	63	0.02 (0.01, 0.2)*	4 (1.1, 14.2)
Use of salt	Not at all	4	73	1	1
	Always	237	376	11.5(4.1, 31.9)*	3.1 (0.9, 10.2)
	Some times	35	59	10.8 (3.6, 32.2)*	2.9 (0.8, 10.3)
BMI	≤17.99 under weight	6	24	1	1
	18-24.99 normal	130	294	1.7 (0.7, 4.4)	1.0 (0.3, 3.3)
	25-29.99 over weight	130	186	2.8 (1.1, 7.0)	0.8 (0.2, 2.8)
	≥30 obese	10	4	10 (2.3, 43.3)*	3.n (0.4, 23.0)

* denotes statistical significance (*p* value < 0.05).

participants in this study were females (56%), who are less smokers and alcohol users compared to males. This study adds to the evidence that the prevalence of hypertension in Ethiopia is on the rise.

This study was not free of limitations. It involves only physical and behavioral measurements but did not used the biochemical tests due to cost and time constraints. Social desirability bias might have been introduced in "khat" chewing, smoking, and alcohol drinking practices especially for women. The blood pressure measurements were taken in a single day. This study also did not measure the effect of "khat" chewing frequency on hypertension. Another limitation is we used systematic sampling which may not guarantee randomness, and those households who were not owners and/or rented small rooms in the compound were not included.

5. Conclusion

This study has found a higher prevalence of hypertension than previously reported in urban populations in the country. Advancing age, regular "khat" chewing, increased income, and working hour in relation to physical exercise were the identified associated factors with hypertension.

Abbreviations

BMI: Body mass index
NCD: Noncommunicable disease
WHO: World Health Organization.

Additional Points

Paper Context. Nowadays, Ethiopia is facing a double burden of both the communicable and noncommunicable diseases. Hypertension, as one of the major killer noncommunicable diseases, little is known about its prevalence and contributing factors in the adult population. An up-to-date and comprehensive assessment of the evidence concerning hypertension in Ethiopia is lacking. A prevalence of hypertension is found in the adults which urges for regular screening and comprehensive health education and promotion activities on regular physical exercise.

Ethical Approval

The study was conducted after obtaining ethical clearance from institutional review board of College of Medicine and Health Sciences, Arba Minch University. An official letter was written from the Department of Public Health to Gamo Zone Health Department and Arba Minch town Health Office. Informed written consent was obtained from respondents after explaining the objective of the study, and the names of the respondents were not included in the data collecting format to keep confidentiality. Individuals who were hypertensive during the study were advised to go to health institutions for further diagnosis and treatment.

Authors' Contributions

BK was the principal investigator of the study leading from the conception, design, and supervising data collection process to the final analysis and preparation of the manuscript. GA and DH participated in the design of the study and reviewed and criticized the whole document, especially on the method and analysis part. GG participated in reviewing the document, responsible for the writeup, and provided critical comments. All authors read and approved the final manuscript.

Acknowledgments

We want to express great thanks to Arba Minch University Public Health Department. We would also like to thank Gamo Zone Health Department and Arba Minch town administration staffs. Finally, we would like to thank the data collectors, supervisors, and study participants.

References

[1] World Health OrganizationAugust 2019, https://www.who.int/news-room/fact-sheets/detail/noncommunicable-diseases.

[2] World Health Organization, *Global Status Report on Noncommunicable Diseases 2014*, World Health Organization, 2014.

[3] Wikipedia, "Hypertension 2019," August2019, https://en.wikipedia.org/wiki/Hypertension.

[4] M. Molla, "Systematic reviews of prevalence and associated factors of hypertension in Ethiopia: finding the evidence," *Science Journal of Public Health*, vol. 3, no. 4, pp. 514–519, 2015.

[5] S. O. Bushara, S. K. Noor, A. A. Ibraheem, W. M. Elmadhoun, and M. H. Ahmed, "Prevalence of and risk factors for hypertension among urban communities of North Sudan: detecting a silent killer," *Journal of Family Medicine and Primary Care*, vol. 5, no. 3, pp. 605–610, 2016.

[6] P. Thawornchaisit, F. de Looze, C. M. Reid et al., "Health-Risk Factors and the Prevalence of Chronic Kidney Disease: Cross-Sectional Findings from a National Cohort of 87 143 Thai Open University Students," *Global Journal of Health Science*, vol. 7, no. 5, pp. 59–72, 2015.

[7] B. Guchiye, *Prevalence and Associated Factors of Hypertension among Workers of Steel Factories*, Addis Ababa University, Akaki, Addis Ababa, 2014.

[8] K. T. Kibret and Y. M. Mesfin, "Prevalence of hypertension in Ethiopia: a systematic meta-analysis," *Public Health Reviews*, vol. 36, no. 1, p. 14, 2015.

[9] Y. F. Gebreyes, D. Y. Goshu, T. K. Geletew et al., "Prevalence of high bloodpressure, hyperglycemia, dyslipidemia, metabolic syndrome and their determinants in Ethiopia: evidences from the National NCDs STEPS Survey, 2015," *PLoS One*, vol. 13, no. 5, article e0194819, 2018.

[10] Federal Democratic Republic of Ethiopia Population Census Commission, *Summary and Statistical Report of the 2007 Population and Housing Census*, Central Statistical Agency, Addis Ababa: Ethiopia, 2008.

[11] Z. A. Anteneh, W. A. Yalew, and D. B. Abitew, "Prevalence and correlation of hypertension among adult population in Bahir Dar city, Northwest Ethiopia: a community based cross-sectional study," *International Journal of General Medicine*, vol. 8, pp. 175–185, 2015.

[12] World Health Organization, "Global Health Observatory (GHO) data," https://www.who.int/gho/ncd/risk_factors/blood_pressure_prevalence_text/en/.

[13] World Health Organization, "A global brief on hypertension: silent killer, global public health crisis," in *World Health Day 2013*, World Health Organization, 2013.

[14] H. M. Ageely, "Health and socio-economic hazards associated with khat consumption," *Journal of Family & Community Medicine*, vol. 15, no. 1, pp. 3–11, 2008.

[15] https://en.wikipedia.org/wiki/Khat.

[16] World Health Organisation, *Steps_instrument WHO approach to chronic diseases risk factor survellance*, World Health Organization, Geneva, Switzerland, 2015.

[17] T. Acharyya, P. Kaur, and M. V. Murhekar, "Prevalence of behavioral risk factors, overweight and hypertension in the urban slums of North 24 Parganas District, West Bengal, India, 2010," *Indian Journal of Public Health*, vol. 58, no. 3, pp. 195–198, 2014.

[18] K. Angaw, A. F. Dadi, and K. A. Alene, "Prevalence of hypertension among federal ministry civil servants in Addis Ababa, Ethiopia: a call for a workplace-screening program," *BMC Cardiovascular Disorders*, vol. 15, no. 1, 2015.

[19] T. P. Helelo, Y. A. Gelaw, and A. A. Adane, "Prevalence and Associated Factors of Hypertension among Adults in Durame Town, Southern Ethiopia," *PLoS ONE*, vol. 9, no. 11, article e112790, 2014.

[20] A. Belachew, T. Tewabe, Y. Miskir et al., "Prevalence and associated factors of hypertension among adult patients in Felege-Hiwot Comprehensive Referral Hospitals, northwest, Ethiopia: a cross-sectional study," *BMC Research Notes*, vol. 11, no. 1, p. 876, 2018.

[21] A. Esaiyas, T. Teshome, and D. Kassa, "Prevalence of hypertension and associate risk factors among workers at Hawassa University, Ethiopia: an institution based cross sectional study," *Journal of Vascular Medicine & Surgery*, vol. 6, no. 1, p. 2, 2018.

[22] H. Asresahegn, F. Tadesse, and E. Beyene, "Prevalence and associated factors of hypertension among adults in Ethiopia: a community based cross-sectional study," *BMC Research Notes*, vol. 10, no. 1, p. 629, 2017.

[23] A. Bayray, K. G. Meles, and Y. Sibhatu, "Magnitude and risk factors for hypertension among public servants in Tigray, Ethiopia: a cross-sectional study," *PLoS One*, vol. 13, no. 10, article e0204879, 2018.

[24] M. E. Lacruz, A. Kluttig, S. Hartwig et al., "Prevalence and incidence of hypertension in the general adult population: results of the CARLA-cohort study," *Medicine*, vol. 94, no. 22, p. e952, 2015.

[25] T. Nwankwo, S. S. Yoon, and V. L. Burt, *Nwankwo, T., Yoon, S. S., & Burt, V. L. (2013). Hypertension among adults in the*

19

Lessons from Hippocrates: Time to Change the Cancer Paradigm

Carlos M. Galmarini ⓘ

Topazium Artificial Intelligence, Paseo de la Castellana 40, 28046 Madrid, Spain

Correspondence should be addressed to Carlos M. Galmarini; cmgalmarini@topazium.com

Academic Editor: Tadeusz Robak

The ultimate goal of all medical activity is to restore patients to a state of complete physical, mental, and social wellbeing. In cancer, it is assumed that this can only be obtained through the complete eradication of the tumor burden. So far, this strategy has led to a substantial improvement in cancer survival rates. Despite this, more than 9 million people die from cancer every year. Therefore, we need to accept that our current cancer treatment paradigm is obsolete and must be changed. The new paradigm should reflect that cancer is a systemic disease, which affects an individual patient living in a particular social reality, rather than an invading organism or a mere cluster of mutated cells that need to be eradicated. This Hippocratic holistic view will ultimately lead to an improvement in health and wellbeing in cancer patients. They deserve nothing less.

1. Introduction

"Advances are made by answering questions; discoveries are made by questioning answers" (Bernhard Haisch 1975) [1].

The ultimate goal of all medical activity is to preserve health in fit people and to cure those who are sick, understanding by this as to restore a state of complete physical, mental, and social wellbeing on them. Our current therapeutic strategy is based on the fact that a cancer cure can only be achieved through the complete eradication of the tumor burden. Based on this and following the concept of the "poisoned arrow" described by Ehrlich, finding the "Achilles heel" of tumors that may be exploited as a specific target while sparing healthy tissues becomes essential [2]. At present, these vulnerabilities are being targeted by local and systemic treatments (Figure 1). This strategy has led to a substantial improvement in survival rates for cancer patients in an unprecedented way [3]. Despite this progress, more than 9 million people still die from cancer every year [4]. In addition, cancer survivors suffer chronic morbidities that impair their quality of life [5, 6]. We must then admit that, in most patients, the "poisoned arrow" strategy (mutated into "magic bullet") is not leading to a cancer cure, that is, restoring cancer patients to a state of complete physical, mental, and social wellbeing, but to a cancer remission, that is, "the temporary absence of manifestations of a particular disease" [7, 8]. Certainly, current treatments prolong the life of cancer patients and improve their quality of life. We cannot vilify these impacts on every patient life. Any additional time gained with the current treatments can mean a lot to a patient with the prospect of dying. However, inducing a remission is not the same as curing cancer. After months or years of remission, cancer will inevitably recur. We can continue looking for other vulnerabilities in tumors, but the problem will persist.

Therefore, the factual question remains unanswered: how can we truly cure cancer? We can only find the answer to that question if we first accept that our current cancer treatment paradigm is obsolete. The evaluation of the present paradigm shows many triumphs in basic and clinical research but, unfortunately, continues to fail in our goal of restoring a state of complete physical, mental, and social wellbeing in most cancer patients. To cure the approximately 18 million people with cancer worldwide, we must shift from this paradigm [4]. It is time to pause and think about the key challenges and future directions in clinical oncology. What do we need to do in order to create a new kind of collective intelligence to truly cure cancer? How can we make cancer research

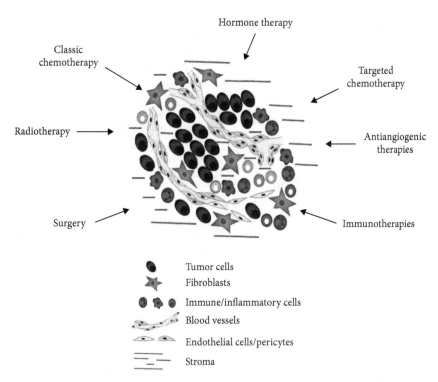

FIGURE 1: Therapeutic approaches currently used in cancer treatment. According to the "tumor-centric" paradigm, a cancer cure is only achieved after the complete eradication of the tumor burden.

smarter? Patients who are dying from cancer cannot wait. There is already enough experimental and clinical evidence to generate a new paradigm based on novel axioms that would allow us to achieve a cure, and not just a remission. This new paradigm would ensure that the right care is delivered to the right patient at the right time. Herein, we describe what we believe should be the axioms of this new cancer paradigm and how it may help to attain our objective of truly curing cancer patients.

2. A Need to Start from Scratch: Lessons from Hippocrates

"Physician must convert or insert wisdom to medicine and medicine to wisdom" (Hippocrates) [9].

Modern medicine is based on the works of Hippocrates (460-370 BC) and his disciples [9, 10]. In essence, Hippocrates claimed that any disease is based on natural causes, and therefore, in order to establish a diagnosis, a prognosis, and a treatment, medicine should be based on detailed observation, reason, and experience. This Hippocratic approach allowed a broader understanding of the causes, context, and clinical course of a particular disease. It is remarkable how much Hippocrates' work can be relevant today. Hippocrates taught us two main lessons: (i) cancer is a systemic ("humoral") disease, i.e., a disease that affects the whole body, and not just a specific organ; (ii) a cancer cure can only be achieved by rebalancing the whole organism through a multidisciplinary, holistic approach, and not just by eradicating the tumor.

3. A New Cancer Paradigm: "For Systemic Diseases, Systemic Methods of Cure"

The aim of cancer treatment should be to restore a state of complete physical, mental, and social wellbeing in cancer patients, and not only to eradicate the tumor burden. Then, we need to move from the paradigm that claims "for extreme diseases, extreme methods of cure" to a new paradigm that may be reformulated as "for systemic diseases, systemic methods of cure". This new paradigm should be based in new axioms that will lead to novel treatment strategies (Table 1).

3.1. Axiom #1: "The Tumor as an Organ-Like Structure, i.e., Another Member of a Complex Organism." "The exacerbations and remissions will be indicated by the diseases, the seasons of the year, the reciprocation of the periods, whether they occur every day, every alternate day, or after a longer period, and by the supervening symptoms" (Hippocrates) [11].

An important breakthrough in cancer biology was the recognition of tumors as abnormal organs acting in the context of an entire organism [12–17]. Tumor metabolism is not necessarily autonomous or self-perpetuating. Tumor nourishment and growth are sustained by the interaction of the tumor with its host. Hormone-dependent breast and prostate cancers constitute examples of the direct interplay between the abnormal organ (tumor) and the organism as a whole. Furthermore, tumors also interact with nearby organs or surrounding tissues, as well as other organs, via glycolysis by-products generated by the specific metabolism of tumors,

TABLE 1: The new cancer treatment paradigm: "for systemic diseases, systemic methods of cure".

Objective:
To restore a state of complete physical, mental, and social wellbeing in cancer patients

Axioms
Tumors as organ-like structures, member of a complex organism
Concomitant resistance
Chronic inflammation
   Local tissue inflammation
   Systemic, low-grade inflammation
Augmented intelligence

Therapeutic approaches
Lifestyle changes
   Daily physical activity
   Healthy diet
   Adequate sleep/wake cycles
Maintenance of concomitant resistance
Use of anti-inflammatory drugs
Restoration of eubiosis
Reprogramming of tissue and tumor metabolism
New schedules of conventional treatments (surgery, radiotherapy, chemotherapy, hormone-therapy, antiangiogenic agents, and immunotherapy)

inflammatory tumor-released cytokines, and other poorly defined circulating components that constitute what is known as the "tumor-derived macroenvironment" [18–20]. Patient mortality is more related to these tumor-induced systemic alterations than to the direct effect of the primary tumor itself or even metastases.

A clear effect of the tumor-derived macroenvironment is the severe suppression of the immune system, resulting in an increased risk of infections and patient mortality [21, 22]. Tumors also activate procoagulatory factors and inhibit fibrinolytic factors, leading to the development of thrombosis, a major complication in cancer patients [23]. Indeed, thromboembolism is estimated to be the second most common cause of cancer-related mortality [24]. In addition, tumor-secreted factors (e.g., TNFα, IFNγ, IL6, and lactate) can disrupt the metabolic functions of the liver and lead to cachexia, which accounts for nearly one-third of cancer deaths [25, 26]. Furthermore, the heightened energetic demand of cancer cells can lead to substantial alterations in hepatic circadian metabolism, with altered insulin levels, glucose intolerance, and deregulated lipid metabolism [20]. Given that these metabolic effects are systemic, it is most likely that tumor-induced metabolic rewiring may also take place in multiple organs, disrupting homeostasis [27, 28]. All these highlight the myriad of complex systemic effects that a tumor can have on its host. As described by Rudolph Virchow (1821-1902), the life of an organism is based on collective features, not individual ones [29]. These features include "abnormal organs" such as tumors, supporting the notion of cancer as a systemic disease: tumors regulate and are regulated by processes that occur both inside and outside the local tumor microenvironment.

3.2. Axiom #2: "Concomitant Resistance (or Game of Thrones)." "What remains in diseases after the crisis is apt to produce relapses" (Hippocrates).

The "societal" organization of cancer may be compared to the behavior of certain species of ants, which form complex organizations known as supercolonies, with the ability to expand their nests over large areas allowing them to achieve ecosystem dominance [30, 31]. Indeed, cancer multiple sites in a patient can be considered as supercolonies; however, unlike ants, these cancer colonies fight against each other for the "iron throne." This phenomenon, first described by Ehrlich and other contemporary investigators, is known as "concomitant resistance" and describes a biological situation in which, upon certain circumstances, a tumor exerts a controlling and inhibitory action on other concomitant tumors, while paradoxically, it continues to grow [32–34]. A similar situation may happen among the different metastatic *foci*, where a main or "leading" metastasis inhibits the growth of the other metastatic colonies. Nowadays, we know that there are four main mechanisms of concomitant resistance: (i) the growth of a tumor might generate a specific antitumor immune response, which even though not strong enough to inhibit its growth, it is capable of preventing the development of small secondary tumors [35, 36]; (ii) tumors produce antiangiogenic molecules that suppress the vascularization and growth of small metastases [37]; (iii) the "athrepsia theory," according to which essential nutrients for tumor growth are mostly consumed by the "main" tumor, makes it difficult for secondary tumors in other sites to grow [32]; (iv) the high metabolic rate of tumors induces the release into the bloodstream of metabolic by-products that further induce a state of dormancy of cancer cells in small metastatic sites. Meanwhile, the primary tumor or main metastasis is protected from their inhibitory effect due to the presence of counteracting amino acids and, therefore, continues to grow [32, 38, 39].

The concomitant resistance model explains the patterns observed in the clinical evolution of some types of cancers. For example, disease recurrence in patients with early breast cancer shows a bimodal pattern, with a broad dominant early peak of relapse at about 1.5-2 years after surgery, followed by a second peak at about 5 years, and then a tapered pattern of relapse extending up to 20 years [40, 41]. According to this evidence, the first peak of relapse is predominantly the result of surgery-promoted growth of dormant micrometastases due to the annihilative effects of surgery on concomitant resistance, while the second peak of relapse is explained by the natural stochastic transitions from dormant to active states [42, 43]. Wound healing and local inflammation induced by surgery might also promote the growth of micrometastases, further enhanced by surgical stress-induced immunosuppression, which helps cancer cells to circumvent immune-mediated rejection at micrometastatic foci [44, 45]. This clinical evolution has also been observed in patients who undergo surgery for primary control of prostate, lung, and pancreatic cancers, as well as osteosarcoma and melanoma [46–50]. A similar situation may develop among the different metastatic foci, where a main or leading metastasis inhibits the growth of other metastatic colonies. For example, liver metastases reappear within the first 2 years in 70% of colorectal cancer patients that underwent resection of liver-limited metastases [51, 52]. Likewise, most cancer patients with multiple metastatic sites who receive treatment with systemic therapies achieve complete or partial responses on a specific site, and after a short period of time, the disease returns in other sites.

3.3. Axiom #3: Chronic Inflammation—"the Source of All Evil."

One of the first researchers to link cancer and inflammation was Virchow, who suggested that irritation of the stroma caused sites of "chronic inflammation" with tumorigenic potential [53]. Years later, Theodor Boveri (1862-1915) provided evidence to support Virchow's ideas, suggesting that tissue inflammation induced chromosomal abnormalities during mitosis, while providing the environmental conditions required by this cancer cells to divide and proliferate [54, 55]. Virchow and Boveri were both right: inflammation promotes tumorigenesis through complex processes that lead to the transformation of healthy cells into cancer cells [56, 57]. Specifically, if inflammation becomes chronic, neutrophils and macrophages remain permanently in the affected tissue, producing reactive oxygen species (ROS) and reactive nitrogen species (RNS), proangiogenic factors (e.g., VEGF), cell-growth-promoting factors (e.g., IL1 and IL6), and immunosuppressive and profibrotic factors (e.g., TGFβ) [58, 59]. ROS and RNS can damage DNA, increasing the frequency of random cancer-inducing mutations [12, 60]. The resulting genetic events can then activate the production of proinflammatory mediators, and the recruitment or activation of more inflammatory cells, thus perpetuating chronic inflammation [61]. Over time, the chronically inflamed tissue may become a cancerous tissue. Once the tumor is established, this vicious circle is closed with the maintenance of chronic inflammation through the constant release of proinflammatory factors by malignant cells [62]. Therefore, carcinogenesis can be seen as the perpetuation of unresolved local inflammation.

3.3.1. The Unseen Enemy: Systemic, Low-Grade Chronic Inflammation.

Alternatively, recent evidence suggests that cancer may also be the result of systemic, low-grade chronic inflammation (SLGCI). In SLGCI, peripheral tissues chronically exhibit high levels of inflammatory factors (C-reactive protein or CRP, TNFα, IL1β, IL6, and IL17) and infiltrated immune cells (macrophages, neutrophils, and T-lymphocytes) without exhibiting structural alterations or loss in their primary functions [63, 64]. It is worth noting that SLGCI plays a fundamental role in the pathogenesis of several noncommunicable and putatively unrelated chronic diseases [65–67]. Moreover, a vicious cycle of sustained SLGCI has been observed in some health conditions of virtually all organs, in parallel with the global adoption of modern environmental and lifestyle changes [67, 68].

The white or visceral adipose tissue plays a role in one of the primary mechanisms involved in the onset of SLGCI. The visceral adipose tissue secretes a wide variety of cytokines and other mediators in order to regulate specific metabolic, endocrine, and immune functions to maintain whole-body homeostasis [69]. Chronic overeating induces severe alterations to this regulatory system. When caloric intake exceeds energy expenditure, insulin levels raise, signaling adipocytes to take up glucose and convert it into an excess of triglycerides and fatty acids, leading to adipocyte hyperplasia and hypertrophy. This induces hypoxia and the subsequent necrosis of white adipose tissue, which is invaded by macrophages, which switch to a proinflammatory phenotype, thereby promoting local inflammation [70, 71]. This tissue damage and the ensuing inflammation promote cellular proliferation via an influx of other immune cells (e.g., neutrophils), proinflammatory mediators (leptin, IL6, Csf1, etc.) and growth factors, tissue remodeling, and angiogenesis. The large amount of fatty acids stored in adipocytes also exacerbates lipoperoxidation, with a considerable increase in ROS and RNS levels. This oxidative burst increases the recruitment of immune cells to the adipose tissue, further promoting inflammation [72]. By contrast, hypertrophic adipocytes reduce the production of anti-inflammatory or insulin-sensitizing factors, such as adiponectin [73]. Furthermore, excess free fatty acids can enter the systemic circulation, reaching other distant organs (e.g., muscle and liver), where they interact with toll-like receptors (TLRs), activate innate immune cells, and initiate the production of proinflammatory mediators (IL6 and MCP1), ultimately bringing inflammation to a systemic level [74, 75]. Altered metabolic states such as dyslipidemia and hyperglycemia can also induce an inflammatory response by activating macrophages through TLRs, which could later reach a systemic level when these cells migrate to insulin-dependent tissues and alter the micro- and macroenvironments of the body through increased cytokine release.

It is possible that, as in obesity, diabetes, and cardiovascular disorders, the unspecific activation of the immune system or SLGCI may also constitute an important risk factor for cancer [76, 77]. Indeed, obesity, overweightness, and diabetes increase cancer risk as well as the likelihood of death from certain types of cancer [78–80]. A clear example of how obesity-related inflammation can induce cancer is pancreatic-ductal adenocarcinoma. In a healthy pancreas, obesity promotes steatosis, inflammation, and fibrosis by modeling a specific microenvironment characterized by the accumulation of hypertrophic adipocytes, which secrete high amounts of cytokines, such as IL1β [81]. This promotes stellate cell activation, increased desmoplasia, neutrophil infiltration, and inflammation, thus promoting tumorigenesis [82]. Once established, malignant cells coopt the inflammatory mechanisms responsible for tissue repair to promote tumor growth and invasion.

3.3.2. The Revenge of the Nerds: The Innate Immune System.

Therefore, rather than being a passive reaction to cancer cells, inflammation seems to play a key active role in carcinogenesis. Innate immune cells, which were always considered as the "nerds" of tumor immunity, are largely responsible for these inflammatory reactions. A common characteristic of innate immune cells is their great phenotypic plasticity. This versatility makes these cells capable of displaying different functions regulated by signaling. For instance, during the early phases of inflammation, these cells will primarily promote the activation of the adaptive immune system, while in the chronic stage, they will suppress the immune reaction and promote tissue repair by activating angiogenesis and initiating stromal generation [83, 84]. Myeloid-derived cells are the main components of the innate immune system and are mainly divided into mononuclear and polymorphonuclear cells [12]. Mononuclear phagocytes include macrophages, which reside in virtually all tissues [85, 86]. Although it is acknowledged that there is a spectrum of intermediate states, macrophages present two major distinct phenotypes: M1, which promotes inflammation, and M2, which suppresses it. On the other hand, polymorphonuclear phagocytes or granulocytes are mainly neutrophils that accumulate in sites of inflammation and disease [87, 88]. Neutrophils can also be divided into two major distinct phenotypes: N1 and N2, which are pro- and anti-inflammatory, respectively [89, 90]. Special consideration should be given to MDSCs, which broadly include immature myeloid progenitors, and monocyte- and granulocyte-like cells, and are characterized by their immunosuppressive ability [90–92].

3.3.3. An Inside Job: Role of the Immune Cells in Tumors. Inflammatory cells are also major cellular components of established tumors [83, 84]. Tumor-associated macrophages (TAMs) are derived from monocytes that are recruited into tumors by chemokines secreted by both malignant and stromal cells. Once in the tumor, TAMs are "conditioned" by the tumor microenvironment towards switching to an M2-like state, in order to display a number of protumoral functions such as promotion of tumor cell proliferation and survival, induction of immunosuppression and angiogenesis, and matrix remodeling and metastasis [84, 93]. Similarly, tumor-associated neutrophils (TANs) are conditioned into N2-like neutrophils promoting tumor formation by producing ROS and RNS species, tumor proliferation factors (e.g., neutrophil elastase), angiogenic factors (e.g., VEGFA), and ECM-degrading enzymes (e.g., MMP9). N2 neutrophils also suppress antitumor immune response by the release of inducible nitric oxide synthase (iNOS), arginase 1, or TGFβ [94, 95]. These functions can be exerted locally, in or around the tumor microenvironment, as well as systemically, in distant organs. The role in cancer of other granulocytes, such as mast cells, eosinophils, and basophils, remains lesser known [85, 96, 97].

3.3.4. Friends as Foes: The Microbiota. Another source of SLGCI is the microbiota [98, 99]. Any imbalance of the microbiota (dysbiosis) may disrupt the symbiotic relationship with its host organism, promoting inflammation and diseases such as hypertension, diabetes, or obesity [100, 101]. Dysbiosis *per se* is also a source of chronic inflammation and carcinogenesis [102, 103]. For example, metagenome-wide association studies in stool samples from patients with colorectal cancer suggest that harmful bacteria in the gut may become more abundant in response to unhealthy lifestyle or deleterious dietary habits. This increases the exposure of the gut epithelium to potentially mutagenic metabolites. On the other hand, the metabolites produced by, for example, fruit and vegetable consumption facilitate the maintenance of the colonic epithelium through inducing a relatively low pH, which helps to reduce amino acid fermentation and pathogen growth. Therefore, depleting these protective metabolites may also promote the development of colon cancer [101, 104, 105].

3.4. Axiom #4: "Augmented Intelligence—the Doctor's Sixth Sense." "One, then, ought to look to the country, the season, the age, and the diseases in which they are proper or not" (Hippocrates).

Treatment decisions are often based on data obtained from a small percentage of patients, i.e., those who take part in clinical trials. This means that clinical information from the majority of patients, who do not take part in clinical trials, is not being used [106]. This is changing with the emergence of artificial intelligence (AI) technologies, which have the ability to work with enormous amounts of data. But AI generates many fears and apocalyptic thoughts due to its potential to replace humans in many different tasks. However, these fears are unjustified, and AI should be viewed as a tool to complement the physician's work, not as a replacement. Then, what can AI add to our human intelligence in healthcare settings? Nowadays, the healthcare world is awash with vast, valuable sources of information. Indeed, improvements in mobile phone technology, sensors, and connectivity generate extraordinarily detailed insights into an individual's health status. AI can assimilate this massive amount of data, while discerning relevant patterns and insights that human intelligence is not capable to detect, allowing the application of real-world healthcare data to an individual's particular healthcare situation. However, AI technology is based on mathematic algorithms that do not have a physician's ability to see the big picture or take into consideration less quantifiable factors that affect a patient's health, let alone to be a substitute for human judgment. Thus, in the coming decades, the traditional role of the physician will be assisted by AI, helping to establish accurate diagnosis and reach wisertreatment decisions (Figure 2).

One of the most interesting areas of research in AI is virtual medicine. The human body is the biggest data platform. A variety of fields have used computational models as virtual surrogates of human physiology. These models can be considered as virtual representations of a subset or the whole of the patient's physiological identity [107]. Patient's data would be made available to the virtual model through integration of electronic health records (EHRs), mobile health (mHealth) devices, telemedicine, electronic patient-reported outcomes (ePROs), and other platforms, tools, or media [108]. Available patient information should include medical history, genetic idiosyncrasies, environmental factors, diet, lifestyle, particular behaviors, preferences, socioeconomic status, location, data recorded by wearable sensors and mHealth devices, and access and adherence to treatment recommendations. MRI and CT scans can also be used to produce a virtual geometric and physiologic view of the patient, reproducing individual anatomy, organ structure, and temporary blood flow. These virtual representations of each individual patient can then be used to tailor prevention,

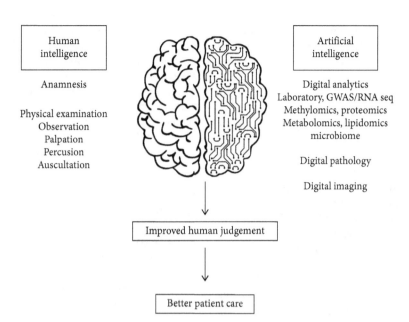

FIGURE 2: A new collective intelligence for a smarter patient care. Artificial intelligence should be viewed as a complementary tool for the physician. With the help of artificial intelligence systems, oncologists will be able to combine its clinical knowledge with massive amounts of data. As a consequence, oncologists will be able to discern new relevant patterns and will gather insights in a way that human intelligence alone cannot do, ultimately improving diagnosis and treatment.

diagnosis, therapeutics, and prognosis for each individual patient [109, 110].

4. Novel Treatment Strategies

It is clear that a cancer cure will not be achieved only by the eradication of the tumor. Indeed, a tumor-centric treatment can never be a solution to a systemic, medical problem. With this in mind, how can we treat cancer patients to truly cure them? We can start by following the example of other therapeutic areas. The clearest is the paradigm shift produced in the treatment of the metabolic syndrome, a cluster of conditions comprising increased blood pressure, high blood sugar, excess body fat around the waist, and increased cholesterol or triglyceride levels. In the past, all these conditions were diagnosed and treated separately, without a global approach. Today, we know that all these markers are related to chronic inflammation, tend to occur together, and increase the risk of heart disease, stroke, and diabetes. Indeed, once established, SLGCI promotes and perpetuates metabolic alterations, establishing a deleterious cycle that promotes pathological processes such as insulin resistance, arteriosclerosis, and endothelial dysfunction. In order to break this cycle, it is necessary to control both the metabolic and inflammatory components simultaneously. These new concepts led to a shift to therapeutic strategies with a more holistic, multidisciplinary approach [111]. Firstly, a person diagnosed with metabolic syndrome or any of its components needs some radical lifestyle changes. A lifelong commitment to a healthy lifestyle includes actions such as being physically active, losing weight, eating a healthy diet, stop smoking, and managing stress. Only with these measures can the development of diabetes or cardiovascular disease be delayed or prevented. If implementing lifestyle changes is not enough, pharmaco-

logical treatments to control blood pressure, cholesterol levels, and blood glucose may also be applied. A similar approach should be used for cancer prevention and treatment, adding to the current strategies, new treatment modalities based on the four axioms that define the new cancer treatment paradigm.

4.1. Evaluation of a Person's Health Status on a Regular Basis. As an old medical adage goes, it is better to prevent a disease than to treat it. This is why the first important step is to educate people so that they can take care of their own health. Simultaneously, primary care should not only include a global clinical analysis and routine imaging/laboratory tests but also include the assessment of SLGCI markers on a regular basis and the characterization of the patient's microbiota whenever possible. The routine analysis of these variables by clinical, imaging, and laboratory tests will allow to determine the levels of chronic inflammation. Therefore, those identified as having a high risk of cancer (among other diseases) based on their level of chronic inflammation can receive early intervention strategies.

4.2. "Mens Sana in Corpore Sano [112]": Lifestyle Changes for a Holistic Approach to Wellbeing. As with other chronic diseases, cancer is linked to unhealthy lifestyles such as smoking, poor diet, lack of physical activity, obesity, sleep deprivation, and alcohol abuse, along with the daily chronic stress imposed by modern life. Thus, current global cancer prevention and treatment strategies should firstly focus on drastically modifying people's lifestyles. Indeed, individuals with a healthy lifestyle appear to have a remarkably lower risk of cancer [113, 114]. This is an enormous social challenge because it involves forcing people to confront their habits, attitudes, and behaviors. In addition to quitting smoking or reducing alcohol intake, there are some basic measures that everybody can apply with impressive results.

4.2.1. Daily Physical Activity.

Physical activity induces a series of adaptive processes that affect tissue metabolism, angiogenesis, and immune regulation [115]. For example, physical activity triggers an intramuscular, inflammatory immune response which induces macrophage differentiation towards a proinflammatory M1 phenotype [116, 117]. Regular physical activity markedly reduces the risk of the primary development of several cancers and might improve clinical outcomes following the diagnosis of a primary tumor [118, 119]. Similarly, there is increasing evidence that supports the role of physical activity in cancer treatment, and it is well accepted that structured, regular physical activity is feasible and well-tolerated in cancer patients [120–122]. Physical activity for as little as 15 minutes a day is associated with a 10% reduced risk in cancer mortality, and every additional 15 minutes of daily physical activity beyond this is associated with an additional 1% reduction in risk [123]. Nevertheless, it is important to stress that response to physical activity prescription is considerably heterogeneous among individual patients, and thus, it should be appropriately prescribed on a case by case basis [124–126].

4.2.2. Healthy Diet.

Different studies have consistently shown a correlation between increased body weight and cancer, with increased mortality rates for all cancers and for cancers at multiple specific sites in obese patients [127–129]. Importantly, adipose-related inflammation and its associated tumorigenic effects have also been observed in one-third of individuals who are not considered to be obese or overweight based on their body mass index [130]. Several studies provide strong evidence that caloric restriction inhibits carcinogenesis [131, 132]. It is calculated that more than 90,000 cancer deaths per year might be avoided if the adult population could maintain a body mass index below 25 throughout their entire life [133–135]. This evidence supports the development of interventions that reduce adipose-related inflammation as a new strategy for cancer prevention and treatment. A modest reduction in fat intake with minimal weight loss represents an easily achievable goal to reduce cancer mortality.

4.2.3. Maintaining a Natural Sleep-Wake Cycle.

Sleep has an impact on a vast array of physiological functions, such as immune function, cognitive ability, and glucose metabolism [27]. When sleep is disturbed or restricted, all these physiological processes are affected. For example, lack of sleep shortness can result in significant changes in a number of circulating proinflammatory cytokine (e.g., IL6 and IL1β) and cortisol levels [136–138]. The effects of sleep deprivation are cumulative. Therefore, over a period of time, sleep debt can lead to a wide range of deleterious health consequences, including SLGCI [139–141]. Sleep shortness can be solved with simple steps (going to sleep and getting up at the same time every day, controlling exposure to light before and during sleep, improving the sleep environment, etc.).

4.3. Interventional Measures.

Once a primary tumor is diagnosed, the therapeutic strategy must be adapted to each patient: this is the only true personalization of medicine. Firstly, we must have new diagnostic tests to evaluate, besides tumor genetics and TME, the degree of interrelation of the tumor with its host organism (e.g., other organs or microbiome), its micro- or macrometastases (concomitant resistance), and the degree of SLGCI. Then, a global approach taking into consideration all these variables must be adopted. For example, we have previously discussed how obesity stimulates pancreatic tumor initiation, growth, and metastasis [142–144]. Thus, the correct strategy to treat this type of patients would be to target not only the tumor but also its original cause, i.e., SLGCI due to obesity. This holistic strategy should include physical activity and diet to reduce obesity and restore normobiosis, combined with treatments to deplete TANs, inactivate PSCs, and inhibit IL1β secretion, so as to prevent obesity-promoted tumor growth and desmoplasia. In preclinical models, this strategy is proved to be successful [143].

4.3.1. Maintenance of the Concomitant Resistance Phenotype.

Novel therapeutic strategies should modulate specific tumor microenvironments to maintain them in a dormant state. Current adjuvant chemotherapy should be administered with different schedules that could be more effective than standard regimens. For example, in surgically treated breast cancer patients, first recurrences tend to occur after 1.5-2 years. Thus, it may be worth to reintroduce specific systemic treatments during that time period in order to eradicate the growing micrometastatic foci; in this sense, the use of oral metronomic chemotherapy appears to be the most interesting schedule as, besides showing antitumor activity, it modulates tumor angiogenesis and immune responses with a moderate toxicity [91, 145]. Oral metronomic chemotherapy should also be used 4-5 years after surgery to prevent the second relapse surge. On the other hand, the use of drugs that alter metabolic stress in cancer cells could be an interesting alternative to modulate the metabolic balance between the primary tumor and its metastases [146]. This could be combined with the administration of metabolic by-products such as m-Tyr. This metabolite was recently shown to exert its antimetastatic effect at low concentrations with no detectable toxic side effects [147]. Surgical stress, besides disrupting concomitant resistance, and inducing immunosuppression and inflammation, also awakens micrometastatic foci from their dormant state [44, 148]. Excessive surgical stress and postoperative complications cause a storm of perioperative cytokines, which has been shown to promote tumor metastasis [149]. Thus, anti-inflammatory drugs may potentially avoid the undesirable effects of surgery. It is interesting to note that some publications showed that in surgically treated breast cancer patients, perisurgical administration of ketorolac dramatically reduced first-peak recurrences [150, 151]. Minimally invasive surgical techniques should also be used to lessen surgical stress.

4.3.2. Treatment with Anti-Inflammatory Drugs.

Therapeutic modulation of chronic inflammation is likely to transform a protumorigenic microenvironment into a healthy microenvironment. For this reason, several commonly used medications, including nonsteroidal anti-inflammatory drugs (NSAIDs), metformin, and statins, represent an additional tool in cancer treatment. For example, COX2 inhibitors are effective cancer chemopreventive agents and have also demonstrated to control cancer-associated chronic inflammation [152, 153]. Effectively counteracting or neutralizing tumor-promoting chronic inflammation can also be achieved by the simultaneous reprogramming of multiple immune response pathways that are activated in cancer. On the basis of the available data, the pathways that currently represent attractive targets for cancer treatment include: (i) trafficking inhibition, depletion, or reprogramming of tumor-associated innate immune cells and (ii) inhibition or sequestration of cytokines or chemokines. All these strategies have an impact on nonredundant mechanisms, and hence, they may be more successful in combination.

4.3.3. Restoration of a Healthy Microbiota. Manipulation of the gut microbiome to restore a protective microbiota (eubiosis) is a goal in patients that show disturbances in microbial composition and functionality (Raman 2013). Diet is the easiest way to restore eubiosis. For example, the consumption of fruits and vegetables promotes the growth of bacterial species that produce butyrate and lactate, which helps to preserve the colonic epithelium through inducing a relatively low pH. This might reduce amino acid fermentation and the growth of cancer-related pathogens [101, 104, 154]. In addition to diet, prebiotics, probiotics, or microbiota transplants may also be used to restore eubiosis, thereby reducing microbially induced genotoxicity and activation of inflammatory, proliferative, and antiapoptotic pathways. Prebiotics are defined as nondigestible substances that produce beneficial physiological effects on the host by stimulating, in a selective manner, the growth and metabolic activity of a limited number of beneficial indigenous bacteria while probiotics are live microorganisms that confer a health benefit on the host. Both prebiotics and probiotics can be used to prevent the onset of dysbiosis when the patient is exposed to predisposing conditions and as therapeutic agents to rebalance an ongoing dysbiosis [155]. Prebiotics act mainly as a specific fuel that indigenous probiotic bacteria can utilize to grow. Most commonly known prebiotics include fructo-oligosaccharide supplements, galacto-oligosaccharides, inulin, lactulose, and breast milk oligosaccharides. Instead, probiotic effects can be categorized as immunological and nonimmunological [156]. Immunological benefits include the activation of local macrophages, an increase in the production of immunoglobulin, the modulation of cytokine profiles, and the induction of hyporesponse to food antigens. Nonimmunological benefits include the digestion process, competition with potential pathogens for nutrients, and intestinal adhesion sites, pH alterations, and bacteriocins production. Currently used probiotics include lactic acid bacteria, bifidobacteria, enterococci, Saccharomyces boulardii, Bacillus spp., and propionibacterias. Finally, fecal microbiota transplantation is the most direct way to change the composition of gut microbiota. This treatment modality can have direct or indirect effects. Different series and case reports have revealed that fecal microbiota transplantation can alleviate various digestive (hepatocarcinoma, gastrointestinal, and pancreatic) and nondigestive (breast and melanoma) cancers linked to intestinal dysbiosis [157]. Additionally, it can be used to counter treatment-associated complications such as radiation enteritis, *C. difficile* infection, or graft-versus-host disease.

5. Back to the Future: Concluding Remarks

There is no doubt that throughout history, the current paradigm has significantly improved cancer care. In addition, nowadays, thanks to recent medical discoveries, patients with cancer live longer and with better quality of life than in the past. But the goal of curing all cancers has not been accomplished yet. We believe that the current paradigm regarding cancer treatment needs significant changes and considerable efforts. Currently, cancer therapy is still based on the millenary paradigm that establishes that in order to achieve a cure, the complete eradication of cancer cells must be achieved. The old philosophical concept of "magister dixit" (said by the teacher, then it is true) has encouraged the faithful fulfillment of the current paradigm despite the fact that, for a long time, no significant improvements have been observed in actual cure (not just remissions) rates, and despite recent scientific and technological advances. Consequently, should we be surprised by this despite the efforts invested in drug discovery and development, pharmacology, and technical devices? Probably not. What should be surprising is the insistence in maintaining a paradigm and axioms that do not work. Nowadays, what seems to matter is not what the medical community knows or does not know regarding a certain fact but rather what it believes or does not believe about it. The real individualization of cancer treatment consists in treating each individual patient following the good general practices of oncology and taking into consideration his/her own particular needs.

Our past reductionist approaches have led us to miss the bigger picture, look in the wrong places, or worse still, not even question if we have the right starting point [158]. According to the Hippocratic view, any treatment modality should consider the patient as a unique physical, mental, and social entity [159]. We need to regain the wisdom of Hippocrates. It is necessary to integrate genetic, biological, clinical, psychological, and social information into a new coherent framework or paradigm to transform it into knowledge and wisdom applied to the clinic that would lead to restoring cancer patients to their fullest physical, emotional, and social capacities. The new paradigm for cancer treatment should be based on this holistic view. As the old masters of medicine said, we must treat patients, not illnesses. We must move away from the "disease" silos and become patient focused [6]. We can start by taking the example of other therapeutic areas. As explained above, the clearest example is the paradigm shift produced in the understanding and treatment of the metabolic syndrome. A similar strategy based on a paradigm shift should be adopted in oncology. Behavioral approaches to control counterproductive lifestyles should be the first measure to prevent or treat cancer [160, 161]. Lifestyle changes do not have to be radical. For instance, simple measures such as eating wholefoods and a plant-based diet, stress management techniques, moderate physical activity, and having social support and being part of a community can slower the progression of localized prostate cancer [162]. These behavioral changes may be combined with pharmacological interventions to reduce SLGCI and the tumor burden.

Big data and AI are redefining cancer research and management [163, 164]. There are many opportunities of how AI can expedite the delivery of new therapeutic options to patients: from computational frameworks that match chemical identity to gene-based descriptors of disease mechanism, to a more unambiguous approach with distributive clinical trials that brings trials to patients (instead of patients to trials). On the other hand, the ability to generate virtual patients from research and clinical data would help to discover and develop novel transformative drugs adapted to the new axioms supporting the innovative paradigm. It should be noted that factual sciences are divided into natural sciences and social sciences. Medicine occupies a special and borderline place between both, and it is very difficult to establish the similarities between a doctor who works through established rules in clinical trials and a family practitioner. The first behavior will be more related to the natural sciences and the latter will be more related to the social sciences, what is known as "the art of medicine." The combination of human and artificial intelligence in a new kind of collective intelligence would allow doctors to incorporate features of the two, i.e., to exercise the art of medicine (social sciences) based on data analysis (natural sciences).

In conclusion, cancer should not be seen as an invading organism or a mere cluster of cancer cells that needs to be eradicated. Instead, a tumor may be better understood as an organ-like structure, acting in the context of a whole organism (a systemic disease) of an individual patient living in a particular social reality. Such a view is more appropriate for understanding complex systems, where some properties of the whole system cannot be inferred from the separate properties of its individual components. Indeed, if one regards the tumor as an organ-like structure within an organism that is a human being (the patient), it seems less outlandish that cancer may be related to homeostatic imbalance, inflammation, or concomitant resistance. These new concepts highlight the notion that even "transient" phenomena can have an impact with lifelong consequences, or in the words of chaos theory, "the ultimate outcome is exquisitely sensitive to the initial conditions." In summary, the understanding of cancer disease based on holistic clinical and pathophysiological concepts will finally lead to an improvement in the health and wellbeing of cancer patients. They deserve nothing less.

References

[1] B. Haisch, *The God Theory, Universes, Zero-Point Fields and What's Behind It All*, Red Wheel/Weiser LLC, San Francisco, 2009.

[2] P. Ehrlich, "Address in pathology, ON CHEMIOTHERAPY: delivered before the Seventeenth International Congress of Medicine," *British Medical Journal*, vol. 2, no. 2746, pp. 353–359, 1913.

[3] E. J. Kort, N. Paneth, and G. F. Vande Woude, "The decline in U.S. cancer mortality in people born since 1925," *Cancer Research*, vol. 69, no. 16, pp. 6500–6505, 2009.

[4] IARC, "Data visualization tool for exploring the cancer global cancer burden," 2019, http://gco.iarc.fr/today/home.

[5] M. M. Hudson, K. K. Ness, J. G. Gurney et al., "Clinical ascertainment of health outcomes among adults treated for childhood cancer," *JAMA*, vol. 309, no. 22, pp. 2371–2381, 2013.

[6] E. M. Jaffee, C. V. Dang, D. B. Agus et al., "Future cancer research priorities in the USA: a Lancet Oncology Commission," *The Lancet Oncology*, vol. 18, no. 11, pp. e653–e706, 2017.

[7] Thesaurus, "Definition of remission," 2019, https://www.dictionary.com/browse/remission.

[8] R. Sullivan, C. S. Pramesh, and C. M. Booth, "Cancer patients need better care, not just more technology," *Nature*, vol. 549, no. 7672, pp. 325–328, 2017.

[9] P. C. Grammaticos and A. Diamantis, "Useful known and unknown views of the father of modern medicine, Hippocrates and his teacher Democritus," *Hellenic Journal of Nuclear Medicine*, vol. 11, no. 1, pp. 2–4, 2008.

[10] S. J. Reiser, "What modern physicians can learn from Hippocrates," *Cancer*, vol. 98, no. 8, pp. 1555–1558, 2003.

[11] M. Scholtz, "Hippocrates' aphorisms," *California and western medicine*, vol. 52, p. 125, 1940.

[12] M. Egeblad, E. S. Nakasone, and Z. Werb, "Tumors as organs: complex tissues that interface with the entire organism," *Developmental Cell*, vol. 18, no. 6, pp. 884–901, 2010.

[13] D. W. Smithers, "Cancer an Attack on Cytologism," *Lancet*, vol. 279, no. 7228, pp. 493–499, 1962.

[14] C. H. Waddington, "Cancer and the theory of organisers," *Nature*, vol. 135, no. 3416, pp. 606–608, 1935.

[15] G. Zajicek, "A new cancer hypothesis," *Medical Hypothesis*, vol. 47, pp. 111–115, 1997.

[16] R. A. Ruggiero and O. D. Bustuoabad, "The biological sense of cancer: a hypothesis," *Theoretical Biology and Medical Modelling*, vol. 3, no. 1, p. 43, 2006.

[17] R. T. Prehn, "The inhibition of tumor growth by tumor mass," *Cancer Research*, vol. 51, no. 1, pp. 2–4, 1991.

[18] W. Al-Zhoughbi, J. Huang, G. S. Paramasivan et al., "Tumor macroenvironment and metabolism," *Seminars in Oncology*, vol. 41, no. 2, pp. 281–295, 2014.

[19] D. Hanahan and R. A. Weinberg, "Hallmarks of cancer: the next generation," *Cell*, vol. 144, no. 5, pp. 646–674, 2011.

[20] S. Masri, T. Papagiannakopoulos, K. Kinouchi et al., "Lung adenocarcinoma distally rewires hepatic circadian homeostasis," *Cell*, vol. 165, no. 4, pp. 896–909, 2016.

[21] J. W. Hadden, "Immunodeficiency and cancer: prospects for correction," *International Immunopharmacology*, vol. 3, no. 8, pp. 1061–1071, 2003.

[22] K. V. I. Rolston and G. P. Bodey, "Infections in patients with cancer," in *Cancer Medicine*, D. W. Kufe, Ed., pp. 1865–1879, Decker, Hamilton, Ontario, 2006.

[23] M. De Cicco, "The prothrombotic state in cancer: pathogenic mechanisms," *Critical Reviews in Oncology/Hematology*, vol. 50, no. 3, pp. 187–196, 2004.

[24] G. J. Caine, P. S. Stonelake, G. Y. H. Lip, and S. T. Kehoe, "The hypercoagulable state of malignancy: pathogenesis and current debate," *Neoplasia*, vol. 4, no. 6, pp. 465–473, 2002.

[25] S. Acharyya, K. J. Ladner, L. L. Nelsen et al., "Cancer cachexia is regulated by selective targeting of skeletal muscle gene products," *The Journal of Clinical Investigation*, vol. 114, no. 3, pp. 370–378, 2004.

[26] R. J. E. Skipworth, G. D. Stewart, C. H. C. Dejong, T. Preston, and K. C. H. Fearon, "Pathophysiology of cancer cachexia: Much more than host–tumour interaction?," *Clinical Nutrition*, vol. 26, no. 6, pp. 667–676, 2007.

[27] J. C. Borniger, W. H. Walker II, Surbhi et al., "A role for hypocretin/orexin in metabolic and sleep abnormalities in a mouse model of non-metastatic breast cancer," *Cell Metabolism*, vol. 28, no. 1, pp. 118–129.e5, 2018, e5.

[28] S. Seton-Rogers, "STAT3 on the brain," *Nature Reviews. Cancer*, vol. 18, no. 8, pp. 468-469, 2018.

[29] R. Virchow, "The Huxley lecture on recent advances in science and their bearing on medicine and surgery: delivered at the opening of the Charing Cross Hospital Medical School on October 3rd," *British Medical Journal*, vol. 2, no. 1971, pp. 1021–1028, 1898.

[30] M. W. Moffett, "Supercolonies of billions in an invasive ant: what is a society?," *Behavioral Ecology*, vol. 23, no. 5, pp. 925–933, 2012.

[31] E. Sunamura, X. Espadaler, H. Sakamoto, S. Suzuki, M. Terayama, and S. Tatsuki, "Intercontinental union of Argentine ants: behavioral relationships among introduced populations in Europe, North America, and Asia," *Insectes Sociaux*, vol. 56, no. 2, pp. 143–147, 2009.

[32] R. A. Ruggiero, J. Bruzzo, P. Chiarella, O. D. Bustuoabad, R. P. Meiss, and C. D. Pasqualini, "Concomitant tumor resistance: the role of tyrosine isomers in the mechanisms of metastases control," *Cancer Research*, vol. 72, no. 5, pp. 1043–1050, 2012.

[33] E. Bashford, J. Murray, and M. Haaland, "General results of propagation of malignant new growths," in *Third Scientific Report on the Investigation of the Imperial Cancer Research Fund*, E. Bashford, Ed., Taylor and Francis, London, 1908.

[34] P. Ehrlich, *Experimentelle Carcinomstudien an Mausen Arb Inst Exp Ther Frankfurt*, vol. 1, pp. 77–103, 1906.

[35] B. N. Bidwell, C. Y. Slaney, N. P. Withana et al., "Silencing of Irf7 pathways in breast cancer cells promotes bone metastasis through immune escape," *Nature Medicine*, vol. 18, no. 8, pp. 1224–1231, 2012.

[36] R. A. Ruggiero, O. D. Bustuoabad, R. D. Bonfil, R. P. Meiss, and C. D. Pasqualini, ""Concomitant immunity" in murine tumours of non-detectable immunogenicity," *British Journal of Cancer*, vol. 51, no. 1, pp. 37–48, 1985.

[37] J. Folkman, "Tumor angiogenesis: therapeutic implications," *The New England Journal of Medicine*, vol. 285, no. 21, pp. 1182–1186, 1971.

[38] S. Benzekry, C. Lamont, D. Barbolosi, L. Hlatky, and P. Hahnfeldt, "Mathematical modeling of tumor-tumor distant interactions supports a systemic control of tumor growth," *Cancer Research*, vol. 77, no. 18, pp. 5183–5193, 2017.

[39] D. R. Montagna, P. Chiarella, R. P. Meiss, and R. A. Ruggiero, "The acceleration of metastases after tumor removal and the paradoxical phenomenon of concomitant tumor resistance," *Journal of Cancer Research and Therapeutics*, vol. 6, pp. 41–51, 2018.

[40] C. M. Galmarini, O. Tredan, and F. C. Galmarini, "Concomitant resistance and early-breast cancer: should we change treatment strategies?," *Cancer Metastasis Reviews*, vol. 33, no. 1, pp. 271–283, 2014.

[41] R. Demicheli, M. W. Retsky, W. J. M. Hrushesky, and M. Baum, "Tumor dormancy and surgery-driven interruption of dormancy in breast cancer: learning from failures," *Nature Clinical Practice. Oncology*, vol. 4, no. 12, pp. 699–710, 2007.

[42] D. G. Baker, T. M. Masterson, R. Pace, W. C. Constable, and H. Wanebo, "The influence of the surgical wound on local tumor recurrence," *Surgery*, vol. 106, no. 3, pp. 525–532, 1989.

[43] S. O. Hofer, D. Shrayer, J. S. Reichner, H. J. Hoekstra, and H. J. Wanebo, "Wound-induced tumor progression: a probable role in recurrence after tumor resection," *Archives of Surgery*, vol. 133, no. 4, pp. 383–389, 1998.

[44] D. Decker, M. Schöndorf, F. Bidlingmaier, A. Hirner, and A. A. von Ruecker, "Surgical stress induces a shift in the type-1/type-2 T-helper cell balance, suggesting downregulation of cell-mediated and up-regulation of antibody-mediated immunity commensurate to the trauma," *Surgery*, vol. 119, no. 3, pp. 316–325, 1996.

[45] J. F. Hansbrough, E. M. Bender, R. Zapata-Sirvent, and J. Anderson, "Altered helper and suppressor lymphocyte populations in surgical patients: A measure of postoperative immunosuppression," *American Journal of Surgery*, vol. 148, no. 3, pp. 303–307, 1984.

[46] R. Demicheli, M. Fornili, F. Ambrogi et al., "Recurrence Dynamics for Non–Small-Cell Lung Cancer: Effect of Surgery on the Development of Metastases," *Journal of Thoracic Oncology*, vol. 7, no. 4, pp. 723–730, 2012.

[47] B. Deylgat, F. van Rooy, F. Vansteenkiste, D. Devriendt, and C. George, "Postsurgery activation of dormant liver micrometastasis: a case report and review of literature," *Journal of Gastrointestinal Cancer*, vol. 42, no. 1, pp. 1–4, 2011.

[48] L. Hanin and M. Zaider, "Effects of surgery and chemotherapy on metastatic progression of prostate cancer: evidence from the natural history of the disease reconstructed through mathematical modeling," *Cancers*, vol. 3, no. 3, pp. 3632–3660, 2011.

[49] W. W. Tseng, J. A. Doyle, S. Maguiness, A. E. Horvai, M. Kashani-Sabet, and S. P. L. Leong, "Giant cutaneous melanomas: evidence for primary tumour induced dormancy in metastatic sites?," *Case Reports*, vol. 2009, no. oct05 1, p. bcr0720092073, 2009.

[50] T. Tsunemi, S. Nagoya, M. Kaya et al., "Postoperative progression of pulmonary metastasis in osteosarcoma," *Clinical Orthopaedics and Related Research*, vol. 407, pp. 159–166, 2003.

[51] G. P. Kanas, A. Taylor, J. N. Primrose et al., "Survival after liver resection in metastatic colorectal cancer: review and meta-analysis of prognostic factors," *Clinical Epidemiology*, vol. 4, pp. 283–301, 2012.

[52] B. Lintoiu-Ursut, A. Tulin, and S. Constantinoiu, "Recurrence after hepatic resection in colorectal cancer liver metastasis -review article," *Journal of medicine and life*, vol. 8, no. Spec Issue, p. 12, 2015.

[53] C. D. Pasqualini, "Experimental oncology. Back to Boveri and Virchow," *Medicina*, vol. 72, no. 6, pp. 530–532, 2012.

[54] T. Boveri, "Concerning the origin of malignant tumours by Theodor Boveri. Translated and annotated by Henry Harris," *Journal of cell science*, vol. 121, Supplement 1, pp. 1–84, 2008.

[55] T. Ried, "Homage to Theodor Boveri (1862-1915): Boveri's theory of cancer as a disease of the chromosomes, and the landscape of genomic imbalances in human carcinomas," *Environmental and Molecular Mutagenesis*, vol. 50, no. 8, pp. 593–601, 2009.

[56] D. G. DeNardo and L. M. Coussens, "Inflammation and breast cancer. Balancing immune response: crosstalk between adaptive and innate immune cells during breast cancer progression," *Breast Cancer Research*, vol. 9, no. 4, p. 212, 2007.

[57] C. Madeddu, G. Gramignano, C. Floris, G. Murenu, G. Sollai, and A. Macciò, "Role of inflammation and oxidative stress in post-menopausal oestrogen-dependent breast cancer," *Journal of Cellular and Molecular Medicine*, vol. 18, no. 12, pp. 2519–2529, 2014.

[58] D. H. Josephs, H. J. Bax, and S. N. Karagiannis, "Tumour-associated macrophage polarisation and re-education with immunotherapy," *Frontiers in Bioscience*, vol. 7, pp. 293–308, 2015.

[59] B. Ruffell and L. M. Coussens, "Macrophages and therapeutic resistance in cancer," *Cancer Cell*, vol. 27, no. 4, pp. 462–472, 2015.

[60] F. Colotta, P. Allavena, A. Sica, C. Garlanda, and A. Mantovani, "Cancer-related inflammation, the seventh hallmark of cancer: links to genetic instability," *Carcinogenesis*, vol. 30, no. 7, pp. 1073–1081, 2009.

[61] N. Antonio, M. L. Bønnelykke-Behrndtz, L. C. Ward et al., "The wound inflammatory response exacerbates growth of pre-neoplastic cells and progression to cancer," *The EMBO Journal*, vol. 34, no. 17, pp. 2219–2236, 2015.

[62] W. H. Fridman, L. Zitvogel, C. Sautès–Fridman, and G. Kroemer, "The immune contexture in cancer prognosis and treatment," *Nature Reviews Clinical Oncology*, vol. 14, no. 12, pp. 717–734, 2017.

[63] H. Kitamura, S. Kimura, Y. Shimamoto et al., "Ubiquitin-specific protease 2-69 in macrophages potentially modulates metainflammation," *The FASEB Journal*, vol. 27, no. 12, pp. 4940–4953, 2013.

[64] S. P. Weisberg, D. McCann, M. Desai, M. Rosenbaum, R. L. Leibel, and A. W. Ferrante Jr., "Obesity is associated with macrophage accumulation in adipose tissue," *The Journal of Clinical Investigation*, vol. 112, no. 12, pp. 1796–1808, 2003.

[65] B. B. Duncan, M. I. Schmidt, J. S. Pankow et al., "Low-grade systemic inflammation and the development of type 2 diabetes: the atherosclerosis risk in communities study," *Diabetes*, vol. 52, no. 7, pp. 1799–1805, 2003.

[66] A. Maxmen, "A reboot for chronic fatigue syndrome research," *Nature*, vol. 553, no. 7686, pp. 14–17, 2018.

[67] S. L. Prescott, "Early-life environmental determinants of allergic diseases and the wider pandemic of inflammatory noncommunicable diseases," *The Journal of Allergy and Clinical Immunology*, vol. 131, no. 1, pp. 23–30, 2013.

[68] J. F. Bach, "The effect of infections on susceptibility to autoimmune and allergic diseases," *The New England Journal of Medicine*, vol. 347, no. 12, pp. 911–920, 2002.

[69] T. Romacho, M. Elsen, D. Röhrborn, and J. Eckel, "Adipose tissue and its role in organ crosstalk," *Acta Physiologica*, vol. 210, no. 4, pp. 733–753, 2014.

[70] B. C. Lee and J. Lee, "Cellular and molecular players in adipose tissue inflammation in the development of obesity-induced insulin resistance," *Biochimica et Biophysica Acta*, vol. 1842, no. 3, pp. 446–462, 2014.

[71] J. M. Olefsky and C. K. Glass, "Macrophages, inflammation, and insulin resistance," *Annual Review of Physiology*, vol. 72, no. 1, pp. 219–246, 2010.

[72] I. Murano, G. Barbatelli, V. Parisani et al., "Dead adipocytes, detected as crown-like structures, are prevalent in visceral fat depots of genetically obese mice," *Journal of Lipid Research*, vol. 49, no. 7, pp. 1562–1568, 2008.

[73] T. Skurk, C. Alberti-Huber, C. Herder, and H. Hauner, "Relationship between adipocyte size and adipokine expression and secretion," *The Journal of Clinical Endocrinology and Metabolism*, vol. 92, no. 3, pp. 1023–1033, 2007.

[74] G. Boden, "Fatty acid-induced inflammation and insulin resistance in skeletal muscle and liver," *Current Diabetes Reports*, vol. 6, no. 3, pp. 177–181, 2006.

[75] T. Suganami, J. Nishida, and Y. Ogawa, "A paracrine loop between adipocytes and macrophages aggravates inflammatory changes," *Arteriosclerosis, Thrombosis, and Vascular Biology*, vol. 25, no. 10, pp. 2062–2068, 2005.

[76] K. A. Gendall, S. Raniga, R. Kennedy, and F. A. Frizelle, "The impact of obesity on outcome after major colorectal surgery," *Diseases of the Colon and Rectum*, vol. 50, no. 12, pp. 2223–2237, 2007.

[77] C. R. Guffey, D. Fan, U. P. Singh, and E. A. Murphy, "Linking obesity to colorectal cancer: recent insights into plausible biological mechanisms," *Current Opinion in Clinical Nutrition and Metabolic Care*, vol. 16, no. 5, pp. 595–600, 2013.

[78] E. E. Calle, C. Rodriguez, K. Walker-Thurmond, and M. J. Thun, "Overweight, obesity, and mortality from cancer in a prospectively studied cohort of U.S. adults," *The New England Journal of Medicine*, vol. 348, no. 17, pp. 1625–1638, 2003.

[79] E. Giovannucci, D. M. Harlan, M. C. Archer et al., "Diabetes and cancer: a consensus report," *CA: a Cancer Journal for Clinicians*, vol. 60, no. 4, pp. 207–221, 2010.

[80] B. Lauby-Secretan, C. Scoccianti, D. Loomis et al., "Body fatness and cancer–viewpoint of the IARC working group," *The New England Journal of Medicine*, vol. 375, no. 8, pp. 794–798, 2016.

[81] J. Incio, H. Liu, P. Suboj et al., "Obesity-induced inflammation and desmoplasia promote pancreatic cancer progression and resistance to chemotherapy," *Cancer Discovery*, vol. 6, no. 8, pp. 852–869, 2016.

[82] K. E. de Visser, A. Eichten, and L. M. Coussens, "Paradoxical roles of the immune system during cancer development," *Nature Reviews Cancer*, vol. 6, no. 1, pp. 24–37, 2006.

[83] M. Egeblad, A. J. Ewald, H. A. Askautrud et al., "Visualizing stromal cell dynamics in different tumor microenvironments by spinning disk confocal microscopy," *Disease Models & Mechanisms*, vol. 1, no. 2-3, pp. 155–167, 2008, discussion 65.

[84] C. E. Lewis and J. W. Pollard, "Distinct role of macrophages in different tumor microenvironments," *Cancer Research*, vol. 66, no. 2, pp. 605–612, 2006.

[85] B. P. Davis and M. E. Rothenberg, "Eosinophils and cancer," *Cancer Immunology Research*, vol. 2, no. 1, pp. 1–8, 2014.

[86] P. J. Murray and T. A. Wynn, "Protective and pathogenic functions of macrophage subsets," *Nature Reviews. Immunology*, vol. 11, no. 11, pp. 723–737, 2011.

[87] S. J. Galli, N. Borregaard, and T. A. Wynn, "Phenotypic and functional plasticity of cells of innate immunity: macrophages, mast cells and neutrophils," *Nature Immunology*, vol. 12, no. 11, pp. 1035–1044, 2011.

[88] C. Nathan, "Neutrophils and immunity: challenges and opportunities," *Nature Reviews. Immunology*, vol. 6, no. 3, pp. 173–182, 2006.

[89] S. B. Coffelt, M. D. Wellenstein, and K. E. de Visser, "Neutrophils in cancer: neutral no more," *Nature Reviews Cancer*, vol. 16, no. 7, pp. 431–446, 2016.

[90] C. Engblom, C. Pfirschke, and M. J. Pittet, "The role of myeloid cells in cancer therapies," *Nature Reviews Cancer*, vol. 16, no. 7, pp. 447–462, 2016.

[91] D. Galmarini, C. M. Galmarini, and F. C. Galmarini, "Cancer chemotherapy: a critical analysis of its 60 years of history," *Critical Reviews in Oncology/Hematology*, vol. 84, no. 2, pp. 181–199, 2012.

[92] D. Marvel and D. I. Gabrilovich, "Myeloid-derived suppressor cells in the tumor microenvironment: expect the unexpected," *The Journal of Clinical Investigation*, vol. 125, no. 9, pp. 3356–3364, 2015.

[93] R. Noy and J. W. Pollard, "Tumor-associated macrophages: from mechanisms to therapy," *Immunity*, vol. 41, no. 1, pp. 49–61, 2014.

[94] D. Di Mitri, A. Toso, J. J. Chen et al., "Tumour-infiltrating Gr-1$^+$ myeloid cells antagonize senescence in cancer," *Nature*, vol. 515, no. 7525, pp. 134–137, 2014.

[95] H. Nozawa, C. Chiu, and D. Hanahan, "Infiltrating neutrophils mediate the initial angiogenic switch in a mouse model of multistage carcinogenesis," *Proceedings of the National Academy of Sciences of the United States of America*, vol. 103, no. 33, pp. 12493–12498, 2006.

[96] P. Andreu, M. Johansson, N. I. Affara et al., "FcRγ Activation Regulates Inflammation-Associated Squamous Carcinogenesis," *Cancer Cell*, vol. 17, no. 2, pp. 121–134, 2010.

[97] R. Carretero, I. M. Sektioglu, N. Garbi, O. C. Salgado, P. Beckhove, and G. J. Hämmerling, "Eosinophils orchestrate cancer rejection by normalizing tumor vessels and enhancing infiltration of CD8$^+$ T cells," *Nature Immunology*, vol. 16, no. 6, pp. 609–617, 2015.

[98] J. C. Clemente, L. K. Ursell, L. W. Parfrey, and R. Knight, "The impact of the gut microbiota on human health: an integrative view," *Cell*, vol. 148, no. 6, pp. 1258–1270, 2012.

[99] A. M. O'Hara and F. Shanahan, "The gut flora as a forgotten organ," *EMBO Reports*, vol. 7, no. 7, pp. 688–693, 2006.

[100] S. V. Lynch and O. Pedersen, "The human intestinal microbiome in health and disease," *The New England Journal of Medicine*, vol. 375, no. 24, pp. 2369–2379, 2016.

[101] J. Wang and H. Jia, "Metagenome-wide association studies: fine-mining the microbiome," *Nature Reviews Microbiology*, vol. 14, no. 8, pp. 508–522, 2016.

[102] A. Couturier-Maillard, T. Secher, A. Rehman et al., "NOD2-mediated dysbiosis predisposes mice to transmissible colitis and colorectal cancer," *The Journal of Clinical Investigation*, vol. 123, no. 2, pp. 700–711, 2013.

[103] B. Hu, E. Elinav, S. Huber et al., "Microbiota-induced activation of epithelial IL-6 signaling links inflammasome-driven inflammation with transmissible cancer," *Proceedings of the National Academy of Sciences of the United States of America*, vol. 110, no. 24, pp. 9862–9867, 2013.

[104] Q. Feng, S. Liang, H. Jia et al., "Gut microbiome development along the colorectal adenoma-carcinoma sequence," *Nature Communications*, vol. 6, no. 1, p. 6528, 2015.

[105] P. Louis, G. L. Hold, and H. J. Flint, "The gut microbiota, bacterial metabolites and colorectal cancer," *Nature Reviews. Microbiology*, vol. 12, no. 10, pp. 661–672, 2014.

[106] S. Russell, "Artificial intelligence: the future is superintelligent," *Nature*, vol. 548, no. 7669, pp. 520-521, 2017.

[107] S. A. Brown, "Building SuperModels: emerging patient avatars for use in precision and systems medicine," *Frontiers in Physiology*, vol. 6, p. 318, 2015.

[108] H. Lippman, "How apps are changing family medicine," *The Journal of Family Practice*, vol. 62, no. 7, pp. 362–367, 2013.

[109] R. Mirnezami, J. Nicholson, and A. Darzi, "Preparing for precision medicine," *The New England Journal of Medicine*, vol. 366, no. 6, pp. 489–491, 2012.

[110] S. R. Steinhubl, E. D. Muse, and E. J. Topol, "The emerging field of mobile health," *Science translational medicine*, vol. 7, no. 283, p. 283rv3, 2015.

[111] Mayo Clinic, "Metabolic syndrome: symptoms and causes," 2019, https://www.mayoclinic.org/diseases-conditions/metabolic-syndrome/symptoms-causes/syc-20351916.

[112] Juvenal, *Book IV: Satires 10-12*, Cambridge University Press, Cambridge, 2014.

[113] H. W. Kohl 3rd, C. L. Craig, E. V. Lambert et al., "The pandemic of physical inactivity: global action for public health," *Lancet*, vol. 380, no. 9838, pp. 294–305, 2012.

[114] J. Myers, M. Prakash, V. Froelicher, D. Do, S. Partington, and J. E. Atwood, "Exercise capacity and mortality among men referred for exercise testing," *The New England Journal of Medicine*, vol. 346, no. 11, pp. 793–801, 2002.

[115] M. E. Kotas and R. Medzhitov, "Homeostasis, inflammation, and disease susceptibility," *Cell*, vol. 160, no. 5, pp. 816–827, 2015.

[116] O. Neubauer, S. Sabapathy, K. J. Ashton et al., "Time course-dependent changes in the transcriptome of human skeletal muscle during recovery from endurance exercise: from inflammation to adaptive remodeling," *Journal of Applied Physiology*, vol. 116, no. 3, pp. 274–287, 2014.

[117] A. Nunes-Silva, P. T. T. Bernardes, B. M. Rezende et al., "Treadmill exercise induces neutrophil recruitment into muscle tissue in a reactive oxygen species-dependent manner. An intravital microscopy study," *PLoS One*, vol. 9, no. 5, article e96464, 2014.

[118] C. M. Friedenreich, H. K. Neilson, M. S. Farris, and K. S. Courneya, "Physical activity and cancer outcomes: a precision medicine approach," *Clinical Cancer Research*, vol. 22, no. 19, pp. 4766–4775, 2016.

[119] S. C. Moore, I. M. Lee, E. Weiderpass et al., "Association of leisure-time physical activity with risk of 26 types of cancer in 1.44 million adults," *JAMA Internal Medicine*, vol. 176, no. 6, pp. 816–825, 2016.

[120] A. S. Fairey, K. S. Courneya, C. J. Field, G. J. Bell, L. W. Jones, and J. R. Mackey, "Randomized controlled trial of exercise and blood immune function in postmenopausal breast cancer

survivors," *Journal of Applied Physiology*, vol. 98, no. 4, pp. 1534–1540, 2005.

[121] O. K. Glass, B. A. Inman, G. Broadwater et al., "Effect of aerobic training on the host systemic milieu in patients with solid tumours: an exploratory correlative study," *British Journal of Cancer*, vol. 112, no. 5, pp. 825–831, 2015.

[122] K. H. Schmitz, K. S. Courneya, C. Matthews et al., "American College of Sports Medicine roundtable on exercise guidelines for cancer survivors," *Medicine and Science in Sports and Exercise*, vol. 42, no. 7, pp. 1409–1426, 2010.

[123] C. P. Wen, J. P. M. Wai, M. K. Tsai et al., "Minimum amount of physical activity for reduced mortality and extended life expectancy: a prospective cohort study," *Lancet*, vol. 378, no. 9798, pp. 1244–1253, 2011.

[124] K. S. Courneya, D. C. McKenzie, J. R. Mackey et al., "Effects of exercise dose and type during breast cancer chemotherapy: multicenter randomized trial," *Journal of the National Cancer Institute*, vol. 105, no. 23, pp. 1821–1832, 2013.

[125] J. P. Sasso, N. D. Eves, J. F. Christensen, G. J. Koelwyn, J. Scott, and L. W. Jones, "A framework for prescription in exercise-oncology research," *Journal of Cachexia, Sarcopenia and Muscle*, vol. 6, no. 2, pp. 115–124, 2015.

[126] H. van Waart, M. M. Stuiver, W. H. van Harten et al., "Effect of low-intensity physical activity and moderate- to high-intensity physical exercise during adjuvant chemotherapy on physical fitness, fatigue, and chemotherapy completion rates: results of the PACES randomized clinical trial," *Journal of Clinical Oncology*, vol. 33, no. 17, pp. 1918–1927, 2015.

[127] E. A. Lew and L. Garfinkel, "Variations in mortality by weight among 750,000 men and women," *Journal of Chronic Diseases*, vol. 32, no. 8, pp. 563–576, 1979.

[128] H. Møller, A. Mellemgaard, K. Lindvig, and J. H. Olsen, "Obesity and cancer risk: a Danish record-linkage study," *European Journal of Cancer*, vol. 30, no. 3, pp. 344–350, 1994.

[129] A. Wolk, G. Gridley, M. Svensson et al., "A prospective study of obesity and cancer risk (Sweden)," *Cancer Causes & Control*, vol. 12, no. 1, pp. 13–21, 2001.

[130] N. M. Iyengar, R. A. Ghossein, L. G. Morris et al., "White adipose tissue inflammation and cancer-specific survival in patients with squamous cell carcinoma of the oral tongue," *Cancer*, vol. 122, no. 24, pp. 3794–3802, 2016.

[131] C. Algire, L. Amrein, M. Zakikhani, L. Panasci, and M. Pollak, "Metformin blocks the stimulative effect of a high-energy diet on colon carcinoma growth in vivo and is associated with reduced expression of fatty acid synthase," *Endocrine-Related Cancer*, vol. 17, no. 2, pp. 351–360, 2010.

[132] A. Tannenbaum and H. Silverstone, "The influence of the degree of caloric restriction on the formation of skin tumors and hepatomas in mice," *Cancer Research*, vol. 9, no. 12, pp. 724–727, 1949.

[133] R. T. Chlebowski, A. K. Aragaki, G. L. Anderson et al., "Low-fat dietary pattern and breast cancer mortality in the women's health initiative randomized controlled trial," *Journal of Clinical Oncology*, vol. 35, no. 25, pp. 2919–2926, 2017.

[134] D. S. Chan, A. R. Vieira, D. Aune et al., "Body mass index and survival in women with breast cancer—systematic literature review and meta-analysis of 82 follow-up studies," *Annals of Oncology*, vol. 25, no. 10, pp. 1901–1914, 2014.

[135] M. Yang, S. A. Kenfield, E. L. van Blarigan et al., "Dietary patterns after prostate cancer diagnosis in relation to disease-specific and total mortality," *Cancer Prevention Research*, vol. 8, no. 6, pp. 545–551, 2015.

[136] E. M. Friedman, "Sleep quality, social well-being, gender, and inflammation: an integrative analysis in a national sample," *Annals of the New York Academy of Sciences*, vol. 1231, no. 1, pp. 23–34, 2011.

[137] F. Kapsimalis, M. Basta, G. Varouchakis, K. Gourgoulianis, A. Vgontzas, and M. Kryger, "Cytokines and pathological sleep," *Sleep Medicine*, vol. 9, no. 6, pp. 603–614, 2008.

[138] A. A. Prather, E. Puterman, E. S. Epel, and F. S. Dhabhar, "Poor sleep quality potentiates stress-induced cytokine reactivity in postmenopausal women with high visceral abdominal adiposity," *Brain, Behavior, and Immunity*, vol. 35, pp. 155–162, 2014.

[139] N. G. Altman, B. Izci-Balserak, E. Schopfer et al., "Sleep duration versus sleep insufficiency as predictors of cardiometabolic health outcomes," *Sleep Medicine*, vol. 13, no. 10, pp. 1261–1270, 2012.

[140] M. Jackowska, M. Kumari, and A. Steptoe, "Sleep and biomarkers in the English Longitudinal Study of Ageing: associations with C-reactive protein, fibrinogen, dehydroepiandrosterone sulfate and hemoglobin," *Psychoneuroendocrinology*, vol. 38, no. 9, pp. 1484–1493, 2013.

[141] Y. Liu, A. G. Wheaton, D. P. Chapman, and J. B. Croft, "Sleep duration and chronic diseases among U.S. adults age 45 years and older: evidence from the 2010 Behavioral Risk Factor Surveillance System," *Sleep*, vol. 36, no. 10, pp. 1421–1427, 2013.

[142] D. Fukumura, J. Incio, R. C. Shankaraiah, and R. K. Jain, "Obesity and cancer: an angiogenic and inflammatory link," *Microcirculation*, vol. 23, no. 3, pp. 191–206, 2016.

[143] J. Incio, J. Tam, N. N. Rahbari et al., "PlGF/VEGFR-1 signaling promotes macrophage polarization and accelerated tumor progression in obesity," *Clinical Cancer Research*, vol. 22, no. 12, pp. 2993–3004, 2016.

[144] M. M. Smits and E. J. van Geenen, "The clinical significance of pancreatic steatosis," *Nature Reviews. Gastroenterology & Hepatology*, vol. 8, no. 3, pp. 169–177, 2011.

[145] E. Pasquier, M. Kavallaris, and N. Andre, "Metronomic chemotherapy: new rationale for new directions," *Nature Reviews. Clinical Oncology*, vol. 7, no. 8, pp. 455–465, 2010.

[146] S. Niraula, R. J. O. Dowling, M. Ennis et al., "Metformin in early breast cancer: a prospective window of opportunity neoadjuvant study," *Breast Cancer Research and Treatment*, vol. 135, no. 3, pp. 821–830, 2012.

[147] G. Gueron, N. Anselmino, P. Chiarella et al., "Game-changing restraint of Ros-damaged phenylalanine, upon tumor metastasis," *Cell Death & Disease*, vol. 9, no. 2, pp. 140–155, 2018.

[148] A. Gottschalk, S. Sharma, J. Ford, M. E. Durieux, and M. Tiouririne, "Review article: the role of the perioperative period in recurrence after cancer surgery," *Anesthesia and Analgesia*, vol. 110, no. 6, pp. 1636–1643, 2010.

[149] T. Hirai, H. Matsumoto, H. Kubota, and Y. Yamaguchi, "Regulating surgical oncotaxis to improve the outcomes in cancer patients," *Surgery Today*, vol. 44, pp. 804–811, 2013.

[150] P. Forget, J. Vandenhende, M. Berliere et al., "Do intraoperative analgesics influence breast cancer recurrence after mastectomy? A retrospective analysis," *Anesthesia and Analgesia*, vol. 110, no. 6, pp. 1630–1635, 2010.

[151] M. Retsky, R. Rogers, R. Demicheli et al., "NSAID analgesic ketorolac used perioperatively may suppress early breast cancer relapse: particular relevance to triple negative subgroup," *Breast Cancer Research and Treatment*, vol. 134, no. 2, pp. 881–888, 2012.

[152] S. M. Grabosch, O. M. Shariff, and C. W. Helm, "Non-steroidal anti-inflammatory agents to induce regression and prevent the progression of cervical intraepithelial neoplasia," *Cochrane Database of Systematic Reviews*, vol. 2, article CD004121, 2018.

[153] A. Mohammed, N. S. Yarla, V. Madka, and C. V. Rao, "Clinically relevant anti-inflammatory agents for chemoprevention of colorectal cancer: new perspectives," *International Journal of Molecular Sciences*, vol. 19, pp. E2332–E2E50, 2018.

[154] G. Zeller, J. Tap, A. Y. Voigt et al., "Potential of fecal microbiota for early-stage detection of colorectal cancer," *Molecular Systems Biology*, vol. 10, no. 11, p. 766, 2014.

[155] M. Raman, P. Ambalam, K. K. Kondepudi et al., "Potential of probiotics, prebiotics and synbiotics for management of colorectal cancer," *Gut Microbes*, vol. 4, pp. 181–192, 2014.

[156] A. Gagliardi, V. Totino, F. Cacciotti et al., "Rebuilding the gut microbiota ecosystem," *International Journal of Environmental Research and Public Health*, vol. 15, article E1679, 2018.

[157] D. Chen, J. Wu, D. Jin, B. Wang, and H. Cao, "Fecal microbiota transplantation in cancer management: current status and perspectives," *International Journal of Cancer*, vol. 145, no. 8, pp. 2021–2031, 2019.

[158] Editorial, "Context: the grey matter of cancer," *Nature Reviews Clinical Oncology*, vol. 14, p. 519, 2017.

[159] A. Sakula, "In search of Hippocrates: a visit to Kos," *Journal of the Royal Society of Medicine*, vol. 77, pp. 682–688, 2016.

[160] K. M. Emmons and G. A. Colditz, "Realizing the potential of cancer prevention - the role of implementation science," *The New England Journal of Medicine*, vol. 376, no. 10, pp. 986–990, 2017.

[161] J. Kerr, C. Anderson, and S. M. Lippman, "Physical activity, sedentary behaviour, diet, and cancer: an update and emerging new evidence," *The Lancet Oncology*, vol. 18, no. 8, pp. e457–e471, 2017.

[162] D. Ornish, G. Weidner, W. R. Fair et al., "Intensive lifestyle changes may affect the progression of prostate cancer," *The Journal of Urology*, vol. 174, no. 3, pp. 1065–1070, 2005.

[163] J. Andreu-Perez, C. C. Poon, R. D. Merrifield, S. T. Wong, and G. Z. Yang, "Big data for health," *IEEE Journal of Biomedical and Health Informatics*, vol. 19, no. 4, pp. 1193–1208, 2015.

[164] R. Bellazzi, "Big data and biomedical informatics: a challenging opportunity," *Yearbook of Medical Informatics*, vol. 9, pp. 8–13, 2014.

20

Practice and Sociodemographic Factors Influencing Self-Monitoring of Blood Pressure in Ghanaians with Hypertension

Kennedy Dodam Konlan [ID],[1] Charles Junior Afam-Adjei,[2] Christian Afam-Adjei,[3] Jennifer Oware,[3] Theresa Akua Appiah,[4] Kennedy Diema Konlan [ID],[5] and Jeremiah Bella-Fiamawle[2]

[1]Department of Social & Behavioural Sciences, School of Public Health, University of Ghana, Legon, Accra, Ghana
[2]Department of Medicine, Nursing Directorate, Korle-Bu Teaching Hospital, Accra, Ghana
[3]Department of Nursing, St. Karol School of Nursing, Aplaku-Accra, Ghana
[4]School of Business, Ghana Institute of Management & Public Administration (GIMPA), Accra, Ghana
[5]Department of Public Health Nursing, School of Nursing and Midwifery, University of Allied Health Sciences, Ho, Ghana

Correspondence should be addressed to Kennedy Dodam Konlan; kennedy.konlan@gmail.com

Academic Editor: Khoa Nguyen

Background. In sub-Saharan Africa, the prevalence of hypertension has assumed epidemic levels and currently accounts for numerous complications such as stroke, heart failure, and kidney damage. Management of hypertension involves both drug and nonpharmacological approaches. Self-monitoring of blood pressure is an important nonpharmacological approach that facilitates early detection of deteriorating blood pressures and complications. *Aims.* We determined the practice and sociodemographic factors influencing self-monitoring of blood pressure among Ghanaians with hypertension. *Methods.* In a cross-sectional design, we recruited four hundred and forty-seven (447) Ghanaians with hypertension receiving care at the hypertensive Outpatient Department (OPD) Clinics of the Medical Department at the Korle-Bu Teaching Hospital (KBTH). The respondents were sampled using a simple random sampling technique of balloting without replacement. A structured questionnaire was used to gather data on the practice of self-monitoring of blood pressure and sociodemographic factors influencing self-monitoring in the respondents. We also measured some anthropometric and haemodynamic indices of the respondents. The data was entered in Microsoft Excel 2010 and exported into SPSS 21.0 to aid with the data analysis. A chi-square test and Student's *t*-test analysis were done to determine the relationship between the practice of self-monitioring and other sociodemographic variables. Data analayses were conducted at a significant level (alpha 0.05) and power of 95% confidence. Thus, $p < 0.05$ was considered statistically significant. *Results.* The practice of self-monitoring of blood pressure was 25.3% with more female respondents claiming to practice self-monitoring as compared to their male counterparts (28.6% vs. 20.7%). Awareness of self-monitoring of blood pressure was associated with increased practice of self-monitoring of blood pressure. Health workers (46.8%), colleague patients (39.8%), relatives/spouses (6.7%), and the media (6.7%) were identified as the sources of information about self-monitoring of blood pressure. Awareness of self-monitoring, level of education, valid health insurance, occupation, income levels, and marital status had a significant relationship with self-monitoring of blood pressure among the respondents. Thus, respondents with higher education, awareness of self-monitoring, valid health insurance, formal employment, and higher income were likely to monitor their blood pressure. *Conclusion.* Several sociodemographic factors influence the practice of self-monitoring of blood pressure in Ghanaians with hypertension. Thus, targeted hypertension education and social-cognitive interventions should focus on these sociodemographic factors so as to improve self-monitoring of blood pressure in order to reduce the complications of hypertension.

1. Introduction

Hypertension, also known as high blood pressure (BP), is now a global public health problem associated with serious health complications [1]. Hypertension is a leading cause of global burden of heart diseases, stroke, renal failure, peripheral vascular disease, and premature mortality and disability [1, 2]. The global burden of hypertension revealed that 25% of adults are living with hypertension and 9.2% of the total mortality is due to hypertension-related events [3]. It is estimated that over a billion people currently suffer from hypertension [1]. This figure is expected to increase to almost two billion in 2025 [1]. Recent studies from Ghana and other sub-Saharan African countries indicate that the prevalence of cardiovascular diseases (CVDs) is increasing at an alarming rate [3, 4].

The current management of hypertension involves pharmacological and nonpharmacological strategies [4, 5]. The pharmacological approach involves using antihypertensive medications such as beta-blockers, beta-blockers with intrinsic sympathomimetic activity, alpha-1 blockers, combined alpha and beta-blockers, vasodilators, and angiotensin II receptor blocker [5, 6]. Nonpharmacological strategies in the management of hypertension include dietary intake moderation or reduction (particularly saturated fats and excess sodium consumption), regular exercise, and avoidance of exposure to active and passive tobacco smoke [6]. Although significant efforts are being made by healthcare providers to control the morbidity and mortality associated with hypertension, it is still considered a major public health problem [7].

Proper management of hypertension requires adherence to management by patients as well as self-monitoring of blood pressure [8]. Self-monitoring of blood pressure refers to the measuring of one's own blood pressure (BP) outside the usual review visit to a general physician (GP), mostly within one's home [2, 6]. It is the practice where a patient voluntarily measures his/her BP using a self-check device, be it manual or electronic [7, 9]. Self-monitoring of blood pressure is crucial in detecting and preventing hypertension-related complications, and it has been shown to improve patient satisfaction and quality of life and also reduce primary care and out-patient and emergency department visits [10]. Most hypertensive patients in Ghana might not be aware of the enormous role of self-monitoring of blood pressure and hence may not practice efficient self-monitoring of blood pressure [11], thus depriving them of the enormous benefits associated with self-monitoring of blood pressure [9].

2. Aim

We determined the practice and sociodemographic factors influencing self-monitoring of blood pressure among Ghanaians with hypertension. In Ghana, complications and mortalities associated with hypertension are still high despite the marked improvement in care [4]. Self-monitoring of blood pressure has been established as one of the effective ways of reducing complications associated with hypertension [10]. Self-monitoring is also useful in getting clients with lifelong conditions involved in their management and the surest way of patient empowerment [9, 11].

3. Method

3.1. Study Design. In this study, we employed a descriptive cross-sectional design. Ghanaians with hypertension receiving care at the Hypertensive Clinic of the Outpatient Department (OPD) of the Medical Department of the Korle-Bu Teaching Hospital (KBTH) were sampled. The philosophical underpinning of the study was the positivist strategy. In adopting the positivist approach to research, which is quantitative, the researcher embarks on the study of the reality by maintaining a distance between him/her and the researcher [12]. Contrary to this approach, researchers who hold the view of interpretivists (qualitative) adopt strategies which will lessen the distance between them and what is being studied [12]. In this study, our view was that self-monitoring of blood pressure and the sociodemographic determinants associated with it can be objectively measured hence the adoption of the positivist approach.

3.2. Setting. The study was conducted at the Korle-Bu Teaching Hospital (KBTH), a resource-constrained health facility in Ghana where there is consistent shortage of staff coupled with increasing patient numbers [13]. Thus, empowerment of patients with hypertension through self-monitoring of blood pressure could be useful in enhancing positive disease outcomes through early detection of uncontrolled blood pressures [10]. The KBTH is located in the southern part of Ghana, and it is the national referral hospital in Ghana. It is the third largest hospital in Africa [13]. The KBTH which was established in 1923 has grown from an initial 200 beds to 2000 beds and 17 clinical and diagnostic departments. The hospital is traditionally known to receive huge numbers of referral cases from across the country with daily average patient attendance of 1,500 with average daily admission of 250 patients [13]. The respondents were selected from the Hypertensive OPD Clinics of the Medical Department at the KBTH. These clinics run for four days in a week from 8am to 2pm. The working days for the clinics were Mondays, Tuesdays, Thursdays, and Fridays. The data collection was done on Fridays.

3.3. Sample Size Determination. The sample size for the study was determined using the Cochran formula for determining the sample size [14]. Thus, the sample size of 385 respondents was required at a desired precision of 0.05 and at an estimated self-monitoring practice rate of 50%. After adding 20% for nonresponse rate, the sample size for the study was estimated to be 461 respondents.

3.4. Selection of Participants and Data Collection. We included male and female hypertensive patients visiting the Hypertensive OPD Clinics of the Medical Department at the KBTH for review post discharge. The inclusion criteria for the selection of the study respondents included Ghanaian hypertensive patients between the ages of 35-65 years, a history of previous admission with hypertension, and being well oriented to time and place with no signs of mental illness.

A simple random sampling technique of balloting without replacement was done using the patients' folders at the Hypertensive OPD Clinics of the Medical Department usually in the morning during waiting time. The patients' folders were numbered, and the corresponding numbers were written on small pieces of paper. The small pieces of paper with the numbers were then placed in a covered container and shaken thoroughly after which thirty (30) papers with corresponding numbers representing patients' folders were selected without replacement. The consent of those selected was obtained, and if they refused to consent, they were replaced by picking other small pieces of paper with the numbers corresponding to specific folders of patients until a total of thirty respondents were selected. The data collection was done on Fridays during a period of fifteen weeks (November, 2018, to March, 2019) excluding public holidays.

A pretested questionnaire was used as the data collection tool. Prior to the data collection, the questionnaire was pretested among hypertensive patients at the Polyclinic of the KBTH. The questionnaire contained sections which asked about the sociodemographic characteristics such as age of respondents, sex of respondents, highest educational level, marital status, occupation, income level, having a valid health insurance, awareness of normal blood pressure, and self-monitoring, as well as the practice of self-monitoring of blood pressure. The data was entered into Microsoft Excel 2010. The data was then exported into the Statistical Package for Social Sciences (SPSS) version 21.0 to aid with the analysis.

3.5. Data Analysis. We analyzed the data using the Statistical Package for Social Sciences (SPSS) version 21.0. During the analysis, we did a gender comparison of sociodemographic variables using Pearson's χ^2 test particularly for the dichotomous variables while using Student's t-test for a continuous variable (age). In determining the association between self-reported practice of self-monitoring of blood pressure and the sociodemographic variables, we used Pearson's χ^2. In this study, $p < 0.05$ was considered statistically significant.

3.6. Ethical Issues. The study data was part of data collected on a protocol titled: Adherence to Management and Quality of Life of Ghanaian Hypertensive on a Structured Health Education Programme (SHEP) approved by the Scientific and Technical Committee and the Institutional Review Board of the Korle-Bu Teaching Hospital (protocol identification number KBTH-IRB/0004/2018). We obtained permission from the Deputy Director of Nursing Service of the Central Outpatient Department prior to data collection. Also, we explained the purpose of the study to each respondent before obtaining written informed consent for the study. Further, we ensured confidentiality of the data collected by assigning unique codes to each response. We also maintained privacy and ensured anonymity throughout the data collection and analysis of the data.

4. Results

A total of four hundred and forty-seven (447) respondents took part in the study. As depicted in Table 1, the majority of the respondents (57.9%) were females with 42.1% being males. The mean age of the respondents was 53.13 ± 7.34 years with the females older than the males (54.13 ± 8.46 versus 51.21 ± 4.83). The majority of the respondents (61.3%) were married with only 4.3%, 11.6%, and 22.6% being single, widowed, and divorced, respectively. The results revealed that the majority of the females (44.4%) had no formal education with only 29 (6.5%) of the respondents reporting having had tertiary education. Further, the study found that 46.5% reported as having low income level with 29.97% of the respondents claiming to have high income levels. Female respondents reported high income level as compared to their male counterparts (41.3% versus 14.4%). Also, the results revealed that only 7.4% of the males had valid health insurance as compared to 63.7% of the females. The majority of the respondents did not have valid health insurance. Also, only 10.1% of the males had formal employment and this was similar among the females where 11.6% reported to have formal employment. With regard to unemployment, 41.3% of the females reported to be unemployed as compared to the 25.5% in males. The majority of the males were artisans/technicians or had vocational training (Table 1).

5. Awareness and Source of Information about Self-Monitoring of Blood Pressure

The majority (59.3%) of the respondents said they were aware of their normal blood pressure even though most of them could not state the said normal blood pressure. Only, 194 (43.4%) of the respondents said they were aware of self-monitoring of blood pressure with majority claiming not to be aware of self-monitoring. On the sources of information about self-monitoring of blood pressure, 90 (46.4%) claimed health workers, 76 (39.2%) cited colleague patients with only 10 (5.7%), and 18 (9.3%) cited spouses and media houses as sources of self-monitoring information (Table 2).

6. Association between Practice of Self-Monitoring of Blood Pressure and Socio-Demographic Factors

The practice of self-monitoring of blood pressure in the respondents was 25.3%. Awareness of self-monitoring of blood pressure was associated with the practice of self-motoring. The study revealed that higher educational qualification was associated with practice of self-monitoring of blood pressure. Respondents with formal employment were likely to self-monitor their blood pressure as compared to their counterparts. Also, having a valid health insurance was associated with the practice of self-monitoring. Further, a high income level was associated with self-monitoring of blood pressure. The results revealed that respondents who were single did more self-monitoring of their blood pressure as compared to married, widowed, and divorced counterparts (Table 3).

TABLE 1: Sociodemographic characteristics of respondents.

Variables	Males, n (%) 188 (42.1%)	Females, n (%) 259 (57.9%)	χ^2, p value
Age (years)	51.21 ± 4.83	54.13 ± 8.46	$<0.001^*$
Marital status, n (%)			
Single	18 (9.6)	1 (0.4)	
Married	90 (47.9)	184 (71)	87.127, $<0.001^*$
Divorced	73 (38.9)	28 (10.8)	
Widowed	7 (3.7)	46 (17.8)	
Highest education, n (%)			
No formal education	90 (47.9)	115 (44.4)	
Junior secondary	38 (20.2)	56 (21.6)	
Senior secondary	22 (11.7)	37 (14.3)	135.238, $<0.001^*$
Vocational/technical	32 (17)	32 (12.4)	
Tertiary	6 (3.2)	19 (7.3)	
Income level, n (%)			
High	27 (14.4)	107 (41.3)	
Middle	29 (15.4)	76 (29.3)	74.478, $<0.001^*$
Low	132 (70.2)	76 (29.3)	
Valid health insurance			
Yes	14 (7.4)	165 (63.7)	143.606, $<0.001^*$
No	174 (92.6)	94 (36.3)	
Occupation			
Formal employment	19 (10.1)	30 (11.6)	
Retired	1 (0.5)	30 (11.6)	
Trading/business	2 (1.1)	60 (23.2)	148.080, $<0.001^*$
Artisan/technician/vocational	118 (62.8)	32 (12.4)	
Unemployed	48 (25.5)	107 (41.3)	

* indicates statistical significance ($p < 0.05$).

TABLE 2: Awareness and source of information about self-monitoring of blood pressure.

Variable	Frequency	Percentage
Awareness of normal BP		
Yes	265	59.3
No	182	40.7
Awareness of SM		
Yes	194	43.4
No	253	56.6
Source of SM information		
Media	30	6.7
Health workers	209	46.8
Relatives/spouse	30	6.7
Colleague patients	178	39.8

7. Summary of Results

The results as shown above indicate that the majority of hypertensive patients who seek care at the KBTH were females. Most of the respondents had low or no formal education with the majority under the low income brackets. The results indicate that the awareness of self-monitoring as well as the practice of self-monitoring of blood pressure was low even though awareness of normal blood pressure was reportedly high. The practice of self-monitoring of blood pressure was low and was associated with awareness of self-monitoring, educational level, valid health insurance, income level, and marital status.

8. Discussion

A total of 447 respondents were involved in the study, and the majority of the respondents were females indicating that more females sought health care rather than males. This finding is in line with the study done by [14, 15] who found out that more females sought health care as compared to males. On the awareness about self-monitoring, 43.4% of the respondents were aware of self-monitoring with the majority not being aware. Only 25.3% of the respondents claimed to be practicing self-monitoring of blood pressure indicating a low level of practice of self-monitoring. This finding is in line with the study by [6, 16] who found out that only 42% of patients among the respondents were measuring their blood pressure. This finding is in contrast with those found by [11, 15] where 88% of the patients were aware and agreed that

TABLE 3: Comparing the association between practice of self-monitoring of BP (SM) and sociodemographic factors in the respondents.

Variable	Total, N (%)	Practice of SM (%)	χ^2, p value
Awareness of SM			49.240, <0.001*
Awareness of SM	194 (43.4)	81 (41.8)	
Not aware of SM	253 (56.6)	32 (12.6)	
Sex of respondent			3.533, 0.06
Male	188 (42.1)	39 (20.7)	
Female	259 (57.9)	74 (28.6)	
Highest education			253.560, <0.001*
No formal education	205 (45.9)	14 (6.8)	
Junior high school	94 (21.0)	11 (11.7)	
Senior high school	59 (13.2)	8 (13.6)	
Vocational/technical	64 (14.3)	10 (15.6)	
Tertiary	25 (5.6)	8 (32)	
Valid health insurance			32.707, <0.001*
Yes	179 (40)	71 (39.7)	
No	268 (60)	42 (15.7)	
Occupation			256.298, <0.001*
Formal employment	49 (11)	17 (34.7)	
Retired	31 (6.9)	4 (12.9)	
Trading/business	62 (13.9)	8 (12.9)	
Artisan/technician	150 (33.6)	39 (26)	
Unemployed	155 (34.7)	8 (5.2)	
Income level			47.34, <0.001*
Low	208 (46.5)	3 (1.4)	
Middle	105 (23.5)	30 (28.6)	
High	134 (30)	80 (59.7)	
Marital status			45.397, <0.001*
Single	19 (4.3)	14 (73.7)	
Married	274 (61.3)	77 (28.1)	
Divorced	101 (22.6)	6 (5.9)	
Widowed	53 (11.9)	16 (30.2)	

* indicates statistical significance ($p < 0.05$).

self-monitoring of blood pressure was important and actually practiced it.

On the source of information about self-monitoring, health workers served as the main source of information. The media and relatives/spouses as a medium for information on self-monitoring were minimal. This result is in line with the study conducted by [16, 17]. Also, [18, 19] in their study supported the view that the availability of information through family/friend/opinion leaders of trusted groups, the media (including radio, public enlightenment programmes, and newspapers), and the doctor/nurse/health worker can affect one's level of awareness on hypertension. Thus, health workers serve as a key source of information to patients, but the potential role of the media in health promotion is yet to be explored especially in developing countries. None of the respondents said they got their information from the internet

despite the increasing internet service availability in Ghana. The need to explore the Internet as a viable means to deliver health educational messages was ought to be emphasized by health providers.

Also, the critical potential of family/spousal support in self-monitoring was found to be low as few of the respondents claimed their family members/spouses helped them with self-monitoring of their blood pressure or even made them aware of it. This finding is in contrast to the findings of [19–21] who observed that family, friends, and churches had powerful influences on patients' long-term management and adoption of healthy lifestyle practice. In a study by [20], 93% of the hypertensive participants reported receiving social support from families while 55% reported receiving social support from friends. Thus, family support remains a crucial need for hypertensive patients if complications of hypertension are to be reduced as they can encourage and support self-monitoring of blood pressure which can eventually reduce the risk of complications.

In our study, we found that the educational level of the respondents was found to be a significant determinant of practice of self-monitoring of blood pressure. The practice of self-monitoring increased marginally with the rising level of education among the respondents. Similar findings have been reported in other studies [16, 20] where the level of formal education was associated with self-monitoring practice in hypertensive patients.

The study found that the practice of self-monitoring of blood pressure increased with increasing self-reported income levels of respondents. Just as found in this study, other studies [16–18] report a positive relationship between the socioeconomic status of patients and the practice of self-monitoring of blood pressure. This could possibly be because of the fact that those within the high income brackets could afford to get blood pressure monitoring devices and thus could practice self-monitoring of their blood pressure at home without any difficulty as compared to their counterparts in the low-income brackets. The respondents in the lower income brackets probably had irregular clinic visits and did not have money to buy the blood pressure gadgets among others hence their low self-monitoring of blood pressure. Similar findings have been reported by some studies which stated that poor attendance to clinics and cost of blood pressure devices were identified by some researchers as a barrier to hypertension self-monitoring [20, 21]. Chronic conditions like hypertension often result in physical disability such as stroke which may decrease one's strength and ability to work. This can reduce the income level of the patient and therefore serve as a source of financial constraint and hence a barrier to hypertensive self-monitoring [15, 17].

The study further found that those who had valid health insurance cards practiced self-monitoring of blood pressure as compared to their counterparts without valid health insurance. It is possible that those with valid health insurance were more likely to be regular in their clinic visitation; hence, they became aware of self-monitoring because it was taught at the OPD by nurses and doctors as compared to their counterparts without valid health insurance. Also, having valid health insurance could reduce the cost of the patient procuring their medications and hence providing alternative income to buy blood pressure devices for self-monitoring. According to [6, 17], resources are needed to support self-monitoring and so a patient's socioeconomic position is of essence when it came to self-monitoring.

9. Limitations of the Study

The study used a cross-sectional design making it difficult to infer causation. Also, since the study depended on a pretested questionnaire which largely depended on the respondents' responses and recall, there is high possibility of recall bias. Further, income levels are usually associated with some social status in society; hence, some of the respondents could claim to be in the high social brackets when actually they are not and vice versa.

Abbreviations

SM: Self-monitoring
CVDs: Cardiovascular diseases
BP: Blood pressure.

Authors' Contributions

KDK contributed to the conception, design, data analysis, and drafting of the manuscript and bears the primary responsibility for the content of the manuscript. CJAA revised the manuscript. CJA, JO, TAA, and JBF were involved in the data collection. KKD was involved in the revision of the manuscript. All the authors read and approved the content of the manuscript.

Acknowledgments

Our profound appreciation to the staff of the Training and Research Unit of the Nursing Directorate, Korle-Bu Teaching Hospital, who assisted during the field work.

References

[1] A. Moran, M. Forouzanfar, U. Sampson, S. Chugh, V. Feigin, and G. Mensah, "The epidemiology of cardiovascular diseases in sub-Saharan Africa: the global burden of diseases, injuries and risk factors 2010 study," *Progress in Cardiovascular Diseases*, vol. 56, no. 3, pp. 234–239, 2013.

[2] T. S. Ferguson, M. K. Tulloch-Reid, N. O. M. Younger et al., "Prevalence of the metabolic syndrome and its components in relation to socioeconomic status among Jamaican young adults: a cross-sectional study," *BMC Public Health*, vol. 10, no. 1, p. 307, 2010.

[3] A. de-Graft Aikins, "Ghana's neglected chronic disease epidemic: a developmental challenge," *Ghana Medical Journal*, vol. 41, no. 4, pp. 154–159, 2007.

[4] S. H. Nyarko, "Prevalence and Sociodemographic Determinants of Hypertension History among Women in Reproductive Age in Ghana," *International Journal of Hypertension*, vol. 2016, Article ID 3292938, 6 pages, 2016.

[5] M. Seyedmazhari, "Pharmacological and non-pharmacological treatment of hypertension: a review article," *ARYA Atherosclerosis*, vol. 3, pp. S217–S221, 2013.

[6] F. Gohar, S. M. Greenfield, D. G. Beevers, G. Y. H. Lip, and K. Jolly, "Self-care and adherence to medication: a survey in the hypertension outpatient clinic," *BMC Complementary and Alternative Medicine*, vol. 8, no. 1, article 4, 2008.

[7] R. A. Adedoyin, C. E. Mbada, M. O. Balogun et al., "Prevalence and pattern of hypertension in a semi-urban community in Nigeria," *European Journal of Cardiovascular Prevention & Rehabilitation*, vol. 15, no. 6, pp. 683–687, 2008.

[8] K. Yeboah, K. K. Dodam, P. K. Affrim et al., "Metabolic syndrome and parental history of cardiovascular disease in young adults in urban Ghana," *BMC Public Health*, vol. 18, no. 1, article 96, 2018.

[9] S. Baral-Grant, M. S. Haque, A. Nouwen, S. M. Greenfield, and R. J. McManus, "Self-Monitoring of Blood Pressure in Hypertension: A UK Primary Care Survey," *International Journal of Hypertension*, vol. 2012, Article ID 582068, 4 pages, 2012.

[10] D. Al Hadithi, A. S. Nazmi, and S. A. Khan, "Self monitoring of blood pressure (SMBP) among hypertensive patients in Muscat- a pilot study," *Journal of Applied Pharmaceutical Science*, vol. 2, no. 9, pp. 155–157, 2012.

[11] T. E. Ambakederemo, I. D. Ebuenyi, and J. Jumbo, "Knowledge and Attitude to Self-Monitoring Of Blood Pressure in a Cardiology Clinic in Nigeria," *IOSR Journal of Dental and Medical Sciences*, vol. 13, no. 5, pp. 63–65, 2014.

[12] J. W. Creswell, "Research design: qualitative, quantitative, and mixed methods approaches," in *Research Design Qualitative Quantitative and Mixed Methods Approaches*, p. 260, Sage Publications, 3rd edition, 2009.

[13] KBTH, *Annual Report of KBTH*, Korle Bu Teaching Hospital, Accra, 2016.

[14] L. G. Glynn, A. W. Murphy, S. M. Smith, K. Schroeder, and T. Fahey, "Interventions used to improve control of blood pressure in patients with hypertension," *Cochrane Database Systematic Review*, vol. 1, no. 3, article Cd005182, 2010.

[15] S. Drayton-Brooks and N. White, "Health promoting behaviors among African American women with faith-based support," *Association of Black Nursing Faculty Journal.*, vol. 15, no. 5, pp. 84–90, 2014.

[16] V. Eugene and P. Bourne, "Hypertensive patients: knowledge, self-care management practices and challenges," *Journal of Behavioral Health*, vol. 2, no. 3, p. 1, 2012.

[17] M. Elkjaer, "E-health: Web-guided therapy and disease self-management in ulcerative colitis. Impact on disease outcome, quality of life and compliance," *Danish Medical Journal*, vol. 59, no. 7, article B4478, 2012.

[18] E. Boulware, S. Flynn, J. Ameling et al., "Facilitators and barriers to hypertension self-management in urban African Americans: perspectives of patients and family members," *Patient Preference and Adherence*, vol. 7, pp. 741–749, 2013.

[19] A. Fex, G. Flensner, A. C. Ek, and O. Soderhamn, "Self-care agency and perceived health among people using advanced

medical technology at home," *Journal of Advanced Nursing,* vol. 68, no. 4, pp. 806–815, 2012.

[20] B. Kaambwa, S. Bryan, S. Jowett et al., "Telemonitoring and self-management in the control of hypertension (TAS-MINH2): a cost-effectiveness analysis," *European Journal Preventive Cardiology,* vol. 21, no. 12, pp. 1517–1530, 2013.

[21] E. L. Knight, R. L. Bohn, P. S. Wang, R. J. Glynn, H. Mogun, and J. Avorn, "Predictors of uncontrolled hypertension in ambulatory patients," *Hypertension,* vol. 38, no. 4, pp. 809–814, 2001.

21

Hypertension and Diabetes Mellitus among Patients at Hawassa University Comprehensive Specialized Hospital, Hawassa, Southern Ethiopia

Andargachew Kassa ⓘ[1] and Endrias Markos Woldesemayat[2]

[1]College of Medicine and Health Sciences, School of Nursing and Midwifery, Hawassa University, Ethiopia
[2]College of Medicine and Health Sciences, School of Public and Environmental Health, Hawassa University, Ethiopia

Correspondence should be addressed to Andargachew Kassa; akandkassa@gmail.com

Academic Editor: Olga Pechanova

Background. The burden of noncommunicable disease (NCD) in Africa is on a remarkable rise exacerbating the poor public health status affected by the existing but yet unsolved communicable disease. In Ethiopia, there is a paucity of evidence regarding prevalence and risk factors to NCD. *Objective*. This study sought to determine the prevalence of risk factors of NCDs, prevalence of DM and HTN, and risk factors associated with diabetes mellitus (DM) and hypertension (HTN). *Method*. This is an institution based cross-sectional study conducted on a sample of 411 clients attending a university-based comprehensive specialized hospital in Southern Ethiopia. The data was collected by using a pretested interviewer-administered questionnaire and observational checklist. Frequency, proportions, bivariate and multivariate logistic regression analysis was conducted using SPSS software version 20. *Result*. We identified 64.2% of the clients had at least one of the risk factors to the NCDs. One-third (33.3%) had physical inactivity, whereas 20.2% had a BMI of $\geq$ 25%. The prevalence of DM and HTN was 12.2% and 10.5%, respectively. The multivariate analysis demonstrated that age $\geq$ 60 years, physical inactivity, higher BMI, and cigarette smoking were risk factors for at least one of the NCDs. *Conclusion*. The prevalence of DM and prevalence of HTN were high. The magnitudes of risk factors to NCDs among the study population were substantial. Higher BMI, physical inactivity, low fruit and vegetable consumption, alcohol use, khat chewing, and cigarette smoking were among the prevailing risk factors identified.

1. Introduction

In the developing world, communicable diseases were the major causes of morbidity and mortality and still, they continued to be the cause. But noncommunicable diseases (NCDs) are on a remarkable rise causing ill health and death for millions. NCD is the cause of 63% of annual global death report, of which 14 million deaths are premature. Unfortunately, 86% of the premature deaths are happening in the middle- and lower-income countries (LMICs) [1]. NCDs are happening as a result of demographic transition characterized by urbanization, industrialization, and the ever-improving life expectancy noted in these countries [2]. The expansion of these catastrophic NCD started exacerbating the existing poor health status of the public and also enticing

the delivery of health care service [2, 3]. The WHO has identified four major NCDs happening in the developing region. These are cardiovascular diseases (CVD), cancer, chronic respiratory diseases, and diabetes (DM) [2].

The common risk factors for these four NCDs are classified into two categories called behavioral and biomedical risk factors. By avoiding the behavioral risk factors such as tobacco use, physical inactivity, unhealthy dietary practice, and alcohol abuse, it is possible to reduce 80% of CVDs and DM. In addition, one-third of all forms of cancers can be prevented by avoiding these risk factors. Unless these behavioral risk factors are avoided, the development of other formidable biomedical risk factors such as increments in blood pressure, blood sugar, blood lipids, and also an abnormal increment in the person's BMI will happen inevitably [1, 2].

The World Health Organization (WHO) estimate to Ethiopia denoted that 34% of the annual death rate is attributable to NCD. The greatest proportion (15%) of these deaths is owing to cardiovascular diseases, where DM accounted for the 2% [2]. One small-scale community-based study conducted in Ethiopia to determine the prevalence of known risk factors for NCD reported 9.3% smoking, 7.1% alcohol use, 38.6% khat use, 27.0% poor dietary practice, and 16.9% poor physical exercise. Other than these behavioral risk factors, 9.3% high blood pressure, 2.6% BMI > 25 kg/m2, 10.7% high cholesterol level, and 7.7% raised triglyceride levels were also among the reported physical and biochemical risk factors [4].

Up until now, there is no nationally representative survey conducted to determine the prevalence of hypertension (HTN) and DM in the country [5]. However, there are few small-scale, community- and institution-based studies reporting the magnitude. Seven community-based studies conducted in Ethiopia revealed prevalence of HTN ranging from 9.9% to 28.3% [6–12]. The other reports from three institution-based studies also revealed a similar proportion among adults with HTN prevalence ranging from 7.7% to 27.3% [13–15]. The prevalence of DM in Ethiopia is only emanating from four institution-based survey studies revealing a range of 0.34%-8% [16–19]. These same studies showed that having DM is a risk factor in developing HTN and vice versa. It also demonstrated that they share similar risk factors. These include age, sex, income, physical inactivity, raised BMI, high salt intake, alcohol use, cigarette smoking, and eating vegetable three or fewer days per week.

The Federal Democratic Republic Ministry of Health (FMOH) of Ethiopia affirmed the fact that NCDs are rising at an alarmingly fast rate [5]. Conducting ongoing representative surveys in the area is vital to planning monitoring and evaluation of the effectiveness of health promotion and NCD preventive programs. Nevertheless, there is a paucity of research evidence reporting magnitudes and risk factors of NCD in the country [4, 5]. This study, therefore, is conducted to assess the prevalence of risk factors of NCD, particularly, of HTN and DM, their magnitude and factors associated with these NCDs among patients attending Hawassa University Comprehensive and Specialized Hospital (HU-CSH).

2. Methods

This institution-based cross-sectional study was conducted in January 2016 among patients attending Hawassa University Comprehensive Specialized Hospital (HU-CSH). This tertiary level Public University Hospital is the biggest in the region. It serves as a last referral destination to more than 15 million people residing in the region. The hospital provides services partially to people coming from the southern borders of the neighboring Oromia Region of Ethiopia. The HU-CSH is located at the SNNPR's capital, Hawassa City Administration, at 275 km distance south to Addis Ababa. The hospital has six outpatient departments (OPD), namely, Internal Medicine OPD, Surgical OPD, Pediatrics OPD, Obstetrics and Gynecology OPD, Special Clinics and Emergency OPD.

We conducted the study mainly on patients receiving service at medical OPD and surgical OPD rooms. During the study period, more than 3,000 people visited the hospital in the specified departments. Of these people, we selected our study participants.

The minimum sample size used in this study was determined using a single population proportion formula. Considering 95 percent confidence interval (CI), alpha level 0.05, a proportion of 0.5%, and 10% nonresponse rate, we determined the minimum sample size of 422 clients. Eleven cases with incomplete data were excluded from the analysis. Therefore, this study is based on 411 patients. Every 8th patient, by using a systematic sampling technique, was included in the study among adult patients attending the selected outpatient department, where K was N/n. In 2014/2016 (2007 Ethiopian Fiscal year), 93,944 OPD patients attended. Patients of at least 18 years old, able to give informed consent and not seriously sick, were included in the study. However, we excluded patients with hearing difficulty, unconscious or with serious mental disability, and pregnant women from the study. Performing of more than 20–30 min of moderate exercises (for instance, hurried walking and/or jogging) for at least four times per week was considered as performing the recommended level of physical activity.

The data were collected by trained nurses using a pretested structured interviewer-administered questionnaire and also observational chart review checklist. The questionnaire was designed to gather the client's sociodemographic data and also variable related risk factors of NCDs such as client's substance use history, questions regarding daily fruit and vegetable consumption status, and client's regular physical exercise history. The observation checklist also contained questions to abstract client's medical diagnosis, treatment, and examination results such as weight and height. The study instrument was prepared by reviewing similar scientific study report [20].

The data collected was first entered, cleaned, and analyzed using the Statistical Package Software for Social Science (SPSS) version 20. By using a univariate descriptive statistical analysis, we determined the frequency and prevalence. The bivariate and multivariate logistic regression analysis model was fitted to determine the Cruds Odds Ratio (COR) and Adjusted Odds Ratio (AOR). All variables with their P value < 0.2 were all taken to the next multivariate analysis model. However, those variables demonstrated statistically significant association at P value < 0.05 in the multivariate analysis were taken to be factors affecting the dependent variables that are DM and HTN diagnosis.

The quality of the study was assured by pretesting of the questionnaire and also a proper translation of the questionnaire originally prepared in English to Amharic and back to English by two scholars of good language command in both languages. To control the effect of confounders, we used the multivariate logistic regression analysis model.

3. Results

3.1. Sociodemographic Characteristics of the Study Participants. Nearly, all expected study participants included in

Table 1: Sociodemographic characteristics of the study participants attending university teaching hospital at Hawassa, Southern Ethiopia, 2016.

Sociodemographic characteristics	Male		Female		Total	
	Freq. (n)	Per. (%)	Freq. (n)	Per. (%)	Freq. (n)	Per. (%)
Age						
18-59	192	82.1	167	94.4	359	87.3
≥ 60	42	17.9	10	5.6	52	12.7
Residence						
Urban	138	59.0	130	73.4	268	65.2
Rural	96	41.0	47	26.6	143	34.8
Occupation						
Employed	59	25.2	42	23.7	101	24.6
Farmer	89	38.0	10	5.6	99	24.1
Housewife	0	0	74	41.8	74	18.0
Student	43	18.4	27	15.3	70	17.0
Other	43	18.4	24	13.6	67	16.3
Marital status						
Currently in marital union	163	69.7	130	73.4	293	71.3
Currently not in marital union	71	30.3	47	26.6	118	28.7
Education						
Literate	146	62.4	100	56.5	246	59.9
Illiterate	88	37.6	77	43.5	165	40.1
Household income						
≥ 1500	135	57.7	94	53.1	229	55.7
< 1500	99	42.3	83	46.9	182	44.3

the current study successfully responded to the interviewer-administered survey instrument. This makes the nonresponse rate very minimal, which is 2.75%. In this cross-sectional survey, a total of 411 patients, 234 men, and 177 women were studied. Of these, 359 (87.3%) were in the age group of 18–59 years, 268 (65.2%) were urban dwellers, 165 (40.1%) were illiterate, 101 (24.6%) were farmers, and 293(71.3%) were currently living in a marital union (Table 1).

3.2. Prevalence of Risk Factors for Hypertension and Diabetes. Concerning the BMI, 83 (20.2%) of the patients had a BMI of at least 25. The majority (98.3) of the patients had been getting vegetables in their daily meals. Alcohol drinking, khat chewing, cigarette smoking, and use of marijuna or Hashish were experienced by 60 (14.6%), 41 (10.0%), 11(2.7%), and 4 (1.0%) patients, respectively. Khat chewing and cigarette smoking were more common among men. However, physical inactivity was more common among women. One hundred fifty-eight (38.4%) of the patients had been experiencing one of these unhealthy lifestyle factors. Patients who experienced 2 and 3 of the unhealthy lifestyle factors constituted 71 (17.3%) and 21 (5.1%), respectively (Table 2).

The pattern of the risk factors among women reduced as age increased. Among men, as age increased up to 35–40 years, the magnitude of risk factors reduced; then the risk factors raised with age, from around 14% among age group 35–45 to more than 24% among 55+ years age group. Figure 1 shows the pattern of risk factors of hypertension and diabetes mellitus by age group and sex (Figure 1).

Among the study participants, the prevalence of hypertension, prevalence of diabetes mellitus, and prevalence of both hypertension and diabetes mellitus were 10.5%, 12.2%, and 3.2, respectively. The prevalence of hypertension and or diabetes mellitus was 19.5% (Table 2). Prevalence of hypertension and/or DM steadily increased from below 10% among 25–34 years age group to nearly 35% among patients in the age group of 55+ years.

In unadjusted regression analysis age, smoking, khat chewing, alcohol drinking, and BMI were associated with having of hypertension. In the multivariate analysis, old age (AOR = 4.0, 95% CI 1.8–9.0), smoking (AOR = 5.0, 95% CI 1.1–23.3), and high BMI (AOR = 5.7, 95% CI 2.7–11.9) maintained the significance in predicting having of hypertension (Table 3).

Concerning diabetes mellitus, exercise, alcohol drinking, khat chewing, and BMI were associated with having diabetes mellitus in unadjusted analysis. In a multivariate logistic regression analysis, only exercise (Adj. OR = 3.0, 95% CI 1.6–5.7) and high BMI (Adj. OR = 4.9, 95% CI 2.5–9.7) were found to predict having diabetes mellitus. Details on factors determining diabetes mellitus are described in Table 4.

4. Discussion

In this study, we found high prevalence DM and HTN. Unhealthy life style was experienced by significant proportion of the study participants. Variables like age, smoking,

TABLE 2: Prevalence of risk factors of HTN and DM, types of chronic diseases, and number of risk factors by patients at HU-CSH, January 2015.

Factors	Male; n (%)	Female; n (%)	Total; n (%)
Types of identified risk factors			
Clients with any of the risk factors	144 (61.5)	120 (67.8)	264 (64.2)
Physical inactivity*	58 (24.8)	79 (44.6)	137 (33.3)
BMI high ≥ 25	40 (17.1)	43(24.3)	83 (20.2)
Alcohol drinking	52(22.2)	8(4.5)	60 (14.6)
Khat chewing*	34 (14.5)	7 (4.0)	41 (10.0)
Smoking cigarette*	11 (4.7)	0 (0.0)	11 (2.7)
Substandard consumption of fruit and or vegetables	3 (1.3)	4 (2.3)	7 (1.7)
Hashish	4 (1.7)	0 (0.0)	4 (1.0)
Type of chronic diseases			
Hypertension and or diabetes mellitus (n = 411)	46 (19.7)	34 (19.2)	80 (19.5)
Diabetes mellitus (n = 411)	26 (11.1)	24 (13.6)	50 (12.2)
Hypertension (n = 411)	26 (11.1)	17 (9.6)	43 (10.5)
Hypertension and diabetes mellitus (n = 411)	6 (2.6)	7 (4.0)	13 (3.2)

Unhealthy lifestyle = BMI >/= 25, BMI = <18, not exercising, not taking fruit/vegetables, alcohol drinking, khat chewing, cigarette smoking, hashish taking; *variables with statistically significant difference by gender.

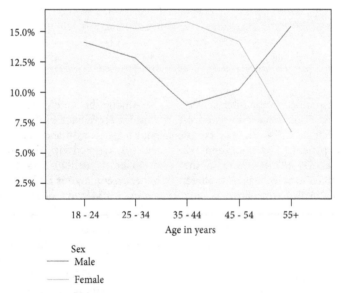

FIGURE 1: Pattern of any of the risk factors of Hypertension and Diabetes by age group and sex among patients at HU-CSH, January 2015.

and BMI were associated with having of hypertension, while exercise and BMI predicted having DM.

The finding of this study revealed a 12.2% prevalence of DM among clients attending the OPD/s of HU-CSH. Four institution-based cross-sectional study reports from Ethiopia reported a prevalence of DM ranging from 0.32% to 8.0%. These are 5.0% among Addis Ababa Police officers [16], 0.34% among patients attending Debre Berhan Hospital [17], 8.0% among Gondar University Hospital [18], and 6.4% among Jimma University Hospital [19]. The latter two studies were conducted on similar university hospitals which are comparable to the current study site. However, they were conducted merely on HIV-infected clients. In contrast to

these study reports and also the global prevalence of DM (8.8%), the prevalence obtained in the current study is higher. The differences noted in these reports might be linked to the type of clients involved in these studies and the peculiar geographic and sociodemographic characteristics. In addition, the methods and settings used in the study were all reasons to justify the observed differences.

Hypertension is the most common reason of physician visit among adults in USA. The estimated prevalence of HTN among US citizens ranges from 29 to 30% [21]. Nearly, in a similar fashion, the existing few institution- and community-based studies from Ethiopia reported comparable prevalence of hypertension. As a literature review from two studies

TABLE 3: Risk factors of hypertension among patients at HU-CSH, January 2015.

Variables		Yes	No	UOR (95% CI)	AOR (95% CI)
Age in years	18-59	30	329		
	≥ 60	13	39	3.7 (1.8 – 7.6)∗	4.0 (1.8 – 9.0)∗
Household income	≥ 1500	30	199		
	< 1500	13	169	0.5 (0.3 – 1.0)	0.9 (0.4 – 1.9)
Smoking	No	39	361		
	Yes	4	7	3.6 (1.1 – 12.1)∗	5.0 (1.1 – 23.3)∗
Khat chewing	No	34	336		
	Yes	9	32	2.8 (1.2 – 6.3)∗	1.3 (0.4 – 4.2)
Alcohol drinking	No	30	321		
	Yes	13	47	3.0 (1.4 – 6.1)∗	1.5 (0.6 – 3.9)
BMI	14 – 25	20	308		
	High	23	60	5.9 (3.1 – 11.4)∗	5.7 (2.7 – 11.9)∗

∗$P < 0.05$, UOR: unadjusted odds ratio, AOR: adjusted odds ratio, CI: confidence interval.

TABLE 4: Risk factors of diabetes mellitus among patients at HU-CSH, January 2015.

Variables		Yes	No	UOR (95% CI)	AOR (95% CI)
Residence	Urban	37	231		
	Rural	13	130	0.6 (0.3 – 1.2)	0.8 (0.4 – 1.7)
Household income	≥ 1500	33	196		
	<1500	17	165	0.6 (0.3 – 1.1)	0.8 (0.4 – 1.7)
Exercise	Yes	24	250		
	No	26	111	2.4 (1.3 – 4.4)∗	3.0 (1.6 – 5.7)∗
Alcohol drinking	No	37	314		
	Yes	13	47	2.3 (1.2 – 4.7)∗	1.4 (0.6 – 3.5)
Khat chewing	No	40	330		
	Yes	10	31	2.7 (1.2 – 5.8)∗	1.7 (0.6 – 4.6)
BMI	14 – 25	25	303		
	Low or high	25	58	5.2 (2.8 – 9.7)∗	4.9 (2.5 – 9.7)∗

∗$P < 0.05$, UOR: unadjusted odds ratio, AOR: Adjusted odds ratio, CI: confidence interval.

denoted, the prevalence of hypertension in Ethiopia ranges from 7.7% to 28.3% [11, 14]. This is in agreement with the WHO report that the fast increment of the magnitudes of NCDs is in the developing countries [1, 2].

In the current study, however, we identified relatively lower prevalence of HTN. This finding is similar to one community-based study conducted in a nearby zone called Sidama Zone, which reported a 9.9% HTN and another institution-based study reported a 13.2% prevalence of HTN among clients attending at Jimma University Referral Hospital [12, 15]. The only small, but logically acceptable figure reported from Ethiopia, HTN prevalence of 7.7%, is from undergraduate Gondar University students. The current study finding, nevertheless, is by far lesser from a report of a study conducted among federal ministry civil servants in Addis Ababa [13].

In this study, we identified prevalence for four substances: alcohol 14.6%, khat chewing 10.7%, cigarette 2.7%, and hashish 1.0%. The prevalence of alcohol in this study is high, but seems to be lower compared to other study reports which reported an average of nearly 50% [22, 23]. Khat is

locally cultivated evergreen shrub containing psychoactive ingredients called cathine and cathinone. It is one of the known risk factors of cardiovascular diseases especially for HTN and ischemic heart diseases. [24, 25]. In another study, the prevalence of khat chewing varied from 13.4% to 41.0% [26]. The existing prevalence of cigarette smoking in Ethiopia is 7.7%. In contrast to the current study finding, these reports seem lower [27, 28]. However, the prevalence identified in the current study still is in a level of significant public health problem.

The prevalence of other risk factors of NCD identified in our study included a 20.2% BMI of ≥ 25, 33.3% physical inactivity, and substandard consumption of fruit and or vegetables of 1.7%. The latter is by far negligible compared to a study conducted in Ethiopia which reported 27.0% and the WHO multinational survey reported 72% prevalence of substandard fruit and vegetable consumption [4, 29]. This finding can be explained by the local production and availability of fruits and vegetables in abundance. However, the proportion of people who are overweight and/or obese with their BMI score ≥ 25 reported in the current study is nearly comparable to the report from Addis Ababa [13], but higher than that in other reports [4, 30].

The level of physical inactivity found in this study is higher than that in other reports [4, 30, 31]. The rapid urbanization, the increasing tendency of using a motor vehicle for daily transportation and communities' abandonment of bicycle use trend, might have contributed to the identified physical inactivity. The higher physical inactivity noted in the current study may also explain the observed higher BMI reported in this same population [32]. As it is shown in Figure 1, the prevalence of any of the risk factors is more common in women of the younger age group. However, it is higher among male in the elderly age group. The higher prevalence of any of the risk factors among women in the younger age group could be due to the fact that physical inactivity and a BMI score of > 25 are more common among women than men.

As age increases, the likelihood of developing HTN also increases. Unfortunately, older age is one of the unavoidable risk factors to developing HTN [9, 12]. The current study also identified older age as one of the risk factors. The likelihood of developing HTN was by fourfold higher than among those aged > 60 years (AOR= 4.0, 95% CI 1.8 -9.0). This finding may serve as an evidence to support interventions promoting the need for regular HTN screening checkup [5, 13]. However, cigarette smoking and higher BMI were among the proven avoidable or modifiable risk factors identified in the current study for increasing the risk of developing HTN by five- and sixfold, respectively. These findings are consistent with other study results reported from Ethiopia and the world [9, 12, 13].

The current study result showed that higher BMI was a factor increasing the likelihood of developing DM. The risk of developing DM as a result of a higher BMI among the study population was five times higher than those with lower BMI. This finding is in agreement with other study reports showing higher BMI as the most important predictor of DM [17, 32]. The chance of developing DM increases by threefold among physically inactive patients. The risk of physical inactivity for developing DM is a well-known risk factor which supports the current study finding [33]. Performing regular exercise along with proper nutrition is the best means to control the BMI within the normal limit and prevent DM [32, 33].

5. Limitation of the Study

This study is the first for the area which may serve to lay a baseline finding pertaining to prevalence of risk factors and associated factors with HTN and DM. However, its cross-sectional nature makes it insufficient to establish a temporal relationship between the factors and the diseases conditions. Participants of the study might not remember to respond accurately to some of the questions. Since we conducted an institution-based study, generalization of the study findings to other setups need a meticulous consideration.

6. Conclusion

The prevalence of DM among clients attending at HU-CSH was high. The prevalence of HTN was also substantial. Higher BMI, physical inactivity, low fruit and vegetable consumption, alcohol use, khat chewing, and cigarette smoking were among the prevailing risk factors identified. Older age, higher BMI, and physical inactivity were among the factors increasing the risks of developing HTN. Having a higher BMI and physical inactivity were factors found increasing the risk of developing DM among the studied population. The magnitudes of DM and HTN are at a considerable level indicating the need for further strengthening the existing preventive works. This study also demonstrated avoidable or modifiable risk factors leading to HTN and DM.

Additional Points

Noncommunicable diseases are the cause of 63% of annual global death report, of which 14 million deaths are premature. Nearly, all (86%) of the premature deaths are happening in the middle- and lower-income countries (LMICs), including Ethiopia. Eighty percent (80%) of the CVD and DM can be prevented by avoiding the behavioral risk factors, such as tobacco use, physical inactivity, unhealthy dietary practice, and alcohol abuse. This study, as its contribution, determined the prevalence of DM and HTN among clients attending to the outpatient departments of the biggest hospital in Southern Ethiopia. In this study, the prevalence of the risk factors and the risk factors association with the development of DM and HTN were all identified. These findings can inform policy makers, clinicians, and researchers to work towards curbing the existing situation by considering the current findings.

Consent

Before the data collection, informed verbal consent was obtained from each study participant. Data were collected and analysed anonymously.

Authors' Contributions

Andargachew Kassa and Endrias Markos Woldesemayat conceived and designed the study. Endrias Markos Woldesemayat led and supervised the data collection and conducted data entry. Endrias Markos Woldesemayat and Andargachew Kassa conducted the data analysis. Andargachew Kassa wrote the 1st draft of the manuscript. Andargachew Kassa and Endrias Markos Woldesemayat interpreted and critically revised the manuscript. Both authors read and approved the final draft of the manuscript.

Acknowledgments

We are highly thankful for Hawassa University for funding the research; all the data collectors and clients willfully participated in the study.

References

[1] WHO, *Global action plan for the prevention and control of non-communicable diseases 2013-2020*, World Health Organization, Geneva, Switzerland, 2013.

[2] WHO, *Global Status Report on Noncommunicable Diseases 2014*, World Health Organization, Geneva, Switzerland, 2014.

[3] M. H. Workneh, G. A. Bjune, and S. A. Yimer, "Diabetes mellitus is associated with increased mortality during tuberculosis treatment: a prospective cohort study among tuberculosis patients in South-Eastern Amhara Region, Ethiopia," *Infectious Diseases of Poverty*, vol. 5, no. 1, p. 22, 2016.

[4] F. Alemseged, A. Haileamlak, A. Tegegn et al., *Risk factors for chronic non-communicable diseases at Gilgel Gibe Field Research Center, Southwest Ethiopia: population based study, 2012*, vol. 22 (special issue), 2012.

[5] FMOH, *Health Sector Transformation Plan (HSTP): 2015-2019*, Federal Ministry of health of Ethiopia (FMOH), Addis Ababa, Ethiopia, 2015.

[6] Z. A. Anteneh, W. A. Yalew, and D. B. Abitew, "Prevalence and correlation of hypertension among adult population in Bahir Dar city, northwest Ethiopia: a community based cross-sectional study," *Journal of General Internal Medicine*, vol. 8, pp. 175–185, 2015.

[7] S. M. Abebe, Y. Berhane, A. Worku, and A. Getachew, "Prevalence and associated factors of hypertension: a crosssectional community based study in Northwest Ethiopia," *PLoS ONE*, vol. 10, no. 4, Article ID e0125210, 2015.

[8] M. D. Mengistu, "Pattern of blood pressure distribution and prevalence of hypertension and prehypertension among adults in Northern Ethiopia: disclosing the hidden burden," *BMC Cardiovascular Disorders*, vol. 14, no. 33, pp. 1–8, 2014.

[9] T. P. Helelo, Y. A. Gelaw, and A. A. Adane, "Prevalence and associated factors of hypertension among adults in Durame Town, Southern Ethiopia," *PLoS ONE*, vol. 9, no. 11, Article ID e112790, 2014.

[10] F. Bonsa, E. K. Gudina, and K. W. Hajito, "Prevalence of hypertension and associated factors in Bedele Town, Southwest Ethiopia," *Ethiopian Journal of Health Sciences*, vol. 24, no. 1, pp. 21–26, 2014.

[11] A. Awoke, T. Awoke, S. Alemu, and B. Megabiaw, "Prevalence and associated factors of hypertension among adults in Gondar, Northwest Ethiopia: a community based cross-sectional study," *BMC Cardiovascular Disorders*, vol. 12, p. 113, 2012.

[12] A. Giday and B. Tadesse, "Prevalence and determinants of hypertension in rural and urban areas of southern Ethiopia," *Ethiopian Medical Journal*, vol. 49, no. 2, pp. 139–147, 2011.

[13] K. Angaw, A. F. Dadi, and K. A. Alene, "Prevalence of hypertension among federal ministry civil servants in Addis Ababa, Ethiopia: a call for a workplace-screening program," *BMC Cardiovascular Disorders*, vol. 15, no. 1, p. 76, 2015.

[14] T. Tadesse and H. Alemu, "Hypertension and associated factors among university students in Gondar, Ethiopia: a cross-sectional study," *BMC Public Health*, vol. 14, no. 1, p. 937, 2014.

[15] E. Kebede Gudina, Y. Michael, and S. Assegid, "Prevalence of hypertension and its risk factors in southwest Ethiopia: a hospital-based cross-sectional survey," *Integrated Blood Pressure Control*, vol. 6, pp. 111–117, 2013.

[16] T. Tesfaye, B. Shikur, T. Shimels, and N. Firdu, "Prevalence and factors associated with diabetes mellitus and impaired fasting glucose level among members of federal police commission residing in Addis Ababa, Ethiopia," *BMC Endocrine Disorders*, vol. 16, no. 1, p. 68, 2016.

[17] T. D. Habtewold, W. D. Tsega, and B. Y. Wale, "Diabetes mellitus in outpatients in Debre Berhan Referral Hospital, Ethiopia," *Journal of Diabetes Research*, vol. 2016, Article ID 3571368, 6 pages, 2016.

[18] S. M. Abebe, A. Getachew, S. Fasika, M. Bayisa, A. G. Demisse, and N. Mesfin, "Diabetes mellitus among HIV-infected individuals in follow-up care at University of Gondar Hospital, Northwest Ethiopia," *BMJ Open*, vol. 6, no. 8, Article ID e011175, 2016.

[19] A. E. Mohammed, T. Y. Shenkute, and W. C. Gebisa, "Diabetes mellitus and risk factors in human immunodeficiency virus-infected individuals at Jimma University Specialized Hospital, Southwest Ethiopia," *Diabetes, Metabolic Syndrome and Obesity: Targets and Therapy*, vol. 8, pp. 197–206, 2015.

[20] M. Fortin, J. Haggerty, J. Almirall, T. Bouhali, M. Sasseville, and M. Lemieux, "Lifestyle factors and multimorbidity: a cross sectional study," *BMC Public Health*, vol. 14, no. 1, article 686, 2014.

[21] B. M. Egan, Y. Zhao, and R. N. Axon, "US trends in prevalence, awareness, treatment, and control of hypertension, 1988–2008," *The Journal of the American Medical Association*, vol. 303, no. 20, pp. 2043–2050, 2010.

[22] A. Derese, A. Seme, and C. Misganaw, "Assessment of substance use and risky sexual behaviour among Haramaya University students," *Science Journal of Public Health*, vol. 2, no. 2, pp. 102–110, 2014.

[23] Z. A. Zein, "Polydrug abuse among Ethiopian university students with particular reference to khat (Catha edulis)," *Journal of Tropical Medicine and Hygiene*, vol. 91, no. 2, pp. 71–75, 1988.

[24] P. Widler, K. Mathys, R. Brenneisen, P. Kalix, and H. Fisch, "Pharmacodynamics and pharmacokinetics of khat: a controlled study," *Clinical Pharmacology & Therapeutics*, vol. 55, no. 5, pp. 556–562, 1994.

[25] M. J. Valente, P. Guedes De Pinho, M. De Lourdes Bastos, F. Carvalho, and M. Carvalho, "Khat and synthetic cathinones: a review," *Archives of Toxicology*, vol. 88, no. 1, pp. 15–45, 2014.

[26] A. Astatkie, M. Demissie, Y. Berhane, and A. Worku, "Prevalence of and factors associated with regular khat chewing among university students in Ethiopia," in *Substance Abuse and Rehabilitation*, vol. 6, pp. 41–50, 2015.

[27] CSA, Demographic and health survey 2011. 2012, CSA (Ethiopia) and ORC Macro: Addis Ababa, Ethiopia and Calverton, Maryland, USA. 2012: Maryland, USA.

[28] G. Tesfaye, A. Derese, and M. Hambisa, "Substance use and associated factors among university students in Ethiopia: a cross-sectional study," *Journal of Addiction*, vol. 10, no. 1155, 2014.

[29] J. N. Hall, S. Moore, S. B. Harper, and J. W. Lynch, "Global variability in fruit and vegetable consumption," *American Journal of Preventive Medicine*, vol. 36, no. 5, p. 8, 2009.

[30] F. Tesfaye, *Epidemiology of Cardiovascular Disease Risk Factors in Ethiopia: The Rural-Urban Gradient*, Umea University: Sweden, 2008.

[31] WHO, "WHO Health Statistics And Information Systems. World Health Survey Results, Ethiopia 2003," http://www.who.int/healthinfo/survey/whseth-ethiopia.pdf.

[32] CDC, "Fact Sheets and Brochures: Adult Obesity," 2010, https://www.cdc.gov/obesity/resources/factsheets.html.

[33] D. K. McCulloch and P. Robertson, "Risk factors for type 2 diabetes mellitus," in *UPTODATE*, D. M. Nathan and J. E. Mulder, Eds., USA, 2013.

22

Acetic Acid-Induced Ulcerative Colitis in Sprague Dawley Rats is Suppressed by Hydroethanolic Extract of *Cordia vignei* Leaves through Reduced Serum Levels of TNF-α and IL-6

George Owusu,[1,2] **David D. Obiri ⓘ,**[1] **George K. Ainooson,**[1] **Newman Osafo ⓘ,**[1]
Aaron O. Antwi ⓘ,[1] **Babatunde M. Duduyemi ⓘ,**[3] **and Charles Ansah ⓘ**[1]

[1]*Department of Pharmacology, Faculty of Pharmacy and Pharmaceutical Sciences, College of Health Sciences, Kwame Nkrumah University of Science and Technology (KNUST), Kumasi, Ghana*
[2]*Department of Pharmacology, School of Medicine and Health Sciences, University for Development Studies, Tamale, Ghana*
[3]*Department of Pathology, School of Medical Sciences, Kwame Nkrumah University of Science and Technology (KNUST), Kumasi, Ghana*

Correspondence should be addressed to David D. Obiri; ddobiri.pharm@knust.edu.gh

Academic Editor: Tadeusz Robak

Background. Ulcerative colitis (UC) is a recurrent inflammatory bowel disease (IBD) that causes long-lasting inflammation on the innermost lining of the colon and rectum. Leaf decoctions of *Cordia vignei* have been used in traditional medicine either alone or in combination with other plant preparations to treat the disease. *Aim*. In this study, we investigated the effect of hydroethanolic extract of *Cordia vignei* leaves (CVE) on acetic acid-induced UC in rats. *Method*. Male Sprague Dawley rats received oral treatment of either saline (10 ml/kg), sulfasalazine (500 mg/kg), or CVE (30-300 mg/kg) daily for 7 days. On day 4, colitis was induced by a single intrarectal administration of 500 μl of acetic acid (4% v/v). Rats were sacrificed on day 8 and colons were collected for histopathological examination. Blood was also collected for haematological assessment. *Results*. CVE significantly ($P < 0.05$) prevented colonic ulceration and reduced the inflammatory score. Serum levels of TNF-α and IL-6 were significantly reduced. Depletion of superoxide dismutase (SOD) and catalase (CAT) activities by acetic acid was significantly inhibited while lipid peroxidation indexed as malondialdehyde (MDA) level in the colon was reduced. However, loss of body weight was not significantly affected by treatment with CVE. *Conclusion*. This data suggest that CVE has a potential antiulcerative effect.

1. Introduction

Ulcerative colitis is a recurrent inflammation of the colon. The clinical symptoms often presented by this disease are diarrhoea, loss of weight, nausea, and abdominal pain which affect quality of life [1]. The pathological features include inflammatory cell infiltration and activation, downstream expression of nuclear factor kappa B- (NF-κB-) dependent proinflammatory mediators such as tumor necrosis factor alpha (TNF-α) and interleukin 6 (IL-6), excessive generation of free radicals such as reactive oxygen species (ROS) and reactive nitrogen species (RNS), depletion of antioxidant capacity of the colon, and loss of mucosal integrity [2]. Although genetic, immunological, and environmental factors are implicated in the pathogenesis of ulcerative colitis, the exact aetiology of the disease still remains elusive [3]. Studies in this area contribute to the attempt to elucidate the causes and development of the disease. Also, the increasing number of cases of ulcerative colitis shows the importance of searching for new compounds that can control or eliminate the disease that severely affects the quality of life of these patients.

Due to resemblance of experimentally induced colitis in animals and ulcerative colitis in humans, the former has become an indispensable tool to study the pathomechanism of the disease and also for screening of novel compounds for their antiulcerative activity [4]. An acetic acid-induced ulcerative colitis model involving intrarectal administration of acetic acid in rats was employed in this study. Currently, conventional drugs that are commonly used in the treatment of colitis include 5-aminosalicylic acid, systemic corticosteroids, immunomodulators, and vitamin E [5]. Since excessive production of reactive oxygen species seems to play an important role in tissue damage and inflammatory process of the disease, administration of natural substances as treatment may be a valuable option for new therapies [6–8]. One plant of interest is *Cordia vignei*. It is a woody plant belonging to the family Boraginacaea. It grows to about 30 cm in diameter and 10 m tall. In traditional medicine, decoctions of the leaves of the plant are used either alone or in combination with other plants to treat inflammatory disorders [9]. An ethnopharmacological survey conducted by Agyare et al. (2017) revealed that the leaves of the plant are traditionally used in Ghana for treatment of prostate cancer [10]. Despite the usefulness of the plant in traditional medicine, scientific investigation of its effects has not been conducted.

This study evaluates the antiulcerative effect of hydroethanolic leaf extract of *Cordia vignei* in rats to provide a scientific data and validate the traditional use. We also determined whether the underlying mechanisms involve protection of antioxidant potential of the colon and/or reduction of the serum levels of principal proinflammatory mediators such as TNF-α and IL-6.

2. Materials

2.1. Plant Collection and Extraction. Fresh leaves of *Cordia vignei* were collected from the Diabaa Forest Reserve (located at longitudes 3° W and 3° 30′ W and latitudes 7° N and 7° 30′ N) in the Dormaa West District of Brong Ahafo region of Ghana. The leaves were authenticated at the herbarium of the Department of Herbal Medicine, Faculty of Pharmacy and Pharmaceutical Sciences, Kwame Nkrumah University of Science and Technology (KNUST), Kumasi, Ghana. A voucher specimen (KNUST/HM1/2017/L003) was kept at the herbarium. The plant material was air dried for seven days. Three and half kilograms (3.5 kg) of the dried material was pulverized into fine powder using a heavy-duty blender (37BL85 (240CB6) Waring Commercial, USA). The fine powder was macerated with 5 l of 70% (v/v) ethanol for 72 h, filtered and concentrated in a rotary evaporator (Rotavapor R-210, BUCHI, Switzerland) at 50°C, and further solidified in an oven (Gallenkamp OMT Oven, Sanyo, Japan). The moist gummy solid extract with a total yield of 11.62% (w/w) was kept in a desiccator for 72 h. For oral administration, the extract was reconstituted as an emulsion in 2% tragacanth and referred to as *Cordia vignei* extract (CVE) in this study.

2.2. Animals. Male Sprague Dawley rats (9-11 weeks old, weighing 200-220 g) were obtained from the Animal House of the Department of Pharmacology, KNUST, and maintained under standard laboratory conditions. All animals were carefully handled in accordance with National Institute of Health Guidelines for the Care and Use of Laboratory Animals (NIH, Department of Health and Human Services; Publication No. 85-23, revised 2011) [11]. All protocols involving the use of animals were approved by the Animal Ethics Committee of Kwame Nkrumah University of Science and Technology.

2.3. Drugs and Chemicals. Sulfasalazine (KAR LABS LTD, New Delhi, India) and ELISA Kit for rat TNF-α and IL-6 (Boster Biological Technology Ltd., CA, USA), acetic acid, and ethyl alcohol (British Drug House, Poole, UK) were purchased.

3. Method

3.1. Induction of Colitis. Rats were randomly selected into 6 groups ($n = 5$) and received daily oral administration of either normal saline (10 ml/kg), sulfasalazine (500 mg/kg), or CVE (30, 100, and 300 mg/kg) from day 0 to day 7. On day 4, colitis was induced by intrarectal administration of 500 μl of acetic acid (4% v/v). Body weights of rats were taken daily. Rats were euthanized on day 8 by cervical dislocation under anaesthesia with 50 mg/kg pentobarbitone (i.p.).

3.1.1. Assessment of Colon Weight-to-Length Ratio. Rats were dissected and their colons were extirpated, opened longitudinally, and rinsed gently under running water to remove the faeces. Colons were placed on nonabsorbent surfaces and weight-to-length ratios were blindly assessed. Extirpated colons were stored at –80°C.

3.1.2. Macroscopic Assessment of Colonic Damage. Macroscopically visible injuries such as thickening, shortening, hyperemia, and necrosis were blindly scored from 0-100% based on increasing order of severity as described by Ballester et al. [12] and Motavallian-Naeini et al. [13]. The mean scores were presented as the Disease Activity Index (DAI) of the colon.

3.1.3. Microscopic Assessment of Colonic Damage. Samples of the distal colons were fixed immediately in 10% formaldehyde, embedded in liquid paraffin, cut into transverse sections of 5 μm thick using a Leica RM 2125 Microtome (Leica Biosystems, Wetzlar, Germany), and then mounted on glass slides and stained with haematoxylin and eosin (H&E). Microscopic changes such as necrosis, fibrosis, hyperemia, epithelial damage, ulceration, infiltration, and submucosal abscesses were scored on a 0-4 scale where 0 denotes no detectable damage and 4 denotes most severe damage [1].

3.1.4. Assessment of Antioxidant Enzymes in the Colon. Colons were homogenized using a Potter-Elvehjem homogenizer (Ultra-Turrax T25, Janke and Kunkel IKA-Labortechnik, Staufen, Germany) on ice-cold Tris-HCl buffer (0.01 M, pH 7.4) to give a 10% homogenate which was used for assays of superoxide dismutase and catalase activity in the colons as described below.

(1) Superoxide Dismutase (SOD). Activity of SOD in the colon was determined as described by Misra and Fridovich (1972) [14] with a slight modification. Briefly, 750 μl ethanol (96% v/v) and 150 μl of ice-cold chloroform were added to

$500 \, \mu l$ of the tissue homogenate and centrifuged at 2000 rpm for 20 min at 25°C. To $500 \, \mu l$ of the supernatant, $500 \, \mu l$ EDTA (0.6 mM) and 1 ml carbonate bicarbonate buffer (0.1 M, pH 10.2) were added. The reaction was initiated by the addition of $50 \, \mu l$ of adrenaline (1.3 mM). Absorbance was measured against a blank at 480 nm for 4 min using the Cecil ultraviolet-visible spectrophotometer (CE 2041, Milton, England).

Percentage inhibition of autoxidation of adrenaline was calculated using the formula:

$$\text{Percentage inhibition} = \left[\frac{\text{Absorbance}_{\text{test}} - \text{Absorbance}_{\text{blank}}}{\text{Absorbance}_{\text{test}}} \right] \times 100.$$

(1)

The enzyme activity was expressed as unit per mg protein. One unit of the enzyme activity was defined as the amount of enzyme that inhibits the autooxidation of adrenaline by 50% at 25°C.

$$\text{Unit of SOD activity/mg protein} = \left[\frac{\% \text{ inhibition}}{50 \times \text{weight of protein}} \right] \times 100.$$

(2)

(2) Catalase. Activity of catalase in the colon was determined by using the procedure described by Sinha [15] with a slight modification. The assay mixture containing 1 ml (0.01 M) phosphate buffer (pH 7.0), $500 \, \mu l$ H_2O_2 (1.18 M), and $400 \, \mu l$ of water was added to $100 \, \mu l$ of the aliquot of the tissue supernatant and incubated at 28°C for 5 min to initiate the reaction. The reaction was terminated by adding 2 ml acetic acid-dichromate mixture comprising a 3 : 1 ratio of glacial acetic acid and 5% potassium dichromate. Absorbance of the chromic acetate formed was measured at 620 nm with Cecil ultraviolet-visible spectrophotometer (CE 2041, Milton, England). One unit of catalase activity was defined as the amount of enzyme needed to cause decomposition of $1 \, \mu mol$ H_2O_2 per min per mg protein at 25°C and pH 7.0. The enzyme activity was expressed in terms of its molar extinction coefficient of $39.4 \, M^{-1} \, cm^{-1}$:

$$\text{mUnitCAT mg/protein} = \left[\frac{\text{Absorbance}_{620 \, nm}}{3.94 \times \text{weight of protein}} \right] \times 1000.$$

(3)

(3) Malondialdehyde (MDA) Level. Levels of malondialdehyde a byproduct of lipid peroxidation in the colon was estimated as described by Heath and Parker [16]. Briefly, 1 ml of the tissue extract was added to a 3 ml mixture of 20% trichloroacetic acid (TCA) and 0.5% thiobarbituric acid (TBA). The mixture was heated at 95°C for 30 min, cooled in an ice bath, and centrifuged at 2,000 rpm for 10 min. Absorbance of the MDA-TBA complex formed was read at 532 nm against the

blank using a UV mini-1240 single beam spectrophotometer (Shimadzu Scientific Instrument, SSI, Kyoto, Japan). The concentration (nmol/mg protein) of MDA was calculated using the MDA extinction coefficient of $1.56 \times 10^{-5} \, M^{-1} \, cm^{-1}$.

3.2. Assay of Serum TNF-α and IL-6. Colitis was induced in rats as described earlier and the rats were euthanized on day 8. Blood samples were collected in clot activator tubes (Add Surgifield Medicals, Middlessex, England) and centrifuged (Heraeus Megafuge 16R, Thermo Scientific) at 3000 rpm for 30 min at 4°C to obtain the serum. The serum was assayed quantitatively for TNF-α and IL-6 by using their respective Picokine ELISA kits as instructed by the manufacturer.

3.3. Haematology. Blood samples were also collected into vacutainer sterile tubes coated with EDTA as an anticoagulant. Full blood count was conducted using the Automated Cell Analyzer (YSTE880-Guangzhou Yueshen Medical Equipment Co. Ltd., China).

3.4. Data Analyses. Body weight change values were normalized as percentage of the body weight taken at the start of the experiment. Time-course curves for body weight were subjected to two-way (treatment × time) ANOVA followed by Bonferroni's post hoc test. GraphPad Prism for Windows version 6.01 was used for all statistical analyses and plotting of graphs. Results were presented as mean ± SEM. $P < 0.05$ was considered statistically significant.

4. Results

4.1. Effect of Hydroethanolic Leaf Extract of Cordia vignei on Body Weight of Acetic Acid-Induced Colitic Rats. Intrarectal injection of acetic acid in rats evoked colonic inflammatory response which became evident as passing of loose stool (with or without occult blood) and loss of body weight. The naïve control rats showed a gradual increase in weight (0-1.07%) throughout the 7 days (Figure 1(a)). In contrast to the naïve control, acetic acid control rats exhibited decrease in body weight from day 2 to day 7 (Figure 1(a)). Body weights of sulfasalazine-treated rats decreased from day 3 to day 4 and then slightly increased from day 5 to day 7 (Figure 1(a)). On the other hand, body weights of CVE-treated rats slightly declined from day 3 to day 7 (Figure 1(a)).

The total change in body weight of rats over the 7 days was calculated as area under the curve (AUC) as shown in Figure 1(b). The AUC for the naïve control over the 7 days was 12.57 ± 1.079. Acetic acid significantly reduced the AUC to 7.495 ± 0.8371 ($P = 0.0059$) compared to naïve control (Figure 1(b)). The AUC of sulfasalazine-treated rats was 8.956 ± 0.7331 ($P = 0.2258$) compared to acetic acid control while the AUC of CVE-treated rats were 8.257 ± 0.56 ($P = 0.4700$), 7.858 ± 0.14 ($P = 0.6800$), and 8.086 ± 0.63 ($P = 0.5885$), respectively, at 30, 100, and 300 mg kg^{-1} compared to acetic acid control (Figure 1(b)).

4.2. Effect of Hydroethanolic Leaf Extract of Cordia vignei on Colon Weight-to-Length Ratio of Acetic Acid-Induced Colitic Rats. Increase in inflammatory cell infiltration, vascular

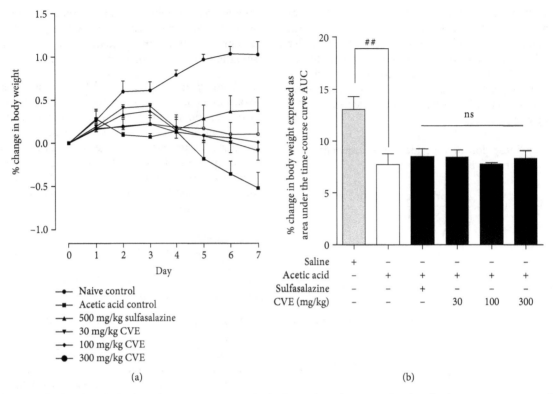

FIGURE 1: Effect of hydroethanolic leaf *Cordia vignei* extract on the body weights of acetic acid-induced colitic rats. Rats received daily oral administration of normal saline (10 ml kg^{-1}), sulfasalazine (500 mg kg^{-1}), or CVE (30-300 mg kg^{-1}) for 7 days. On day 4, rats were challenged with 500 μl acetic acid. Changes in weight were calculated and presented as *mean ± SEM*.[##]$P < 0.005$ (acetic acid control *vs.* naïve control), ns: not significant (acetic acid control vs. treatment group) using t test.

permeability, and oedema of the colon contributes to the increase in weight/length ratio of the colon [17]. The naïve control rats had mean colon weight/length ratio of 0.07 ± 0.01 g/cm which was significantly increased to 0.67 ± 0.05 ($P = 0.0001$) in the acetic acid control rats (Figure 2). Sulfasalazine reduced this mean colon weight/length ratio to 0.32 ± 0.06 g/cm ($P = 0.0022$) compared to acetic acid control rats. Similarly, CVE significantly reduced the mean colon weight/length ratio to 0.48 ± 0.06 ($P = 0.0411$) and 0.45 ± 0.05 g/cm ($P = 0.0116$), respectively, at doses 100 and 300 mg kg^{-1} albeit insignificant (0.6 ± 0.03; $P = 0.3740$) at 30 mg/kg (Figure 2).

4.3. Effect of Hydroethanolic Leaf Extract of Cordia vignei on Macroscopic Score of Colons of Acetic Acid-Induced Colitic Rats. The naïve control rats did not show any sign of colitis (Figure 3(a)). Intrarectal administration of acetic acid evoked a colonic inflammation characterized by increased neutrophil infiltration, massive necrosis of mucosal and submucosal layers, submucosal ulceration, increase in vascular dilation, and oedema (Figure 3(b)). In contrast to the disease control rats, sulfasalazine-treated rats showed mild colonic inflammation with less infiltration and ulceration (Figure 3(c)). Similarly, rats treated with CVE exhibited moderate colonic inflammation with less infiltration and ulceration as shown in Figures 3(d)–3(f), respectively, for 30–300 mg kg^{-1}.

Visible signs of colonic inflammation such as thickening, shortening, hyperemia, and necrosis were quantified as a Dis-ease Activity Index (DAI) ranging between 0 and 100% in ascending order of severity (Figure 3(g)). Naïve control rats had DAI of 0%. In contrast to the naïve control rats, acetic acid control rats showed very severe colonic inflammation characterized by hyperemia, thickening, shortening, and oedema with DAI of 92.26 ± 6.09%. Sulfasalazine significantly reduced the DAI to 44.00 ± 5.81% while the extract significantly and dose dependently protected the rats from severe colonic ulceration. DAI of the CVE-treated groups were 61.78 ± 2.46%, 55.98 ± 8.08%, and 49.288 ± 6.95%, respectively, administered at 30, 100, and 300 mg/kg^{-1} CVE (Figure 3(g)).

4.4. Effect of Cordia vignei Leaf Extract on Colon Histopathology of Acetic Acid-Induced Colitic Rats. Colons of naïve control rats exhibited no observable histopathologi-cal changes (Figure 4(a)). Conversely, colons of acetic acid control rats showed necrosis and abscesses in the colonic mucosa with infiltration of inflammatory cells into the sub-mucosa (Figure 4(b)). Treatment of rats with sulfasalazine significantly prevented the colonic injury. There was mild infiltration and abscesses (Figure 4(c)). CVE-treated rats' colons exhibited reduced colonic inflammation. There was mild infiltration and abscesses in the mucosa. Epithelial cell loss and gross colonic injury were significantly reduced at doses 30-300 mg kg^{-1} (Figure 4(d)–4(f)).

On quantification, the mean histopathological score of the colons of naïve control rats was 0.0 ± 0.0 (Figure 4(g)).

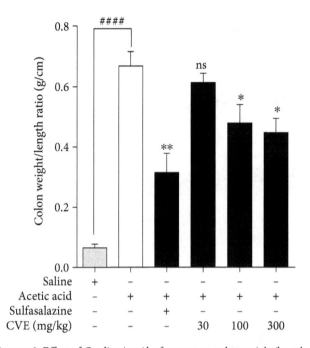

FIGURE 2: Effect of *Cordia vignei* leaf extract on colon weight/length ratio of acetic acid-induced colitic rats. Colitis was induced in rats as described in Method. Rats were sacrificed on day 8 and colon weight-to-length ratios were assessed. Results were presented as mean ± SEM. $^{\#\#\#\#}P < 0.0001$ (acetic acid control *vs.* naïve control); $^{*}P < 0.05$, $^{**}P < 0.01$, and ns not significant (acetic acid control *vs.* treatment group) using t test.

In contrast to the naïve control, colons of acetic acid control rats exhibited severe inflammation with a significant increase in the histopathological score of 3.820 ± 0.12 ($P = 0.0001$). Sulfasalazine significantly reduced this mean score to 1.604 ± 0.24 ($P = 0.0001$) while CVE treatment ameliorated acetic acid-induced colon damage and significantly reduced inflammatory score to 2.54 ± 0.26 ($P = 0.0019$), 2.26 ± 0.35 ($P = 0.0030$), and 2.162 ± 0.32 ($P = 0.0030$) at doses 30, 100, and 300 mg kg^{-1}, respectively, when compared to acetic acid control (Figure 4(g)).

4.5. Effect of Hydroethanolic Extract of Cordia vignei Leaves on Activity of Superoxide Dismutase and Catalase on Colons of Acetic Acid-Induced Colitic Rats

4.5.1. Superoxide Dismutase. The mean activity of superoxide dismutase (SOD) in the tissue of naïve animals was 12.02 ± 1.65 U/mg protein (Figure 5(a)). Intrarectal administration of acetic acid significantly reduced the mean SOD activity (U/mg protein) in the tissue to 2.55 ± 0.07 U/mg ($P = 0.0007$). Sulfasalazine significantly increased SOD activity (U/mg protein) to 9.02 ± 1.62 ($P = 0.0063$). Similarly, treatment of rats with CVE significantly increased the mean SOD activity (U/mg protein) to 6.68 ± 0.72 ($P = 0.0035$), 7.26 ± 0.94 ($P = 0.0038$), and 8.28 ± 1.05 ($P = 0.00190$, respectively, at doses 30, 100, and 300 mg kg^{-1} (Figure 5(a)).

4.5.2. Catalase. The mean CAT activity (nmol/min/mg protein) of naive control rats was 10.12 ± 1.64 (Figure 5(b)). Acetic acid significantly reduced CAT activity to $2.64 \pm$ 0.39 nmol/min/mg protein ($P = 0.0022$). Sulfasalazine significantly increased the mean CAT activity (nmol/min/mg protein) to 7.20 ± 1.33 ($P = 0.0110$) compared to the acetic acid control group. Treatment of rats with 30, 100, and 300 mg kg^{-1} CVE significantly increased CAT activity (nmol/min/mg protein) to 6.30 ± 0.74 ($P = 0.0023$), 6.82 ± 1.23 ($P = 0.0119$), and 7.54 ± 1.41 ($P = 0.0099$), respectively, (Figure 5(b)).

4.5.3. Malondialdehyde (MDA) Levels. There was an insignificant mean MDA level of 1.68 ± 0.58 nmol/mg protein in naïve control rats (Figure 5(c)). Acetic acid significantly increased the mean MDA level to 66.86 ± 4.32 nmol/mg protein ($P = 0.0001$) compared to the naïve control. Sulfasalazine decreased the mean MDA level to 32.64 ± 3.78 nmol/mg protein ($P = 0.0003$) compared to acetic acid control. CVE also reduced the mean MDA level to 48.79 ± 4.93 ($P = 0.0247$), 42.41 ± 4.37 ($P = 0.0041$), and 38.03 ± 4.26 ($P = 0.0014$) nmol/mg protein at 30, 100, and 300 mg kg^{-1}, respectively, compared to acetic acid control.

4.6. Effect of Hydroethanolic Extract of Cordia vignei Leaves on Levels of TNF-α and IL-6 in the Serum of Acetic Acid-Induced Colitic Rats

4.6.1. TNF-α Concentration. The TNF-α concentration in the serum of naive control rats was 16.34 ± 3.79 pg ml^{-1} (Figure 6(a)). Acetic acid significantly increased serum TNF-α concentration (pg ml^{-1}) to 84.32 ± 3.06 ($P = 0.0002$). Sulfasalazine significantly reduced this TNF-α level (pg ml^{-1}) to 37.40 ± 7.24 ($P = 0.0040$). Treatment of rats with CVE significantly reduced serum TNF-α concentration (pg ml^{-1}) to 63.02 ± 5.77 ($P = 0.0311$), 48.94 ± 4.57 ($P = 0.0030$), and 46.03 ± 4.26 ($P = 0.0019$), respectively, at doses 30, 100, and 300 mg kg^{-1} (Figure 6(a)).

4.6.2. IL-6 Concentration. The mean concentration of IL-6 in serum of the naïve control group was 3.68 ± 1.07 pg ml^{-1} and was significantly increased to 36.55 ± 2.40 ($P = 0.0002$) in the acetic acid control rats (Figure 6(b)). Sulfasalazine significantly reduced this concentration to 10.47 ± 3.23 ($P = 0.0029$) while CVE significantly reduced the serum concentrations of IL-6 to 24.12 ± 2.47 ($P = 0.0225$), 21.10 ± 4.15 ($P = 0.032$) and 19.72 ± 3.26 ($P = 0.0142$), respectively, at 30, 100, and 300 mg kg^{-1} (Figure 6(b)).

4.7. Effect of Hydroethanolic Extract of Cordia vignei Leaves on Haematological Parameters of Acetic Acid-Induced Colitic Rats.
All the blood parameters of the naïve control rats were within the range of normal blood values of healthy rats (Table 1). Intrarectal administration of acetic acid did not cause any significant change in blood values compared to the naïve control. Sulfasalazine did not cause any significant change in all the blood parameters that were assessed. CVE caused a significant ($P < 0.0077$) reduction of lymphocyte level at 100 mg kg^{-1} albeit insignificant at 30 or 300 mg kg^{-1} compared to acetic acid control.

Also, CVE significantly ($P < 0.05$) reduced neutrophil levels at 100–300 mg kg^{-1}, albeit, insignificant at 30 mg kg^{-1} compared to acetic acid control.

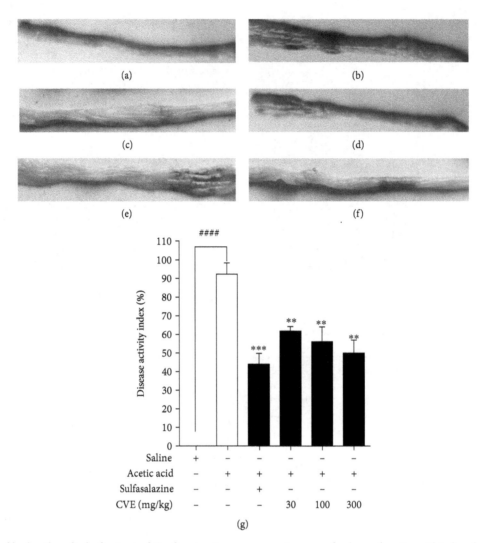

FIGURE 3: Effect of hydroethanolic leaf extract of *Cordia vignei* on macroscopic score of colons of acetic acid-induced colitic rats. Colitis was induced as described in Method. Rats were euthanized on day 8 and the colons were excised, longitudinally opened, washed, and examined (a–f). Colons were scored from 0-100% in ascending order of severity of inflammation (g). Results were presented as mean ± SEM. ####$P < 0.0001$ (acetic acid control *vs.* naïve control); **$P < 0.01$; ***$P < 0.001$ (acetic acid control *vs.* treatment group) using *t* test.

Male Sprague Dawley rats ($n = 5$) were orally treated with either normal saline ($10 \, ml \, kg^{-1}$), sulfasalazine ($500 \, mg \, kg^{-1}$), or CVE (30-$300 \, mg \, kg^{-1}$) from day 0 to day 7. On day 4, colitis was induced as described in methods. Rats were euthanized on day 8 and blood samples were collected from the jugular vein for full blood count using automated cell analyzer. Mean blood values were statistically compared using *t* test. Results were presented as mean ± SEM. *$P < 0.05$ and **$P < 0.01$ (acetic acid control vs. treatment group).

5. Discussion

Ulcerative colitis experimentally induced by intrarectal administration of low concentration (usually 3-5%) of acetic acid is a well-recognized model for the study of inflammatory bowel disease [1]. Though acetic acid-induced ulcerative colitis and human inflammatory bowel disease may differ in aetiology, the two diseases share common pathophysiological features as well as sensitivity to drug treatment. For example,

colonic changes such as mucosal ulceration, weight loss, hemorrhage, and inflammation which occur following intrarectal administration of acetic acid in rodents are also common in human IBD [18]. Also, influx of inflammatory cells such as neutrophils into the injured colon, rupture of colonic barrier, release of inflammatory mediators such as cytokines, arachidonic acid metabolites, and production of reactive oxygen species (ROS) which results in oxidative damage are common in both diseases [6].

In this study, intrarectal administration of acetic acid significantly reduced the body weight of rats. Loss of weight in colitis is due to deficiency of nutrients resulting from reduced appetite, food aversion or malabsorption, and rapid loss of body fluid through colorectal bleeding and diarrhoea. Also, TNF-α and IL-6 contribute immensely to loss of body weight in colitis by releasing neuropeptides that suppress appetite and precipitate cachexia [19]. Though serum levels of both TNF-α and IL-6 were significantly reduced by sulfasalazine and the extract, loss of body weight was not significantly

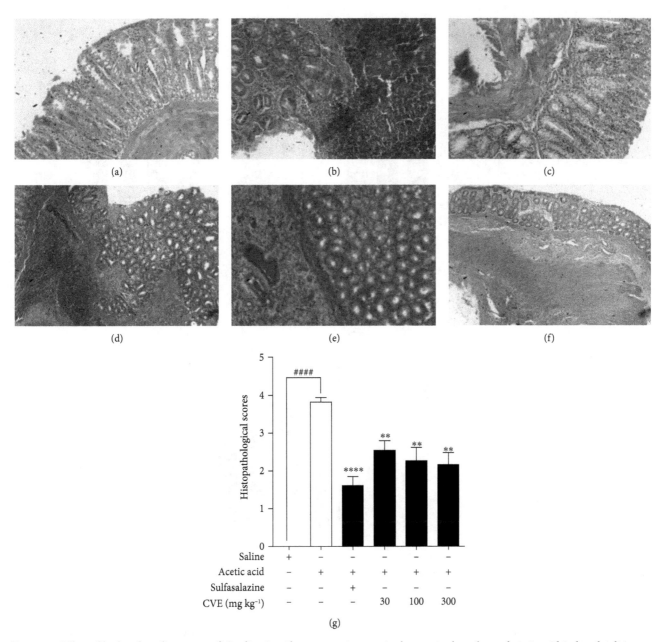

FIGURE 4: Effect of hydroethanolic extract of *Cordia vignei* leaves on microscopic changes in the colons of acetic acid-induced colitic rats. Colitis was induced as described in Method. Colons were fixed in 10% formaldehyde, sectioned (5 μm thick), and stained with H&E. Representative photomicrographs shown are colons of naïve control rats (a), acetic acid control rats (b), sulfasalazine-treated rats(c), and 30-300 mg kg^{-1} CVE-treated rats (d–f, respectively). Microscopic changes were quantified based on severity of damage (*g*). Results were presented as mean ± SEM. $^{####}P < 0.0001$ (acetic acid control vs. naïve control); $^{**}P < 0.01$; $^{****}P < 0.0001$ (acetic acid control vs. treated group).

affected by both agents in this study. Therefore, the weight loss could result from loss of body fluid through diarrhoea and bleeding.

Macroscopic examination of the colon revealed a significant increase in colon weight/length ratio of rats. This is due to severe tissue oedema, necrosis, goblet cell hyperplasia, and inflammatory cell infiltration [20, 21]. The macroscopic examination of intestinal content of CVE-treated rats showed well-formed fecal pellets without visible blood or mucus stains, and this could be due to uncompromised mucus layer and inhibition of excessive blood loss which

are indicative of therapeutic success of potential antiulcerative agents [22–24]. The mucus layer is well known to enhance the repair of the chemically induced epithelial damage and also prevents diarrhoea and loss of blood through faeces [25]. It is therefore not surprising that preservation of mucus layer by CVE ameliorated colonic ulceration and reduced inflammatory score.

Histopathological assessment revealed that treatment of rats with *Cordia vignei* extract preserved the functional cytoarchitecture of the entire colonic mucosa and inhibited inflammatory cell infiltration, congestion, ulceration,

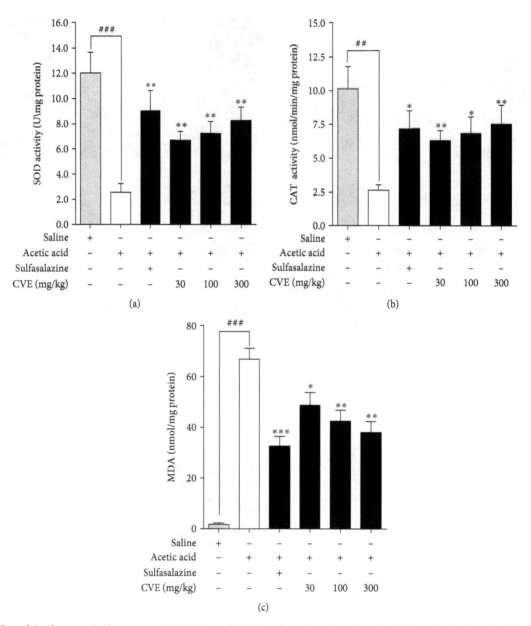

FIGURE 5: Effect of *Cordia vignei* leaf extract on SOD, CAT, and MDA on the colons of acetic acid-challenged rats. Rats ($n = 5$) orally received normal saline (10 ml kg^{-1}), sulfasalazine (500 mg kg^{-1}), or CVE (30-300 mg kg^{-1}) daily for 7 days. On day 4, rats were challenged with 500 μl acetic acid (4% v/v). Rats were sacrificed on day 8 and the colons were homogenized and centrifuged. The supernatant was used for the assay of activity of SOD (a) and CAT (b) and levels of MDA (c). Results were presented as mean ± SEM and statistically compared using student's t test. $^{####}P < 0.0001;^{###}P < 0.001;^{##}P < 0.01$ (acetic acid control *vs.* naïve control); $^{*}P < 0.05$; $^{**}P,<0.01$, $^{***}P < 0.001$ (acetic acid control *vs.* treatment group).

erosions, necrosis, and hyperplasia caused by acetic acid. This is also indicative of the ability of the extract to protect the animals and reduce progression of the disease.

In healthy rats, superoxide dismutase (SOD) and catalase (CAT) play important roles as protective antioxidant enzymes. In ulcerative colitis, levels of these enzymes in colonic tissues become exhausted as a consequence of oxidative damage caused by free radicals [26]. SOD protects the cells against ulcerative damage by mediating dismutation of superoxide anion and preventing lipid peroxidation. SOD also prevents leukocyte rolling and adhesion in colonic tissues [27]. CAT, which is concentrated in subcellular organ-

elles of peroxisomes, catalyzes the conversion of hydrogen peroxide, a cytotoxic compound to water and oxygen [27]. Malondialdehyde (MDA) is a byproduct of lipid peroxidation occurring in the tissue. In ulcerative colitis, levels of MDA in the plasma increases significantly and this is used as important diagnoses of patients with inflammatory bowel disease [6]. Since lipid peroxidation occurs during oxidative stress, natural products with antioxidant activity are beneficial [28]. Significant inhibition of MDA levels and increased SOD and CAT activities in the colons by CVE is indicative of its antioxidant potential which is important in its anti-inflammatory effect.

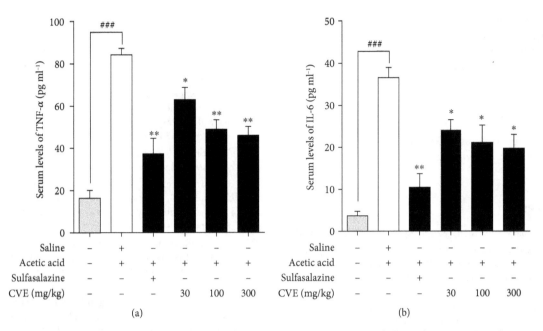

FIGURE 6: Effect of *Cordia vignei* leaf extract on serum levels of TNF-α and IL-6 in acetic acid-challenged rats. Rats ($n = 5$) were orally treated with normal saline (10 ml kg^{-1}), sulfasalazine (500 mg kg^{-1}), or CVE (30-300 mg kg^{-1}) daily for 7 days. On day 4, rats were challenged with 500 μl of acetic acid (4% v/v). Rats were sacrificed on day 8 and serum levels of TNF-α (a) and IL-6 (b) were assessed by ELISA. Results were presented as mean ± SEM. $^{###}P < 0.001$ (acetic acid control *vs.* naïve control); $^{*}P < 0.05$, $^{**}P < 0.01$ (acetic acid control *vs.* treatment group).

TABLE 1: Effect of hydroethanolic leaf extract of *Cordia vignei* on haematological parameters of acetic acid-induced colitic rats.

Treatment (group)	WBC ($\times10^3/\mu$l)	RBC ($\times106/\mu$l)	HGB (g/dl)	LYMP (%)	NEUT (%)	HCT (%)	PLT ($\times103/\mu$l)
Nonacetic	11.32 ± 1.03	10.56 ± 095	14.51 ± 0.77	69.5 ± 3.33	7.5 ± 0.57	45.72 ± 4.32	593 ± 14.38
Acetic acid	13.47 ± 0.97	8.87 ± 1.18	13.61 ± 0.89	57.8 ± 3.96	8.9 ± 1.12	42.4 ± 1.80	631 ± 20.01
Sulfasalazine	12.71 ± 1.02	6.95 ± 0.88	12.92 ± 1.25	51.9 ± 2.96	6.7 ± 0.69	49.31 ± 2.89	583 ± 36.88
30 mg/kg CVE	10.32 ± 1.07	7.46 ± 0.64	11.95 ± 0.86	61.7 ± 6.26	7.3 ± 0.45	48.66 ± 4.58	667 ± 20.77
100 mg/kg CVE	11.61 ± 1.52	6.71 ± 0.67	12.94 ± 1.00	42.2±1.94**	5.7 ± 0.46*	43.12 ± 2.50	580 ± 17.01
300 mg/kg CVE	12.14 ± 0.99	7.18 ± 0.68	13.67 ± 0.90	47.3 ± 2.34	6.2 ± 0.16*	44.90 ± 1.79	624 ± 16.40

Tumor necrosis factor alpha (TNF-α) and interleukin 6 (IL-6) play essential roles in the pathophysiology of inflammatory bowel disease [29, 30]. They modulate mucosal immune system, alter epithelial integrity, and orchestrate neutrophil and macrophage infiltration and activation which result in colonic injury. TNF-α is involved in increased endothelia cell permeability, pyrexia, algesia, cachexia, and leukocyte production and activation to generate more prostaglandins (PGs). IL-6 stimulates production of acute-phase proteins and activation of the complement system thereby releasing C3 and C5. C5 and C3 are involved in neutrophil chemotaxis and activation of leukocytes to release more mediators and activation of mast cells to release histamine and heparin. Recently, TNF-α, IL-6, COX-2, and their upstream signal regulator, NF-κB, have become new promising anti-inflammatory targets for the treatment of IBD [31]. In this study, elevation of TNF-α and IL-6 levels in the control rats as opposed to the reduced levels in the CVE-treated rats is suggestive of antiulcerative potential of the extract. Also, treatment of rats with CVE which significantly

inhibited TNF-α and IL-6 elevation and prevented depletion of SOD and CAT levels resulted in gross protection of colons.

These findings are similar to those reported by Aleisa et al. [1], Gautam et al. (2012) [2], Lopes et al. (2014) [32], and Nartey et al. [33] in which *Gymnema sylvestre*, *Antrocaryon micraster*, *Terminalia chebula*, *Solanum cernuum*, and *Cassia sieberiana* extracts attenuated acetic acid-induced ulcerative colitis in rats by inhibiting various physical, haematological, and biochemical markers such as body weight loss, colon density, TNF-α and IL-6 expressions, neutrophil infiltration, and oxidative stress although in this research, loss of body weight was not significantly affected by CVE.

6. Conclusion

The findings of the present study are indicative of the preventive ability of *Cordia vignei* leaf extract against the damaging effect of acetic acid-induced colitis in Sprague Dawley rats through inhibition of TNF-α and IL-6 activities. Also, SOD and CAT activities in the colons were increased. The results may be useful in future clinical trials of the *Cordia vignei* leaves or its bioactive constituents as natural, safe and effective treatment of patients with inflammatory bowel disease.

Acknowledgments

We are grateful to Messrs Gordon Daaku and Fulgencios Somkang for their technical assistance during this research.

References

[1] A. M. Aleisa, S. S. al-Rejaie, H. M. Abuohashish, M. S. Ola, M. Y. Parmar, and M. M. Ahmed, "Pretreatment of Gymnema sylvestre revealed the protection against acetic acid-induced ulcerative colitis in rats," *BMC Complementary and Alternative Medicine*, vol. 14, no. 1, 2014.

[2] M. K. Gautam, S. Goel, R. R. Ghatule, A. Singh, G. Nath, and R. K. Goel, "Curative effect of Terminalia chebula extract on acetic acid-induced experimental colitis: role of antioxidants, free radicals and acute inflammatory marker," *Inflammopharmacology*, vol. 21, no. 5, pp. 377–383, 2013.

[3] I. Loddo and C. Romano, "Inflammatory bowel disease: genetics, epigenetics, and pathogenesis," *Frontiers in Immunology*, vol. 6, no. 2015, p. p551, 2015.

[4] E. Mizoguchi, D. Nguyen, and D. Low, "Animal models of ulcerative colitis and their application in drug research," *Drug Design, Development and Therapy*, vol. 7, pp. 1341–1357, 2013.

[5] G. Tahan, E. Aytac, H. Aytekin et al., "Vitamin E has a dual effect of anti-inflammatory and antioxidant activities in acetic acid-induced ulcerative colitis in rats," *Canadian Journal of Surgery*, vol. 54, no. 5, pp. 333–338, 2011.

[6] A. A. Ali, E. N. Abd al Haleem, S. A. H. Khaleel, and A. S. Sallam, "Protective effect of cardamonin against acetic acid-induced ulcerative colitis in rats," *Pharmacological Reports*, vol. 69, no. 2, pp. 268–275, 2017.

[7] M. M. Pastrelo, C. C. Dias Ribeiro, J. W. Duarte et al., "Effect of concentrated apple extract on experimental colitis induced by acetic acid," *International Journal of Molecular and Cellular Medicine*, vol. 6, no. 1, pp. 38–49, 2017.

[8] T. Tian, Z. Wang, and J. Zhang, "Pathomechanisms of oxidative stress in inflammatory bowel disease and potential antioxidant therapies," *Oxidative Medicine and Cellular Longevity*, vol. 2017, Article ID 4535194, 18 pages, 2017.

[9] H. M. Burkill, *The Useful Plants of West Tropical Africa*, Royal Botanic Gardens, Kew, 2004, http://www.aluka.org/.

[10] C. Agyare, V. Spiegler, A. Asase, M. Scholz, G. Hempel, and A. Hensel, "An ethnopharmacological survey of medicinal plants traditionally used for cancer treatment in the Ashanti region, Ghana," *Journal of ethnopharmacology*, vol. 212, pp. 137–152, 2018.

[11] National Institute of Health (NIH), *Guide for the Care and Use of Laboratory Animal Use and Care*, National Academic Press, Washinton D.C., 8th Ed edition, 2011, http://www.nap.edu/.

[12] I. Ballester, A. Daddaoua, R. López-Posadas et al., "The bisphosphonate alendronate improves the damage associated with trinitrobenzenesulfonic acid-induced colitis in rats," *British Journal of Pharmacology*, vol. 151, no. 2, pp. 206–215, 2007.

[13] A. Motavallian-Naeini, S. Andalib, M. Rabbani, P. Mahzouni, M. Afsharipour, and M. Minaiyan, "Validation and optimization of experimental colitis induction in rats using 2, 4, 6-trinitrobenzene sulfonic acid," *Research in Pharmaceutical Sciences*, vol. 7, no. 3, pp. 159–169, 2012.

[14] H. P. Misra and I. Fridovich, "The role of superoxide anion in the autoxidation of epinephrine and a simple assay for superoxide dismutase," *Journal of Biological Chemistry*, vol. 247, no. 10, pp. 3170–3175, 1972.

[15] A. K. Sinha, "Colorimetric assay of catalase," *Analytical Biochemistry*, vol. 47, no. 2, pp. 389–394, 1972.

[16] R. L. Heath and L. Packer, "Photoperoxidation in isolated chloroplasts: I. Kinetics and stoichiometry of fatty acid peroxidation," *Archives of Biochemistry and Biophysics*, vol. 125, no. 1, pp. 189–198, 1968.

[17] G. A. Soliman, G. A. Gabr, F. I. al-Saikhan et al., "Protective effects of two Astragalus species on ulcerative colitis in rats," *Tropical Journal of Pharmaceutical Research*, vol. 15, no. 10, pp. 2155–2163, 2016.

[18] R. M. Hartmann, M. I. Morgan Martins, J. Tieppo, H. S. Fillmann, and N. P. Marroni, "Effect of Boswellia serrata on antioxidant status in an experimental model of colitis rats induced by acetic acid," *Digestive Diseases and Sciences*, vol. 57, no. 8, pp. 2038–2044, 2012.

[19] S. Hunschede, R. Kubant, R. Akilen, S. Thomas, and G. H. Anderson, "Decreased appetite after high-intensity exercise correlates with increased plasma interleukin-6 in normal-weight and overweight/obese boys," *Current Developments in Nutrition*, vol. 1, no. 3, p. e000398, 2017.

[20] H. S. el-Abhar, L. N. A. Hammad, and H. S. A. Gawad, "Modulating effect of ginger extract on rats with ulcerative colitis," *Journal of Ethnopharmacology*, vol. 118, no. 3, pp. 367–372, 2008.

[21] M. M. Harputluoglu, U. Demirel, N. Yücel et al., "The effects of Gingko biloba extract on acetic acid-induced colitis in rats," *The Turkish Journal of Gastroenterology: the official journal of Turkish Society of Gastroenterology*, vol. 17, no. 3, pp. 177–182, 2006.

[22] S. S. Al-Rejaie, H. M. Abuohashish, M. M. Ahmed, A. M. Aleisa, and O. Alkhamees, "Possible biochemical effects following inhibition of ethanol-induced gastric mucosa damage by Gymnema sylvestrein male Wistar albino rats," *Pharmaceutical Biology*, vol. 50, no. 12, pp. 1542–1550, 2012.

[23] R. H. Duerr, "Update on the genetics of inflammatory bowel disease," *Journal of Clinical Gastroenterology*, vol. 37, no. 5, pp. 358–367, 2003.

[24] B. E. Sands, "Therapy of inflammatory bowel disease," *Gastroenterology*, vol. 118, no. 2, pp. S68–S82, 2000.

[25] A. S. Awaad, A. M. Alafeefy, F. A. S. Alasmary, R. M. el-Meligy, and S. I. Alqasoumi, "Anti-ulcerogenic and anti-ulcerative colitis (UC) activities of seven amines derivatives," *Saudi Pharmaceutical Journal*, vol. 25, no. 8, pp. 1125–1129, 2017.

[26] S. V. Rana, S. Sharma, K. K. Prasad, S. K. Sinha, and K. Singh, *The Indian Journal of Medical Research*, vol. 139, no. 4, pp. 568–571, 2014.

[27] D. E. B. Baldo and J. E. Serrano, "Screening for intestinal anti-inflammatory activity of Alpinia galanga against acetic acid-induced colitis in mice (Mus musculus)," *Journal of Medicinal Plants Studies*, vol. 4, no. 1, pp. 72–77, 2017.

[28] C. E. Rosas, L. B. Correa, and M. G. Henriques, "Neutrophils in rheumatoid arthritis: a target for discovering new therapies based on natural products," in *Role of Neutrophils in Disease Pathogenesis*, pp. 89–118, IntechOpen Limited, London, UK, 2017.

[29] Q. Guan and J. Zhang, "Recent advances: the imbalance of cytokines in the pathogenesis of inflammatory bowel disease," *Mediators of Inflammation*, vol. 2017, Article ID 4810258, 8 pages, 2017.

[30] Z. H. Nemeth, D. A. Bogdanovski, P. Barratt-Stopper, S. R. Paglinco, L. Antonioli, and R. H. Rolandelli, "Crohn's disease and ulcerative colitis show unique cytokine profiles," *Cureus*, vol. 9, no. 4, p. e1177, 2017.

[31] M. F. Neurath, "Cytokines in inflammatory bowel disease," *Nature Reviews Immunology*, vol. 14, no. 5, pp. 329–342, 2014.

[32] L. C. Lopes, J. E. de Carvalho, M. Kakimore et al., "Pharmacological characterization of Solanum cernuum Vell.: 31-norcycloartanones with analgesic and anti-inflammatory properties," *Inflammopharmacology*, vol. 22, no. 3, pp. 179–185, 2013.

[33] E. T. Nartey, M. Ofosuhene, and C. M. Agbale, "Anti-ulcerogenic activity of the root bark extract of the African laburnum "Cassia sieberiana" and its effect on the anti-oxidant defence system in rats," *BMC Complementary and Alternative Medicine*, vol. 247, no. 1, p. 247, 2012.

[34] A. Sofowora, *Medicinal Plants and Traditional Medicine in Africa*, Spectrum Books Ltd., Ibadan, 2nd edn edition, 1993.

[35] D. L. Pavia, M. G. Lampman, and G. S. Kriz, *Introduction to Spectroscopy*, Thomson Learning Berkshire House, London, UK, 3 ed edition, 2001.

[36] N. D. M. Lakshmi, B. Mahitha, and T. Madhavi, "Phytochemical screening and FTIR analysis of Clitoria ternatea leaves," *International Journal of Scientific & Engineering Research*, vol. 6, no. 2, pp. 287–290, 2015.

23

The Contributive Role of IGFBP-3 and Mitochondria in Synoviocyte-Induced Osteoarthritis through Hypoxia/Reoxygenation Injury

Daniel Gululi[ID],[1] **Guy-Armel Bounda**[ID],[2,3,4] **Jianping Li**[ID],[1] **and Haohuan Li**[ID][1]

[1]Department of Orthopaedics, Renmin Hospital of Wuhan University, Wuhan, 430060 Hubei, China
[2]Department of Clinical Pharmacy, School of Basic Medicine and Clinical Pharmacy, China Pharmaceutical University, 24# Tong Jia Xiang, Nanjing, 210009 Jiangsu, China
[3]Sinomedica Co., Ltd., 677# Nathan Road, Mong Kok, Kowloon, Hong Kong
[4]Gabonese Scientific Research Consortium B.P. 5707, Libreville, Gabon

Correspondence should be addressed to Daniel Gululi; gululidaniel@gmail.com and Haohuan Li; lihaohuan@whu.edu.cn

Academic Editor: Albert S Mellick

Osteoarthritis (OA), one of the most common joint disorders, is characterized by chronic progressive cartilage degradation, osteophyte formation, and synovial inflammation. OA lesions are not only located in articular cartilage but also in the entire synovial joint. Nevertheless, most of the early studies done mostly focused on the important role of chondrocyte apoptosis and cartilage degeneration in the pathogenesis and progress of OA. The increased expression of hypoxia-inducible factors (HIF-1α and HIF-2α) is known to be the cellular and biochemical signal that mediates the response of chondrocytes to hypoxia. The role of the synovium in OA pathogenesis had been poorly evaluated. Being sensitive to hypoxia/reoxygenation (H/R) injury, fibroblast-like synoviocytes (FLS) play an essential role in cartilage degradation during the course of this pathology. Insulin-like growth factor binding protein 3 (IGFBP-3) acts as the main carrier of insulin-like growth factor I (IGF-I) in the circulation and remains the most abundant among the six IGFBPs. Synovial fluids of OA patients have markedly increased levels of IGFBP-3. We aim to discuss the interconnected behavior of IGFBP-3 and synoviocytes during the course of osteoarthritis pathogenesis, especially under the influence of hypoxia-inducible factors. In this review, we present information related to the essential role that is played by IGFBP-3 and mitochondria in synoviocyte-induced osteoarthritis through H/R injury. Little research has been done in this area. However, strong evidences show that the level of IGFBP-3 in synovial fluid significantly increased in OA, inhibiting the binding of IGF-1 to IGFR 1 (IGF receptor-1) and therefore the inhibition of cell proliferation. To the best of our knowledge, this is the first paper providing a comprehensive explanatory contribution of IGFBP-3 and mitochondria in synovial cell-induced osteoarthritis through hypoxia/reoxygenation mechanism.

1. Introduction

Osteoarthritis (OA), also known as degenerative joint disease or osteoarthrosis, is the most common form of arthritis and the leading source of physical disability with severely impaired quality of life in people in industrialized nations [1]. OA was first differentiated from other forms of joint disease at the beginning of the 20th century, on the basis of the hypertrophic changes seen in bone [2], encouraging scientists to focus more on osteology with the aim of providing further insights into the disease [3]. Osteoarthritis, although derived from the Greek words *osteon* for bone, *arthron* for joint, and the suffix *-itis* for inflammation, the site of the most pronounced structural alterations is not the bone but the joint cartilage, and severe inflammation is seen in only few patients [1]. Biochemical processes involving tissues, ligaments, bones, and muscles

Healthy   Osteoarthritis

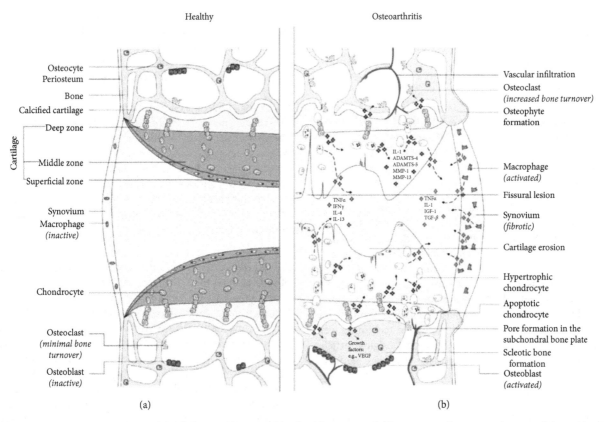

(a)   (b)

FIGURE 1: Schematic representation of the differences between (a) a healthy joint and (b) an osteoarthritic joint (*reprinted from Glyn-Jones et al. [5] and reused with permission from Elsevier under license number 4820090120408*). (a) In a healthy condition, chondrocytes produce substances that provide lubrication and reduce friction during joint articulation. (b) In osteoarthritic state, the joint changes pathologically due to alterations of multiple cell types and there is activation of synovial macrophages. Abbreviations: ADAMTS = a disintegrin and metalloproteinase with thrombospondin-like motifs; IL = interleukin; MMP = matrix metalloproteinase; TNF = tumor necrosis factor; IFN = interferon; IGF = insulin-like growth factor; TGF = transforming growth factor; VEGF = vascular endothelial growth factor.

eventually intertwine and collectively damage all joint compartments [1], resulting in a cascade of events including alterations of the synovium on both morphologic and biochemical levels as shown in Figure 1 and very well depicted by Glyn-Jones et al. in one of their relevant publications [1, 4, 5]. Generally, the process of joint destruction can always be evaluated for the pathogenesis ("typing"), for its extent ("staging"), and for the degree of the most extensive focal damage ("grading") [1]. While the "typing" of the disease is either idiopathic ("primary") or posttraumatic ("secondary"), its "grading" and "staging" have been much under debate [1]. This ongoing debate has brought forth proposal of several systems by eminent scientists or research groups including Pritzker and colleagues [6], Outerbridge [7], Otte [8], and Gelse et al. [9].

Systemic and local biomechanical factors affect the likelihood for a joint to develop OA [3]. Strong and irrefutable evidences show that osteoarthritis is a disease with a variety of pathophysiologic drivers leading to multiple phenotypes including inflammatory OA, cartilage-driven OA, traumatic/acute OA, and bone-driven OA [10]. In some cases, patients may present an overlap of more than one phenotype during the clinical course of their pathology. However, let us note that each OA phenotype may potentially be treated differently, and this might pave the way for methodologies of developing stratified medicines and phenotypical regimens

for OA patients. Although estimates of the OA prevalence and incidences have varied across studies, there is an undeniable fact that adults are the most affected [11].

The quest to understand the pathophysiology of OA had previously focused on cartilage and periarticular bone studies as OA had been principally regarded to be a disease of cartilage. Hypoxia-inducible factors (HIF) play a key role in the breakdown of cartilage during OA. Findings show that the expression of HIF-1α and HIF-2α is significantly upregulated in osteoarthritic cartilages to mediate the response of chondrocytes to hypoxia [12–15]. However, nowadays, mounting and undeniable findings allow us to scientifically and clinically acknowledge that OA does not only affect the cartilage but the whole joint, including cartilage, bone, and synovium, with each of these components playing a critical role in the pathogenesis and the course of the disease [16]. Synovial fluids of OA patients have markedly increased levels of insulin-like growth factor binding protein 3 (IGFBP-3) [17]. The investigation of synoviocytes' behavior during the course of osteoarthritis pathogenesis has become an area of interest for many scientists.

This review presents general knowledge on OA and the sources and functions of reactive oxygen species/oxidative stress in the synovium. It highlights the impact of synovitis in OA, with evidence implicating synovial cell responses to cytokines in the pathogenesis of OA. We will discuss recent development in the best of our understanding of the role of IGFBP-3 in synoviocyte-induced OA under hypoxia/reoxygenation conditions.

2. Methods

A comprehensive literature review was conducted in order to identify studies and analyze findings that discuss the pathogenic role of IGFBP-3 in synoviocyte-induced OA in a hypoxic state. The methodology used here was adapted from the one previously used by Leonardi et al. [18].

2.1. Search Strategy. We performed an electronic search by looking into several databases including MEDLINE and Embase via OvidSP, Scopus, and Google Scholar, from inception up to January 31, 2020. Electronic search strategy consisted of keywords such as "osteoarthritis AND IGFBP-3" and "Osteoarthritis and Hypoxia/Reoxygenation OR hypoxy-inducible factor" with the following limits activated: synoviocytes and mitochondria. Related publication links from the relevant papers and references of identified citations were manually used to further retrieve additional original articles that were not captured by the primary electronic searches. The search and selection of papers were restricted to documents written in English.

2.2. Selection of Studies. Any published study or paper in English was considered for inclusion especially if in addition to "osteoarthritis" one or more of the following keywords, "IGFBP-3," "Fibroblast-like synoviocytes," "hypoxia/reoxygenation," and "hypoxia-inducible factors," constituted the main focus of the study. Eligible studies were considered if they included a randomized control cohort and case cohort. In case a study was included in more than one publication, only the available full-text publication was considered.

2.3. Eligibility Assessment and Data Extraction. The first two authors (DG and GAB) independently performed the literature search and carried out the data extraction. Agreement by consensus was used to solve any discrepancies between the two authors. Study design, research objectives, osteoarthritis state, and study findings were the main features of data extraction performed by the two authors.

3. Results

3.1. Number of Retrieved Publications. The primary and secondary searches identified 624 articles. Titles of all articles were reviewed, search results were screened, and 110 duplicates were removed. However, 481 publications were excluded for several reasons: articles not published in English, published papers from non-peer-reviewed journals, abstract and posters from conference presentations, editorials, studies without control cases, papers with no access to full text, case reports, clinical trial protocols, studies with wrong comparator, and studies focusing on concepts other than synoviocytes, IGF binding protein 3, and hypoxia-inducible factors. Afterwards, we identified 33 articles, which we considered deemed relevant for the focus on this specific topic.

3.2. Major Joint Tissues Involved in Osteoarthritis. According to the American College of Rheumatology (ACR) criteria, OA is clinically characterized by joint pain, tenderness, crepitus, stiffness and limitation of movement with occasional effusion, and variable degrees of local inflammation [19]. The pain in OA is frequently activity related; and constant pain usually becomes a feature later in the disease [20]. The OA-related pain is not simply attributable to the structural changes in the affected joint but a result of intermovement between structural change, peripheral and central pain processing mechanisms. Additionally, damage to cartilage, chondrocytes, and menisci gives debris to the synovium that in turn initiates the recruitment of inflammatory mediators, which again increase responsiveness to synovial nerve endings to heighten OA pain.

3.2.1. Types of Synovial Joints. The human body is composed of several types of joints. According to their structural classification, they are divided in three types, namely, fibrous, cartilaginous, and synovial joints. However, based on the degree of the movement permitted, they are categorized as synarthrosis (immoveable), amphiarthrosis (slightly moveable), and diarthrosis (freely moveable) [21]. Sutures, gomphoses, and syndesmoses are the three types of fibrous joints. They are joints where the adjacent bones are strongly and directly connected to each other by fibrous connective tissue. The cartilaginous joints are subdivided into two, namely, synchondrosis and symphysis. They lack a joint cavity and involve bones that are joined together by either hyaline cartilage (synchondrosis) or fibrocartilage (symphysis) [21, 22]. Identified as the most common type of joints, synovial joints are associated as the most weight-bearing joints [22]. As intricate structures, these joints are composed of articular cartilage, synovial membranes, ligaments, and an articular capsule that is characterized by the presence of a lubricating synovial fluid. Structurally, they are the most complex and are most likely to develop uncomfortable and crippling dysfunctions. Each of the different types of synovial joints allows for specialized movements that permit different degrees of motion [21]. Based on the anatomical structure of the joints and the synergy of their movement, synovial joints are subclassified into six types: pivot (between C1 and C2 vertebrae), hinge (elbow, knee), condyloid (wrist), saddle (trapeziometacarpal joint), plane (between tarsal bones), and ball and socket (shoulder, hip) [22]. Their mobility makes the synovial joints especially important to the quality of life. The bones of a synovial joint are covered by a layer of hyaline cartilage that lines the epiphyses of joint ends of bone with a smooth and slippery surface [21].

3.2.2. Clinical Features of OA by Joint Site. Classically described as slowly progressive and the most common form of arthritis, OA is an irreversible disease of articular joints leading to pain and loss of joint function. Based on clinical features, the cause and prevalence of osteoarthritis at different joints differ from one site to another (Table 1). Each site-joint osteoarthritis often presents its own distinct features [23, 24].

TABLE 1: Clinical features of OA by joint site.

Site-joint OA	Characteristics	Ref.
Knee OA	Knee osteoarthritis is very common, comprising the largest proportion of all cases and affecting 12.4 million (33.6%) adults over the age of 65. There are five phenotypes: (a) minimal joint disease phenotype, (b) strong muscle phenotype, (c) nonobese and weak muscle phenotype, (d) obese and weak muscle phenotype, and (d) depressive phenotype.	[23, 25]
Hip OA	Hip osteoarthritis stands for 13% in osteoarthritic patients and a major cause of pain and disability in the elderly population. Three different subtypes (normotrophic, hypertrophic, and atrophic) of hip OA have been considered nowadays.	[24, 26]
Shoulder OA	Shoulder OA is the final diagnosis in 5% of those who report shoulder pain, affecting up to 32.8% of patients over the age of sixty years. Its prevalence increases with age, and women appear to be more susceptible than men.	[24, 27]
Hand OA	Hand OA affects 26% of women and 13% of men over the age of 71.	[28].
Ankle OA	Ankle OA has a prevalence of less than 1% of the world's adult population. Approximately 30% of ankle OA cases are idiopathic and affect a relatively younger population as compared with other OA joint afflictions.	[24, 29]
Elbow OA	OA is far less common at the elbow than at the other upper limb joints and even seems rare. Symptomatic elbow OA is a relatively rare condition that comprises only up to 2% of patients with elbow arthritis and almost exclusive to males. According to the joint side involved, the elbow OA can be categorized as humeroradial OA and humeroulnar OA.	[24, 30]
Lumbar spine OA	Lumbar spine osteoarthritis (OA) is very common, with estimates of prevalence ranging from 40 to 85%. Facet joint osteoarthritis (FJOA) is a common disease widely prevalent in older adults causing low back and lower extremity pain.	[31, 32]
Temporomandibular joint OA	Little focus is given to the incidence of temporomandibular joint (TMJ) OA, although it may lead to dental malocclusion and reduced health-related quality of life. In an age group of 9-90 years, the percentage of TMJ OA ranges from 28% to 38% and the incidence increases with advancing age.	[33, 34]

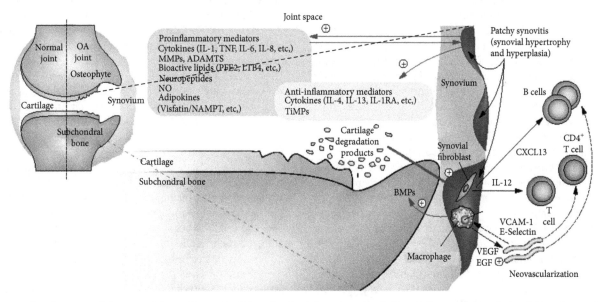

FIGURE 2: Involvement of the synovial membrane in OA pathophysiology (*reprinted from Sellam and Berenbaum* [4] *and reused with permission from Nature Springer under license no. 4820091329692*). The type A synoviocytes phagocytosed the cartilage breakdown products that are released into the synovial fluid, amplifying synovitis. This process will lead to the production of anti-inflammatory substance and to the formation of osteophytes via the bone morphogenetic protein (BMP). Abbreviations: CCL2: CC-chemokine ligand 2; CXCL13: CXC-chemokine ligand 13; EGF: endothelial growth factor; GM-CSF: granulocyte-macrophage colony-stimulating factor; IL-1Ra: IL-1 receptor antagonist; LIF: leukemia inhibitory factor; LTB4: leukotriene B4; NAMPT: nicotinamide phosphoribosyl transferase; NO: nitric oxide; NGF: nerve growth factor; PGE2: prostaglandin E2; TIMP: tissue inhibitor of metalloproteinase; TNF: tumor necrosis factor; VCAM-1: vascular cell adhesion molecule 1; VEGF: vascular endothelial growth factor.

3.3. Role of Synovium in the Pathology of Osteoarthritis. The synovium is a major part of the joint; therefore, its inflammation plays an essential role in the course of the disease. Undeniable evidences of the role of synovitis in OA are now widely accepted and available in medical literature. Sellam and Berenbaum, in one of their OA-related papers, have well summarized the evidence of the role of synovitis in OA. The findings showed that the role of synovium inflammation

TABLE 2: Major histopathological features of the four patterns of OA-associated synoviopathy in comparison to each other and to normal synovium (adapted from Oehler et al. [38]).

	Normal	Hyperplastic synoviopathy	Inflammatory synoviopathy	Fibrotic synoviopathy	Detritus-rich synoviopathy
Villous hyperplasia	−	++(+)	++(+)	++(+)	++(+)
Synovial lining—proliferation	−	+	++	++	++(+)
Synovial lining—activation	−	+	++	+	+
Fibrinous exudate	−	−	(+)	+	++(+)
Capsular fibrosis	−	−	(+)	+++	+++
(Macromolecular) cartilage and bone debris	−	−	(+)	−	+++
Granulocytic infiltrate	−	−	−	−	+
Lymphoplasmocellular infiltrate—diffuse	−	−	++	(+)	+(+)
Lymphoplasmocellular infiltrate—aggregates/follicles	−	−	++	(+)	(+)
Stage of the disease		Early stage	Early and late stage	Late stage	Late stage

Note: −: negative; +: positive; ++: moderate; +++: excessive; (+): activated. Bold data indicate key diagnostic criteria.

can be undeniably proven from five levels of evidence: (i) clinical, (ii) imaging, (iii) histological, (iv) molecular, and (v) biological markers [4]. Type A synoviocytes (macrophage-like cells) and type B synoviocytes (synovial fibroblast) are the two major types of cells found within the synovium. The responsibility of the former type of cells lies in the fight against pathogens by producing and releasing specific substances, which in turn are involved in the inflammation and cartilage degradation [35]. Over the course of the pathology, they either exhibit a proinflammatory M1 phenotype (early stage) or anti-inflammatory M2 phenotype (latter stage) [36]. Synovial fibroblasts, along with other cell types such as chondrocytes, are presumably responsible for hyaluronan secretion. They are proven for acting as a barrier that keeps synovial fluid in the joint capsule [35]. These two types of synoviocytes both function as integral players in their physiological state and power to maintain a healthy environment. In OA progression, the alteration of their cellular functions may result from a pivotal role of synovitis in OA pathogenesis [4]. In synovitis, upregulated factors such as interleukin (IL), matrix metalloproteinases (MMPs), and a disintegrin and metalloproteinase with thrombospondin motifs (ADAMTs) induce the production of anti-inflammatory mediators. Moreover, there is formation of osteophytes via bone morphogenetic protein (BMPs) (Figure 2) [4].

Synovitis has long been an indicator of rheumatoid arthritis; research findings have now proven its participation and impact in OA [35]. Synovitis is considered to be associated at any stage in OA pathogenesis and therefore considered as a predictor of disease progression [4]. Since the past decade, undisputable evidence shows synovitis to be associated with greater symptoms such as pain and degree of joint dysfunction and may promote more rapid cartilage degeneration in OA [6, 37]. In OA synovial specimens, scientists have identified four patterns of OA-associated "synoviopathy" including (i) hyperplastic, (ii) fibrotic, (iii) detritus-rich, and (vi) inflammatory (Table 2) [38].

3.4. Pivotal Role of Mitochondria in Osteoarthritis Pathogenesis through H/R Injury. Known as the powerhouse of the cell, a mitochondrion is a platform of cell signaling and decision-maker of cell death. It modulates cell metabolism, reactive oxygen species (ROS) genesis, cell apoptosis, and Ca^{2+}. Mitochondria perform oxidative phosphorylation (OXPHOS) via election transport chain (ETC) reaction to synthesize ATP [39]. Ischemia-reperfusion (I-R) and hypoxia/reoxygenation (H/R) mechanisms are two distinct mechanisms that alter mitochondrial functions. These two expressions are sometimes interchangeably used by researchers and scientific writers. However, they are two distinct pathophysiological phenomena, although the clinical outcome from these two distinct events might look the same, resulting in cell death (Figure 3) [39]. Hypoxia is a condition in which the body or one of its regions is deprived of adequate oxygen supply while ischemia is a reduction of blood supply to tissues, causing a limitation of oxygen and glucose required for the metabolism. Ischemia always results in hypoxia; however, hypoxia can occur without ischemia. Outcomes of such insults are variable depending on the type and severity of the insult [40]. For instance, when ischemia is severe and prolonged, the loss of ATP and metabolic alterations induce an inevitable cell necrosis. However, if ischemia is short and transient, activation of prosurvival signals increases myocardial tolerance against subsequent ischemia [40].

Mitochondrial function serves as a key effector in the pathways and a mediator for the protective effect that short periods of hypoxia-reoxygenation and some drugs provide against tissue injury caused by subsequent prolonged hypoxia-reoxygenation (preconditioning) [41]. They induce an array of alterations in mitochondrial metabolic function, and therefore, these changes in mitochondrial structure integrity are widely believed to be important pathogenic factors that underlie ischemic cell injury in various tissues [41]. During hypoxia at mitochondrial permeability transition

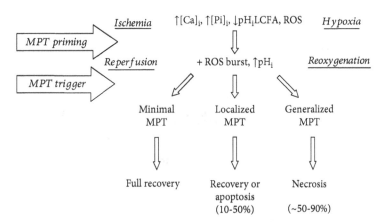

FIGURE 3: MPT and cell fate during ischemia-reperfusion and hypoxia/reoxygenation (*adapted from Weiss et al.* [39]). MPT occurs during ischemia or hypoxia injury. Cytosolic Ca^{2+} becomes elevated and is driven into the matrix. During mitochondria depolarization, accumulated matrix Ca^{2+} flows down its electrochemical gradient back into the cytoplasm. Cell fate depends on the degree of mitochondria depolarization. Abbreviations: Ca: calcium; LCFA: long-chain fatty acids; MPT: mitochondrial permeability transition; Pi: inorganic phosphate; ROS: reactive oxygen species.

(MPT) priming phase, accumulation of intracellular $Ca2^{2+}$, long-chain fatty acid (LCFA), ROS, and inorganic phosphate (P_i) promotes mitochondrial permeability transition pore (MPTP), which is a high conductance channel in the inner mitochondrial membrane (IMM) (Figure 3).

Because O_2 is used as a substrate by mitochondria, during hypoxia their respiration is inhibited. However, during reoxygenation, rapid restoration of respiration results in increased mitochondrial ROS production [41]. Oxidative stress and especially O_2^- cause synovial cell apoptosis in vitro through mitochondrial injury [42]. Likewise, NO reduces the survival and induces cell death of OA synoviocytes by regulating mitochondrial functionality [43]. However, high NO levels can induce synovial cell apoptosis only when cell capacities to repair DNA damage are exceeded [a], through activation of caspase-3, caspase-9, and MAPK and upregulation of COX-2 expression [44]. In the IMM, there is a high conductance channel known as the mitochondrial permeability transition pore (MPTP), and an increased ROS production and calcium dysregulation are likely to contribute to its opening [45]. Several published data reported that there are four types of K^+ channels localized in the IMM: ATP-sensitive K^+ channel (K_{ATP} channel), Ca^{2+}-activated K^+ channel (K_{Ca} channel), voltage-gated Kv1.3 K^+ channel, and twin-pore domain TASK-3 K^+ channel [46]. Findings have claimed that the ATP-activated K^+ channels (K_{ATP}) and Ca^{2+}-activated K^+ channels (K_{Ca}) are present in the IMM and display changes in activity during H/R injury [47, 48].

ROS and reactive nitrogen species (RNS) have been associated in the process of matrix and cell component degradation in OA and may play a critical role in the pathogenesis of OA. Human chondrocytes cultured from OA patients express inducible nitric oxide synthase (iNOS) and produce significant amounts of NO [1], even though the mechanisms by which NO could contribute to OA pathogenesis are still hypothetical and still under investigation from various clinical and laboratory perspectives. Neuronal NOS (nNOS), endothelial NOS (eNOS), and inducible NOS (iNOS) are the three recognized isoforms of NOS [49]. The existence of mitochondrial NOS (mtNOS) is still a subject of debate as no specific gene for mtNOS has yet been validated [50]. The essential participation of iNOS expression and the subsequent increase of NO in the pathogenesis of OA are corroborated by *in vivo* experiments demonstrating that specific inhibition of iNOS results in decreased production of catabolic factors such as IL-1β, MMPs, and peroxynitrite [51]. OA synoviocytes produced low nitrite levels spontaneously under basal normoxic conditions, and studies revealed that under H/R conditions, there is an induction of NO metabolism in OA synoviocytes, which is shown by increased iNOS expression and nitrite production [52–54]. Thus, RNS and ROS are two key areas in which scientists could offer deeper investigation in order to elucidate the pathogenesis and molecular biology of OA.

3.5. Role of IGFBP-3 in Synoviocyte-Induced Osteoarthritis

3.5.1. Overview of IGF and IGFBP Family. The insulin-like growth factor (IGF) signaling pathway is a well-defined system playing an essential role in regulating proliferation, differentiation, and apoptosis in mammalian organisms [55]. This system involves the complex coordination of growth factors (IGF-I and IGF-II), cell surface receptors (IGF-IR, IGF-IIR, and the insulin receptor (IR)), high-affinity binding proteins (IGFBP-1 to 6), IGFBP proteases, and several low-affinity IGFBP-related proteins (IGFBP-rP1 to 10) [55] (Figure 4). IGF-I plays specialized roles at different stages of life. Until pubertal life stage, IGF-1 stimulates the linear growth of bones by increasing the proliferation of epiphyseal chondrocytes and remodeling processes within the growth plate cartilage. At adulthood stage, its role is crucial for maintaining homeostasis in articular cartilage, by stimulating the production of matrix proteins through chondrocytes, counteracting their degradation, and preventing cell death [56, 57].

The bioactivity of IGF is not only dependent on interaction with IGFRs but also by the multifunctional family of

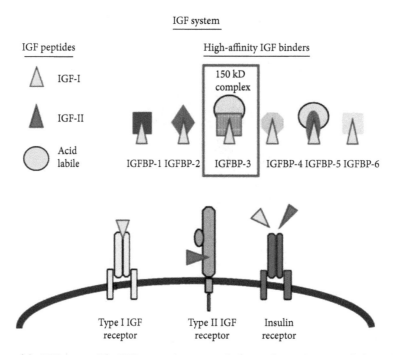

FIGURE 4: Schematic diagram of the IGF system. The IGF system is composed of several constituents including IGF-I, IGF-II, their respective receptors, and insulin receptor. In addition, there are 6 high-affinity binding proteins. IGFBP-3 binds to IGF-1 in complex with acid labile subunit. Abbreviations: IGF: insulin-like growth factor; IGFBP: insulin-like growth factor binding protein (*reused with permission from Garza [59], author of the dissertation entitled "Insulin-like growth factor binding protein-3 (IGFBP-3) plays an essential role in cellular senescence: molecular and clinical implications"*).

IGFBPs. Based on their primary structure and their post-translational modifications, IGFBPs are differentially tissue targeted. Among the six known IGFBPs, IGFBP-2, IGFBP-3, and IGFBP-4 are known to be secreted by articular cartilage or chondrocytes, with IGFBP-3 being the predominant one and responsible for carrying 75% of IGF-I and IGF-II in the heterotrimeric ternary complex with an acid-labile subunit [58].

3.5.2. IGFBP-3 in Synoviocyte-Induced Osteoarthritis through H/R Injury. Among the high-affinity binding proteins of the IGF system, IGFBP-3 remains the best and extensively studied protein. Strong evidence exists to support the striking versatility of action of this protein, based on the fact that IGFBP-3 can not only act as a modulator of IGF action but also as an independent ligand to promote intracellular signaling [60]. The activity of IGFBP-3 has been studied to a certain extent as this protein has been implicated in the pathogenesis of a number of different pathologies including osteoarthritis [61], asthma [62], cancer [49], fetal trisomy 21 [63], and depressive disorder [64].

Traditionally considered not associated with transient episodes of ischemia and/or hypoxia, osteoarthritis is nowadays receiving great attention as a clinical manifestation of I-R and/or H/R injury [17, 54, 65]. Hypoxia is recognized as an important feature of the joint microenvironment, especially in the perpetuation of joint destruction in OA [54].

Highly sensitive cells to H/R, FLS are considered associated with cartilage degradation during osteoarthritis pathogenesis [17]. Hypoxia-inducible factor (HIF) family members (HIF-1α, 2α, and 3α) are the principal mediators

of hypoxic response. Transcription of HIF-1α is highly expressed in OA cartilage, particularly in the late stage of the disease. The expression of HIF-1α and its target genes *Glut-1* and *PGK-1* in OA cartilage is associated with the progression of articular cartilage degeneration [12, 13]. On the other hand, HIF-1α is also a pivotal regulator in cartilage engineering allowing chondrocytes to maintain their function as professional secretory cells in the hypoxic growth plate [66–68]. In osteoarthritic cartilage, the transcription factor HIF-1α is involved in the upregulation of microsomal prostaglandin E synthase 1 (mPGES-1) and may therefore play an important role in the metabolism of OA cartilage [69]. HIF-2α is a key component for hypoxic induction of the human articular chondrocyte phenotype [70]. Evidences suggested that articular cartilage destruction might also be associated with the fact that HIF-2α directly induces the higher expression of catabolic factors including matrix metalloproteinases (MMP1, MMP3, MMP9, MMP12, and MMP13), aggrecanase-1 (ADAMTS4), nitric oxide synthase-2 (NOS2), and prostaglandin-endoperoxide synthase-2 (PTGS2) [14, 66]. Thus, these findings support its implication in OA through cartilage breakdown to be a critical evidence of the participation of this protein in OA pathogenesis [14]. Sound evidence has also indicated that H/R injury participates in various signaling cascade episodes including increased expression of tumor necrosis factor-(TNF-) α-induced IGFBP-3, downregulation of the expression of IGF-1, and release of intracellular ROS, eventually leading to apoptosis (Figure 5) [71].

In hypoxic conditions, HIF-1 activates transcription of the proapoptotic protein IGFBP-3, which blocks IGF-1

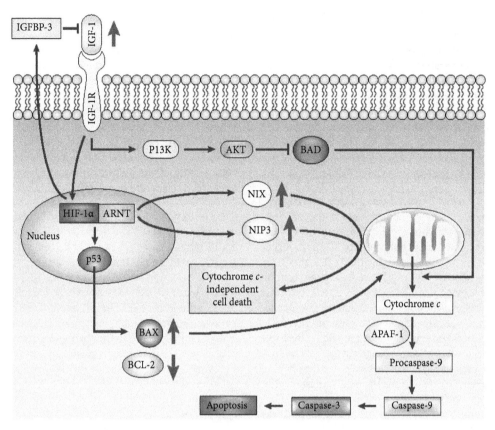

FIGURE 5: Hypoxia regulation of the cell death pathway (*reprinted from Harris* [72] *and reused with permission from Springer Nature under license number 4820081324341*). HIF-1 (a complex of HIF-1α and ARNT) activates transcription of many proapoptotic genes including IGFBP-3. HIF-1 activates the transcriptional activity of p53 and induces transcription of BAX. In turn, BAX promotes release of cytochrome *c* and promotes apoptosis via cascade reactions. Abbreviations: APAF-1: apoptotic protease-activating factor-1; ARNT: aryl hydrocarbon receptor nuclear translocator; HIF: hypoxia-inducible factor; IGF-1: insulin-like growth factor-1; IGF-1R: IGF-1 receptor; IGFBP-3: IGF binding protein 3; PI3K: phosphatidylinositol 3-OH kinase.

signaling. HIF-1 also activates expression of NIP3 and NIX, which in turn induce a mitochondrial-pore permeability transition and cell death. Studies showed that, compared to healthy subjects, synovial fluids of OA patients have markedly increased levels of IGFBP-3 [61]. Moreover, the increased level of IGFBP-3 in OA has been reported to be directly associated with the severity of the disease. In another study, Zhang and coworkers investigated the regulating effects of IGFBP-3 in inflammation and apoptosis, and conclusive evidence showed that the inflammatory response was reduced by the blockage of the NF-κB pathway and induction of apoptotic in OA FLS by IGFBP-3 [61]. The implication of IGFBP-3 in OA pathogenesis has also been studied under different signaling pathways. For instance, published data showed that IGFBP-3 induced chondrocyte apoptosis through nuclear-mitochondrial translocation of Nur77 [72].

Investigation of the implications of IGFBP-3 in OA pathogenesis under H/R mechanism is becoming an area of interest for scientists nowadays. In a study conducted by Zhang et al., the findings revealed that the expression of IGFBP-3 in FLS was upregulated under H/R conditions; pretreatments with TNF-α before H/R significantly increased the expression of IGFBP-3 [61]. In addition, other results showed that

H/R significantly increased the levels of various factors including CCL5, interleukin-1b (IL-1β), and interleukin-6 in cell-free culture supernatants and promoted TNF-α-induced expression of inflammatory cytokines [17]. Overall, findings suggest that under H/R, IGFBP-3 may promote the permeability of the mitochondrial membrane and release of ROS, triggering inflammation in FLS and therefore inducing osteoarthritis.

4. Discussion

4.1. Main Findings. As we used the same search strategy and considered the principal focus on the essential role of IGF binding protein 3 in fibroblast-like synoviocyte-induced osteoarthritis pathogenesis, as well as hypoxia/reoxygenation injury, we found that there are few studies conducted that focus on this specific topic. Although several original studies highlighted their primary focus on either IGF binding protein 3, or synovial cells in osteoarthritis, or on hypoxia and synoviocytes, only two papers had investigated the relation between IGFBP-3, synoviocytes, and hypoxia/reoxygenation in osteoarthritis. However, there was a high proportion of relevant studies that included the investigation of chondrocytes and IGF binding proteins. While the medical literature stated an undeniable evidence of the involvement of cells such as chondrocytes in osteoarthritis pathogenesis, researches regarding fibroblast-like synoviocyte role in osteoarthritis are still comparatively few. Moreover, the pivotal role of hypoxia/reoxygenation injury in this musculoskeletal disorder has become an area of great interest. Overall, evidence from the scientific literature strongly supports that osteoarthritis is a musculoskeletal disorder affecting the whole joint, and the synovium plays a key role in osteoarthritis pathogenesis.

4.2. Signaling Pathways Involved in Synoviocyte-Induced Osteoarthritis and Future Research Direction.

In osteoarthropathies, most of the research has paid more attention to the chondrocytes in terms of understanding the OA pathogenesis. Recently, several reports had indicated that synovitis is the major characteristic of OA and that reducing the number of osteoarthritis synoviocytes (OAS) is one of the key factors for curing the disease. In the quest to understand the mechanisms and nature of signaling pathways involved in synoviocyte-induced OA, several proteins and transcripts have gone through investigations throughout the years. Findings showed that various signaling pathways are involved in synoviocyte-induced OA, including hypoxia signaling [17], NF-κB signaling pathway [73, 74], eicosanoid pathway [75], IL-6/STAT3 signaling pathway [76], Wnt/β-catenin pathway [77], and hedgehog signaling [78].

Liang and colleagues investigated the influence of vasoactive intestinal peptide (VIP) recombinant plasmid on synoviocytes. Findings suggested that VIP recombinant plasmid could inhibit the proliferation of synoviocytes, improve the pathological symptoms of OA disease, and produce a therapeutic effect on OA via the NF-κB signaling pathway [73]. In another study, authors found that follistatin-like protein 1 (FSTL1) functions as an essential proinflammatory factor in the pathogenesis of OA by activating the first pathway and enhancing synoviocyte proliferation [74]. Recently, researchers have assessed the implication of arachidonic acid, linoleic acid, and 20 oxylipins in synovial fluid from 58 knee OA patients and 44 controls. Results showed that levels of three lipoxins (LXs) in synovial fluid were associated with knee OA. The expression of 11,12-DHET and 14,15-DHET was statistically upregulated in affected compared to unaffected knees of people with unilateral disease. In addition, their expression and the expression of 8,9-DHET were also associated with knee OA radiographic progression in the over 3.3 years of follow-up of 87 individuals [75]. Through the IL-6/STAT3 signaling pathway, Li and colleagues investigated the role of lncRNA gastric cancer-associated transcript 3 (GACAT3) in OA [56]. Researchers found that, compared with normal synoviocytes, GACAT3 was significantly highly expressed in OA synoviocytes [76]. In addition, GACAT3 could influence the proliferation of OA synoviocytes. Researchers have investigated the role of this signaling pathway in TMJ OA and facet joint OA. Findings showed that mediators and downstream effectors of Wnt/β-catenin signaling are increased in OA as well other forms of arthritis, suggesting that the Wnt/β-catenin signaling pathway plays

a direct role in OA pathogenesis through bone and joint pathology and synovial tissue [77].

Recent advances in osteoarthritis synoviocytes have enabled comprehensive analysis of various cells, proteins, and signaling pathways involved in this musculoskeletal disorder. The association of fibroblast-like synoviocytes in osteoarthritis pathogenesis is a strong and clear evidence that cannot be undermined today. In addition, mitochondria role through hypoxia/reoxygenation mechanism is an area that needs to be highly considered in further researches. Outcomes from these investigations shall definitively provide better, suitable, and targeted therapy to orthopedic patients.

4.3. Limitations.

Retrieved papers included diversified types of osteoarthritis, which again varied across the studies. In addition, variation in setting and study population/samples are two main factors that limited the comparability. Publication bias was not assessed, meaning that several published studies we retrieved might have been data reporting only positive findings of IGFBP-3, FLS, and H/R on osteoarthritis pathogenesis. Although this paper has some limitations, it stands as the first study that brings an explanatory contribution role of IGF binding protein 3 and mitochondria in synoviocyte-induced osteoarthritis through hypoxia/reoxygenation injury.

5. Conclusions

OA is an invalidating disease characterized by progressive cartilage degradation. Research findings suggested that OA is a disease with a variety of pathophysiologic drivers leading to multiple phenotypes. Increasing undeniable evidence is now at hand proving that OA is not just a cartilage problem but of the entire joint tissue. Studies have shown the essential role of hypoxia-inducible factors into the course of the disease. Moreover, hypoxia plays a vital role in OA pathogenesis as hypoxia amplifies the NF-κB pathways by inducing synovitis. Strong evidences show that the level of IGFBP-3 in synovial fluid significantly increased in OA, inhibiting the binding of IGF-1 to IGFR 1 and therefore the inhibition of cell proliferation. Published papers related to the implication of the insulin-like growth factor (IGF) signaling pathway as a complete system or including its associated receptors and proteins in inflammatory joint disorders are available in the medical literature. Although some of these papers have shared undeniable knowledge in the light of the mechanistic pathogenesis of the pathology, they often either focus on chondrocytes [72], osteoblast [79], or usually rheumatoid arthritis [80]. Even where IGFBP-3 is put in exert, little is known regarding its pivotal role at the different stages of the disease [17]. Scientists from interdisciplinary background are using novel techniques such as bioinformatics to add to the field the knowledge regarding potential therapy target in order to understand OA development [81]. To the best of our analysis and in the light of the knowledge presented and discussed in this review, compared with other papers, the novelty of our submission lies in the highlights made on the exploration of inflammation mechanisms leading to OA pathogenesis. Although the exact mechanism of OA pathogenesis, which is surely complex, remains poorly understood, there is no doubt that synovitis is counted to be one of the key pathogenic events during the course of the disease. Our paper not only discusses in depth the implication of hypoxic factors but also highlights the insulin-like growth factor binding protein-3–synoviocyte interaction and interconnectivity in osteoarthritis. Further investigations are needed to strengthen the undeniable evidence of IGFBP-3 and synovial cell interconnectivity in osteoarthritis pathogenesis through H/R injury.

Authors' Contributions

D.G. and H.L. conceptualized the paper. D.G. and G.A.B. wrote the manuscript. D.G., G.A.B., J.L., and H.L. revised the manuscript. H.L. supervised the entire manuscript. All authors have read and agreed to the published version of the manuscript.

Acknowledgments

This research was funded by the National Natural Science Foundation of China under Grant No. 81171760 and the Natural Science Foundation of Hubei Province under Grant No. ZRMS2017000057.

References

[1] T. Aigner and N. Schmitz, *Pathogenesis and Pathology of Osteoarthritis*, 2010.

[2] J. E. Goldthwaite, "The treatment of disabled joints resulting from the so-called rheumatoid diseases," *The Boston Medical and Surgical Journal*, vol. 136, no. 4, pp. 79–84, 1897.

[3] J. Rogers, L. Shepstone, and P. Dieppe, "Is osteoarthritis a systemic disorder of bone?," *Arthritis and Rheumatism*, vol. 50, no. 2, pp. 452–457, 2004.

[4] J. Sellam and F. Berenbaum, "The role of synovitis in pathophysiology and clinical symptoms of osteoarthritis," *Nature Reviews Rheumatology*, vol. 6, no. 11, pp. 625–635, 2010.

[5] S. Glyn-Jones, A. J. R. Palmer, R. Agricola et al., "Osteoarthritis," *Osteoarthritis Lancet*, vol. 386, no. 9991, pp. 376–387, 2015.

[6] K. P. H. Pritzker, S. Gay, S. A. Jimenez et al., "Osteoarthritis cartilage histopathology: grading and staging," *Osteoarthritis and Cartilage*, vol. 14, no. 1, pp. 13–29, 2006.

[7] R. E. Outerbridge, "The etiology of chondromalacia patellae," *The Journal of bone and joint surgery. British volume*, vol. 43, pp. 752–757, 1961.

[8] P. Otte, "Die konservative behandlung der hüft-und kniearthrose und ihre gefahren," *Anual Chronicles of German Medicine*, vol. 20, pp. 604–609, 1969.

[9] K. Gelse, S. Söder, W. Eger, T. Diemtar, and T. Aigner, "Osteophyte development-molecular characterization of differentiation stages," *Osteoarthritis and Cartilage*, vol. 11, no. 2, pp. 141–148, 2003.

[10] P. G. Conaghan, "Parallel evolution of OA phenotypes and therapies," *Nature Reviews Rheumatology*, vol. 9, no. 2, pp. 68–70, 2013.

[11] K. D. Allen and Y. M. Golightly, "State of the evidence," *Current Opinion in Rheumatology*, vol. 27, no. 3, pp. 276–283, 2015.

[12] K. Yudoh, H. Nakamura, K. Masuko-Hongo, T. Kato, and K. Nishioka, "Catabolic stress induces expression of hypoxia-inducible factor (HIF)-1 alpha in articular chondrocytes: involvement of HIF-1 alpha in the pathogenesis of osteoarthritis," *Arthritis Research & Therapy*, vol. 7, no. 5, pp. 225–R914, 2005.

[13] D. Pfander, T. Cramer, and B. Swoboda, "Hypoxia and HIF-1? in osteoarthritis," *International Orthopaedics*, vol. 29, no. 1, pp. 6–9, 2005.

[14] S. Yang, J. Kim, J. H. Ryu et al., "Hypoxia-inducible factor-2alpha is a catabolic regulator of osteoarthritic cartilage destruction," *Nature Medicine*, vol. 16, no. 6, pp. 687–693, 2010.

[15] M. Hirata, F. Kugimiya, A. Fukai et al., "C/EBPβ and RUNX2 cooperate to degrade cartilage with MMP-13 as the target and HIF-2α as the inducer in chondrocytes," *Human Molecular Genetics*, vol. 21, no. 5, pp. 1111–1123, 2012.

[16] G. S. Man and G. Mologhianu, "Osteoarthritis pathogenesis - a complex process that involves the entire joint," *Journal of Medicine and Life*, vol. 7, no. 1, pp. 37–41, 2014.

[17] S. Zhou, H. Wen, W. Cai, Y. Zhang, and H. Li, "Effect of hypoxia/reoxygenation on the biological effect of IGF system and the inflammatory mediators in cultured synoviocytes," *Biochemical and Biophysical Research Communications*, vol. 508, no. 1, pp. 17–24, 2019.

[18] M. Leonardi, C. Hicks, F. El-Assaad, E. El-Omar, and G. Gondous, "Endometriosis and the microbiome: a systematic review," *BJOG : An International Journal of Obstetrics and Gynaecology*, vol. 127, no. 2, pp. 239–249, 2019.

[19] S. L. Kolasinski, T. Neogi, M. C. Hochberg et al., "2019 American College of Rheumatology/Arthritis Foundation guideline for the management of osteoarthritis of the hand, hip, and knee," *Arthritis Care and Research*, vol. 72, no. 2, pp. 149–162, 2020.

[20] D. T. Felson, "Developments in the clinical understanding of osteoarthritis," *Arthritis Research & Therapy*, vol. 11, no. 1, p. 203, 2009.

[21] TeachMe Anatomy, *Classification of joints*July 2020, https://teachmeanatomy.info/the-basics/joints-basic/classification-of-joints/.

[22] Rice University, *Synovial joints In Anatomy and Physiology*May 2019, https://opentextbc.ca/anatomyandphysiology/chapter/9-4-synovial-joints.

[23] J. Knoop, M. van der Leeden, C. A. Thorstensson et al., "Identification of phenotypes with different clinical outcomes in knee osteoarthritis: data from the osteoarthritis initiative," *Arthritis Care Res (Hoboken)*, vol. 63, no. 11, pp. 1535–1542, 2011.

[24] J. Cushnaghan and P. Dieppe, "Study of 500 patients with limb joint osteoarthritis. I. Analysis by age, sex, and distribution of symptomatic joint sites," *Annals of the Rheumatic Diseases*, vol. 50, no. 1, pp. 8–13, 1991.

[25] C. M. Borkhoff, G. A. Hawker, H. J. Kreder, R. H. Glazier, N. N. Mahomed, and J. G. Wright, "The effect of patient's sex on physician's recommendations for total knee arthroplasty," *CMAJ*, vol. 178, no. 6, pp. 681–687, 2008.

[26] M. C. Castaño-Betancourt, F. Rivadeneira, S. Bierma-Zeinstra et al., "Bone parameters across different types of hip osteoarthritis and their relationship to osteoporotic fracture risk," *Arthritis and Rheumatism*, vol. 65, no. 3, pp. 693–700, 2013.

[27] R. J. Meislin, J. W. Sperling, and T. P. Stitik, "Persistent shoulder pain: epidemiology, pathophysiology, and diagnosis," *The American Journal of Orthopedics*, vol. 34, 12 Suppl, pp. 5–9, 2005.

[28] Y. Zhang, J. Niu, M. Kelly-Hayes, C. E. Chaisson, P. Aliabadi, and D. T. Felson, "Prevalence of symptomatic hand osteoarthritis and its impact on functional status among the elderly: the Framingham study," *American Journal of Epidemiology*, vol. 156, no. 11, pp. 1021–1027, 2002.

[29] C. L. Saltzman, M. L. Salamon, G. M. Blanchard et al., "Epidemiology of ankle arthritis: report of a consecutive series of 639 patients from a tertiary orthopaedic center," *The Iowa Orthopaedic Journal*, vol. 25, pp. 44–46, 2005.

[30] D. Stanley, "Prevalence and etiology of symptomatic elbow osteoarthritis," *Journal of shoulder and elbow surgery*, vol. 3, no. 6, pp. 386–389, 1994.

[31] A. P. Goode, T. S. Carey, and J. M. Jordan, "Low back pain and lumbar spine osteoarthritis: how are they related?," *Current rheumatology reports*, vol. 15, no. 2, p. 305, 2013.

[32] A. C. Gellhorn, J. N. Katz, and P. Suri, "Osteoarthritis of the spine: the facet joints," *Nature Reviews Rheumatology*, vol. 9, no. 4, pp. 216–224, 2013.

[33] X. D. Wang, J. N. Zhang, Y. H. Gan, and Y. H. Zhou, "Current understanding of pathogenesis and treatment of TMJ osteoarthritis," *Journal of Dental Research*, vol. 94, no. 5, pp. 666–673, 2015.

[34] M. F. Mani and S. S. Sivasubramanian, "A study of temporomandibular joint osteoarthritis using computed tomographic imaging," *biomedical journal*, vol. 39, no. 3, pp. 201–206, 2016.

[35] R. Monemdjou, H. Fahmi, and M. Kapoor, "Synovium in the pathophysiology of osteoarthritis," *Therapy*, vol. 7, no. 6, pp. 661–668, 2010.

[36] M. Hesketh, K. B. Sahin, Z. E. West, and R. Z. Murray, "Macrophage phenotypes regulate scar formation and chronic wound healing," *International Journal of Molecular Sciences*, vol. 18, no. 7, p. 1545, 2017.

[37] C. R. Scanzello and S. R. Goldring, "The role of synovitis in osteoarthritis pathogenesis," *Bone*, vol. 51, no. 2, pp. 249–257, 2012.

[38] S. Oehler, D. Neureiter, C. Meyer-Scholten, and T. Aigner, "Subtyping of osteoarthritic synoviopathy," *Clinical and Experimental Rheumatology*, vol. 20, no. 5, pp. 633–640, 2002.

[39] J. N. Weiss, P. Korge, H. M. Honda, and P. P. Ping, "Role of the mitochondrial permeability transition in myocardial disease," *Circulation Research*, vol. 93, no. 4, pp. 292–301, 2003.

[40] E. Murphy and C. Steenbergen, "Preconditioning: the mitochondrial connection," *Annual Review of Physiology*, vol. 69, no. 1, pp. 51–67, 2007.

[41] X. Liu and G. Hajnóczky, "Altered fusion dynamics underlie unique morphological changes in mitochondria during hypoxia–reoxygenation stress," *Cell Death and Differentiation*, vol. 18, no. 10, pp. 1561–1572, 2011.

[42] S. Galleron, D. Borderie, C. Ponteziere et al., "Reactive oxygen species induce apoptosis of synoviocytes in vitro. α-Tocopherol provides no protection," *Cell Biology International*, vol. 23, no. 9, pp. 637–642, 1999.

[43] B. Cillero-Pastor, M. A. Martin, J. Arenas, M. J. López-Armada, and F. J. Blanco, "Effect of nitric oxide on mitochondrial activity of human synovial cells," *BMC Musculoskeletal Disorders*, vol. 12, no. 1, p. 42, 2011.

[44] D. V. Jovanovic, F. Mineau, K. Notoya, P. Reboul, J. Martel-Pelletier, and J. P. Pelletier, "Nitric oxide induced cell death in human osteoarthritic synoviocytes is mediated by tyrosine kinase activation and hydrogen peroxide and/or superoxide formation," *The Journal of Rheumatology*, vol. 29, no. 10, pp. 2165–2175, 2002.

[45] F. Di Lisa, M. Canton, R. Menabo, N. Kaludercic, and P. Bernardi, "Mitochondria and cardioprotection," *Heart Failure Reviews*, vol. 12, no. 3-4, pp. 249–260, 2007.

[46] A. Szewczyk, W. Jarmuszkiewicz, and W. S. Kunz, "Mitochondrial potassium channels," *IUBMB Life*, vol. 61, no. 2, pp. 134–143, 2009.

[47] Y. Cheng, X. Gu, P. Bednarczyk, F. Wiedemann, G. Haddad, and D. Siemen, "Hypoxia increases activity of the BK-channel in the inner mitochondrial membrane and reduces activity of the permeability transition pore," *Cellular Physiology and Biochemistry*, vol. 22, no. 1-4, pp. 127–136, 2008.

[48] W. Xu, Y. Liu, S. Wang et al., "Cytoprotective role of Ca2+-activated K+ channels in the cardiac inner mitochondrial membrane," *Science*, vol. 298, no. 5595, pp. 1029–1033, 2002.

[49] D. N. Granger and P. R. Kvietys, "Reperfusion injury and reactive oxygen species: the evolution of a concept," *Redox Biology*, vol. 6, pp. 524–551, 2015.

[50] T. Zaobornyj and P. Ghafourifar, "Strategic localization of heart mitochondrial NOS: a review of the evidence," *American Journal of Physiology. Heart and Circulatory Physiology*, vol. 303, no. 11, pp. H1283–H1293, 2012.

[51] J. P. Pelletier, V. Lascau-Coman, D. Jovanovic et al., "Selective inhibition of inducible nitric oxide synthase in experimental osteoarthritis is associated with reduction in tissue levels of catabolic factors," *The Journal of Rheumatology*, vol. 26, no. 9, pp. 2002–2014, 1999.

[52] C. Chenevier-Gobeaux, C. Simonneau, H. Lemarechal et al., "Hypoxia induces nitric oxide synthase in rheumatoid synoviocytes consequences on NADPH oxidase regulation," *Free Radical Research*, vol. 46, no. 5, pp. 628–636, 2012.

[53] S. Hooshmand, S. Juma, D. A. Khalil, P. Shamloufard, and B. H. Arjmandi, "Women with osteoarthritis have elevated synovial fluid levels of insulin-like growth factor (IGF)-1 and IGF-binding protein-3," *Journal of Immunoassay & Immunochemistry*, vol. 36, pp. 284–294, 2014.

[54] C. Chenevier-Gobeaux, C. Simonneau, H. Lemarechal et al., "Effect of hypoxia/reoxygenation on the cytokine-induced production of nitric oxide and superoxide anion in cultured osteoarthritic synoviocytes," *Osteoarthritis and Cartilage*, vol. 21, no. 6, pp. 874–881, 2013.

[55] V. Hwa, Y. M. Oh, and R. G. Rosenfeld, "The insulin-like growth factor-binding protein (IGFBP) superfamily 1," *Endocrine Reviews*, vol. 20, pp. 761–787, 1999.

[56] E. Schoenle, J. Zapf, C. Hauri, T. Steiner, and E. R. Froesch, "Comparison of in vivo effects of insulin-like growth factors I and II and of growth hormone in hypophysectomized rats," *Acta Endocrinologica*, vol. 108, no. 2, pp. 167–174, 1985.

[57] S. B. Trippel, M. T. Corvol, M. F. Dumontier, R. Rappaport, H. H. Hung, and H. J. Mankin, "Effect of somatomedin-C/insulin-like growth factor I and growth hormone on

cultured growth plate and articular chondrocytes," *Pediatric Research*, vol. 25, no. 1, pp. 76–82, 1989.

[58] X. Chevalier and J. A. Tyler, "Production of binding proteins and role of the insulin-like growth factor I binding protein 3 in human articular cartilage explants," *British Journal of Rheumatology*, vol. 35, no. 6, pp. 515–522, 1996.

[59] A. E. Garza, *Insulin-like growth factor binding protein-3 (IGFBP-3) plays an essential role in cellular senescence: molecular and clinical implications*, Virginia Commonwealth University Scholars Compass, Theses and dissertations, Richmond, Virginia, 2010, July 2019, https://scholarscompass.vcu.edu/cgi/viewcontent.cgi?article=1069&context=etd.

[60] I. P. Morales, "The insulin-like growth factor binding proteins in uncultured human cartilage. Increases in insulin-like growth factor binding protein 3 during osteoarthritis," *Arthritis and Rheumatism*, vol. 46, no. 9, pp. 2358–2367, 2002.

[61] X. L. Zhang, H. H. Li, Y. P. Cao, F. Peng, and J. P. Li, "Insulin-like growth factor binding protein 3 inhibits inflammatory response and promotes apoptosis in fibroblast-like synoviocytes of osteoarthritis," *International Journal of Clinical and Experimental Pathology*, vol. 10, pp. 3024–3032, 2017.

[62] H. Lee, S. R. Kim, Y. Oh, S. H. Cho, R. P. Schleimer, and Y. C. Lee, "Targeting insulin-like growth factor-I and insulin-like growth factor-binding protein-3 signaling pathways. A novel therapeutic approach for asthma," *O Biologico*, vol. 50, no. 4, pp. 667–677, 2014.

[63] R. Sifakis, R. Akolekar, D. Kappou, N. Mantas, and K. H. Nicolaides, "Maternal serum IGF-I, IGFBP-1 and IGFBP-3 at 11-13 weeks in trisomy 21 and trisomy 18 pregnancies," *European Journal of Obstetrics, Gynecology, and Reproductive Biology*, vol. 157, no. 2, pp. 166–168, 2011.

[64] S. Mahmood, A. Evinová, M. Škereňová, I. Ondrejka, and J. Lehotský, "Association of EGF, IGFBP-3 and Tp53 gene polymorphisms with major depressive disorder in Slovak population," *Central European journal of public health*, vol. 24, no. 3, pp. 223–230, 2016.

[65] Y. Zhang, S. Zhou, W. Cai et al., "Hypoxia/reoxygenation activates the JNK pathway and accelerates synovial senescence," *Molecular Medicine Reports*, vol. 22, no. 1, pp. 265–276, 2020.

[66] F. J. Zhang, W. Luo, and G. H. Lei, "Role of HIF-1α and HIF-2α in osteoarthritis," *Joint Bone Spine*, vol. 82, no. 3, pp. 144–147, 2015.

[67] L. Bentovim, R. Amarilio, and E. Zelzer, "HIF1 is a central regulator of collagen hydroxylation and secretion under hypoxia during bone development," *Development*, vol. 139, no. 23, pp. 4473–4483, 2012.

[68] E. Aro, R. Khatri, R. Gerard-O'Riley, L. Mangiavini, J. Myllyharju, and E. Schipani, "Hypoxia-inducible factor-1 (HIF-1) but not HIF-2 is essential for hypoxic induction of collagen prolyl 4-hydroxylases in primary newborn mouse epiphyseal growth plate chondrocytes," *The Journal of Biological Chemistry*, vol. 287, no. 44, pp. 37134–37144, 2012.

[69] C. Grimmer, D. Pfander, B. Swoboda et al., "Hypoxia-inducible factor 1α is involved in the prostaglandin metabolism of osteoarthritic cartilage through up-regulation of microsomal prostaglandin E synthase 1 in articular chondrocytes," *Arthritis and Rheumatism*, vol. 56, no. 12, pp. 4084–4094, 2007.

[70] J. E. Lafont, S. Talma, and C. L. Murphy, "Hypoxia-inducible factor 2alpha is essential for hypoxic induction of the human articular chondrocyte phenotype," *Arthritis and Rheumatism*, vol. 56, no. 10, pp. 3297–3306, 2007.

[71] A. L. Harris, "Hypoxia–a key regulatory factor in tumour growth," *Nature Reviews. Cancer*, vol. 2, no. 1, pp. 38–47, 2002.

[72] Z. Wei and H. H. Li, "IGFBP-3 may trigger osteoarthritis by inducing apoptosis of chondrocytes through Nur77 translocation," *International Journal of Clinical and Experimental Pathology*, vol. 8, no. 12, pp. 15599–15610, 2015.

[73] Y. Liang, S. Chen, Y. Yang et al., "Vasoactive intestinal peptide alleviates osteoarthritis effectively via inhibiting NF-κB signaling pathway," *Journal of Biomedical Science*, vol. 25, no. 1, p. 25, 2018.

[74] S. Ni, K. Miao, X. Zhou et al., "The involvement of follistatin-like protein 1 in osteoarthritis by elevating NF-κB-mediated inflammatory cytokines and enhancing fibroblast like synoviocyte proliferation," *Arthritis Research & Therapy*, vol. 17, no. 1, p. 91, 2015.

[75] A. M. Valdes, S. Ravipati, P. Pousinis et al., "Omega-6 oxylipins generated by soluble epoxide hydrolase are associated with knee osteoarthritis," *Journal of Lipid Research*, vol. 59, no. 9, pp. 1763–1770, 2018.

[76] X. Li, W. Ren, Z. Y. Xiao, L. F. Wu, H. Wang, and P. Y. Guo, "GACAT3 promoted proliferation of osteoarthritis synoviocytes by IL-6/STAT3 signaling pathway," *European Review for Medical and Pharmacological Sciences*, vol. 22, no. 16, pp. 5114–5120, 2018.

[77] Y. C. Zhou, T. Y. Wang, J. L. Hamilton, and D. Chen, "Wnt/β-catenin signaling in osteoarthritis and in other forms of arthritis," *Current Rheumatology Reports*, vol. 19, no. 9, p. 53, 2017.

[78] J. S. Rockel, C. Yu, H. Whetstone et al., "Hedgehog inhibits β-catenin activity in synovial joint development and osteoarthritis," *The Journal of Clinical Investigation*, vol. 126, no. 5, pp. 1649–1663, 2016.

[79] N. Maruotti, A. Corrado, and F. P. Cantatore, "Osteoblast role in osteoarthritis pathogenesis," *Journal of Cellular Physiology*, vol. 232, no. 11, pp. 2957–2963, 2017.

[80] H. S. Lee, S. J. Woo, H. W. Koh et al., "Regulation of apoptosis and inflammatory responses by insulin-like growth factor binding protein 3 in fibroblast-like synoviocytes and experimental animal models of rheumatoid arthritis," *Arthritis & Rhematology*, vol. 66, no. 4, pp. 863–873, 2014.

[81] W. Cai, H. Li, Y. Zhang, and G. Han, "Identification of key biomarkers and immune infiltration in the synovial tissue of osteoarthritis by bioinformatics analysis," *Peer J*, vol. 8, p. e8390, 2020.

24

Point-of-Care Ultrasound (POCUS) in the Field of Diabetology

X. Vandemergel ⓘ

Department of Endocrinology and Diabetology, EpiCURA, Belgium

Correspondence should be addressed to X. Vandemergel; vandemergel@hotmail.fr

Academic Editor: Maria Gazouli

Ultrasound is increasingly used in daily clinical practice to improve the efficiency of the clinical examination. In this article, we reviewed its various possible uses in the field of diabetology. The ultrasonic evaluation of the carotid arteries (plaques and intima media thickness) allows improving the assessment of the cardiovascular risk. Steatosis can be detected relatively easily on liver ultrasound. Ultrasound also allows a more sensitive detection of lipohypertrophy resulting in glycemic fluctuations and thus increasing the risk of hypoglycemia than the clinical examination. Finally, muscle ultrasound appears to be a promising tool to assess the nutritional status and its consequences (e.g., falls).

1. Introduction

Diabetes is a systemic disease. Its global prevalence is estimated to be 9.3% (463 million people), rising to 10.2% by 2030 [1], being a major public health issue. Patients with type 1 or type 2 (T2D) diabetes (DP) are at risk for micro- and macrovascular complications [2]. The management of DP is therefore multifactorial and requires, in addition to sometimes restrictive treatments, regular monitoring and screening examination (fundus examination, electrocardiogram, detection of microalbuminuria, dental follow-up, and vaccination). The multiplicity of examinations regularly decreases the patient's compliance. For example, in the study by Murchison et al., the rate of adherence to the follow-up recommendations in the context of ocular examinations was disappointingly low regardless of the age and ethnic group, ranging from 35% to 65% depending on the severity of retinopathy [3]. Moreover, epidemiological evidence suggests that T2D patients are at significantly higher risk for many types of cancer, including liver, pancreas, endometrium, breast, and colorectal cancers [4, 5]. This association requires a careful clinical examination of DP and a close follow-up with appropriate cancer screening as recommended for all individuals depending on their age and sex. While technological advances have been made in recent years in terms of self-monitoring or treatment (smartphone applications, subcutaneous glucose monitoring, and insulin pumps) [6–8], the

tools used during the quarterly or semiannual consultations by diabetologists have not changed much. Indeed, a stethoscope, reflex hammer, tuning fork, and monofilament are still the basis for the examination. While the clinical examination remains a fundamental step in the clinical approach, it should be kept in mind that it does not significantly contribute to the diagnosis, even when a stethoscope is used. In a prospective study conducted in 80 medical outpatients with new or previously undiagnosed conditions published in 1992, Peterson et al. [9] have shown that the anamnesis alone allowed making a diagnosis in 80% of cases while the physical examination alone allowed making a diagnosis in only 12% of cases. In a similar study conducted in patients with cardiovascular diseases, Sandler [10] had reported that 56%, 17%, and 23% of diagnoses were made based on patient history, physical examination, and laboratory tests, respectively. Tools allowing improving the performance of our clinical examinations are thus needed.

1.1. Introduction of Ultrasound in Medicine and Advent of POCUS. Cardiologists have integrated ultrasound (US) in their daily practice since 1954 [11], followed four years later by gynecologists [12], and it took until 1979 for the first publication of a radiological study assessing the interest of US in patients with right upper quadrant pain and gallstones [13]. In recent years, a new generation of clinicians have implemented the use of US in their daily practice such as in emergency medicine (as well as in war and disaster medicine) and in intensive care units [14–16] and more recently in other specialties such as internal general medicine [17] and rheumatology [18].

Point-of-care ultrasonography (POCUS), i.e., ultrasonography performed and interpreted by the clinician at the bedside or in the ambulatory setting, has emerged thanks to multiple factors including technology improvement and the fact that the US equipment has become more compact, with an enhanced image quality, and is equipped with software to facilitate result interpretation. It offers several advantages: it is noninvasive and nonirradiating and is performed at the bedside and it allows saving time [17].

Furthermore, trained and young physicians are significantly more competent and attentive when using US. In a study, first-year medical students who used POCUS obtained better results in identifying heart abnormalities than board-certified cardiologists who used a bedside cardiovascular physical examination, with, respectively, 75% and 49% of cases identified by students and cardiologists (using only a stethoscope) [19]. In another study, the authors have shown that medical students who used POCUS estimated more accurately the liver size than board-certified internists who performed a physical examination [20].

Only a few studies have investigated the interest of POCUS in diabetology. However, as we will see, diabetology is a specialty in which POCUS could find a special place to improve the diagnostic efficiency and to simplify the management and decision-making.

1.2. Some Technical Considerations. US is defined as a frequency higher than the upper audible limit of human hearing, i.e., greater than 20,000 Hz (20 kHz). The frequency of diagnostic US is in the range of 1 million hertz (MHz). Lower-frequency US has a better penetration, but a lower resolution. Higher-frequency US provides higher quality images, but it does not allow visualizing the deep structures. A typical transabdominal or cardiac probe has a frequency in the range of 2-5 MHz, whereas probes used for the superficial structures such as the carotids, thyroid, or muscles have a frequency in the range of 10-15 MHz. Three modes may be used for image analysis: (1) the B mode (real-time analysis of a structure), (2) the M mode which is a diagnostic US presentation of the temporal changes in echoes in which the depth of echo-producing interfaces is displayed along one axis and time (T) is displayed along the second axis and the motion (M) of the interfaces is recorded toward and away from the transducer, and finally (3) the Doppler mode to analyze the blood flow.

2. Assessment of the Cardiovascular Risk

DP are at high risk of cardiovascular diseases (CVD) [21]. Their risk of incident coronary heart disease or ischemic stroke is increased by 2-4 and their risk of mortality by 1.5-3.6 compared to nondiabetic subjects (NDS) [22]. T2D is also a major risk factor for heart failure, peripheral arterial insufficiency, and microvascular complications, affecting patients' quality of life and life expectancy. In DP, the life expectancy is

estimated to be reduced by 4 to 8 years compared to that in NDS [23]. Traditional risk factors such as aging, hypertension, hyperlipidemia, or smoking have been shown to only moderately refine the CV risk [24, 25], and the use of calculators is needed to improve the risk prediction. However, at least 110 different CV risk score calculators are currently used and 45 exclusively in DP [26]. Due to differences in databases and diverse mathematical algorithms and to the different combinations of CVD endpoints, there is considerable variability in the scores obtained. It is important to keep in mind that the validation of these scores is limited to the characteristics of the studied population. In contrast, invasive procedures such as coronary angiography or coronary computed tomography angiography can be used to determine the presence and severity of coronary artery disease (CAD) but with potential adverse effects and high costs. Determining more precisely the CV risks of DP is crucial to identify which patients are likely to benefit from preventive treatment. For example, in the Ascend trial, administering low-dose aspirin to all DP improved CVD prevention while it increased the risk of hemorrhage [27]. Therefore, noninvasive and inexpensive indices of subclinical and silent atherosclerosis with more than moderate predictive capacity are required. Carotid ultrasonography (CU) is a promising tool to achieve it. CU may show atherosclerotic changes including intima media thickening (IMT or carotid intima media thickness (CIMT)) and plaque formation which allows analyzing the plaque structure, stenosis, or vessel occlusion. The CIMT is a well-described surrogate marker for CVD. The carotids are evaluated using a high-frequency (10-14 MHz) linear probe. In B mode, the carotid wall is visualized as three layers (Figure 1(a)). The two layers closer to the vascular lumen are defined as the "intima media" complex, and the thickness of the intima-media complex is defined as the CIMT [28]. The CIMT is classically measured near a carotid bifurcation, and US devices equipped with automatic IMT measurement software have recently become widely used to reduce interexaminer errors and the examination duration [28]. Plaques (Figure 1(b)) are defined as a focal wall thickening > 50% (or 0.5 mm) of the surrounding IMT or a CIMT > 1.5 mm [29]. The plaques are assessed based on their echogenicity, heterogeneity, and structure. The plaques may be characterized by their presence or absence, location, thickness, number, irregularity (smooth, irregular, or ulcerated), and echodensity (echolucent or echogenic) [29]. Many studies have shown that CU may be used to measure coronary atherosclerosis and myocardial ischemia [30, 31]. In a study by Akazama et al. conducted in 322 DP, 92% of patients with CAD had plaques compared to 54% of patients without CAD [32]. In the ARIC trial, Nambi et al. have reported that the prediction of the CAD risk could be improved by adding information on the CIMT and plaques to traditional risk factors [33]. In their study, 10% of patients had diabetes. When the CIMT was >75th percentile and plaques were present in men, a dramatic elevation of the number of CV events was observed. Indeed, the adjusted incidence rate of coronary heart disease per 1000 person years was 24.7 in patients with a CIMT >75th percentile and plaque versus 7.2 in patients with a CIMT <25th percentile without plaque. They have also

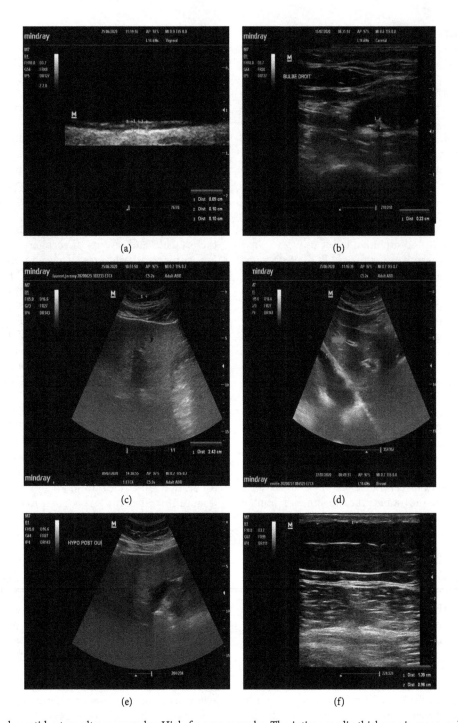

FIGURE 1: (a) Normal carotid artery ultrasonography. High-frequency probe. The intima media thickness is measured at three points. (b) Visualization of a plaque of 0.23 mm thickness located near the carotid bifurcation. High-frequency probe. (c) Liver echography with determination of the skin capsular distance (2.43 cm). Low-frequency curvilinear probe. (d) Normal liver echography showing the portal veins (horizontal arrow), the diaphragm, and a homogeneous parenchyma. Low-frequency curvilinear probe. (e) Nonalcoholic steatohepatitis. This picture shows a rapid ultrasound attenuation. The vessels are attenuated, and the posterior liver is not seen. (f) Measurement of the rectus femoris (1) and vastus intermedius (2) thickness. High-frequency linear probe.

shown that taking into account the presence of plaques in addition to the CIMT significantly improved the risk of reclassification by 9.9% in the overall population and by 21.7% in the intermediate-risk group. It should be noted that a higher number of subjects were reclassified into a lower-risk group than into a higher-risk group. Regardless of the

CIMT, the presence of plaques was associated with a higher incidence of coronary heart disease. The US assessment of carotid plaques has been shown to have a higher diagnostic accuracy than the CIMT for predicting future myocardial infarction. In addition, the absence of carotid plaque was more reassuring, with a low 10-year rate of myocardial infarction (4.0%). In another study [34], the authors have shown that after a 10-year follow-up, based on the US assessment of the carotid arteries, a first clinical event was identified in 3% of subjects with an initially normal US examination, in 32% of patients with IMT thickness, and in 62% of patients with an asymptomatic carotid plaque. In DP without apparent CVD, Irie et al. [35] have also shown that a maximum IMT was significantly associated with the presence of coronary artery stenosis.

Plaque features are also a valuable tool to assess the CV risk. The presence of a lipid-rich core, calcification, and ulceration is associated with a higher risk. In a large study including 582 DP who underwent CU, Vigili de Kreutzenberg et al. have found a prevalence of plaques of 82%. The plaque was echolucent in 16% of cases, heterogeneous in 43% of cases, and echogenic in 22% of cases while 19% of patients had no plaque. The presence of a plaque was associated with incident major CV events with a hazard ratio varying depending on the plaque features (1.97 (0.93-3.44) for echolucent plaques, 3.1 (2.09-4.23) for heterogeneous plaques, and 3.71 (2.09-5.59) for echogenic plaques) [36].

Therefore, CU appears to be a promising tool to assess the CV risk, but further studies are needed to validate the previous findings, particularly in the diabetic population.

2.1. Steatohepatitis. Nonalcoholic fatty liver disease (NAFLD) and T2D are common disorders that often coexist and can act synergistically to drive adverse outcomes. The reported prevalence of NAFLD in DP ranges from 29.6% to 87.1% [37, 38]. The presence of both NAFLD and T2D increases the risk for developing complications of diabetes (including both macro- and microvascular complications) as well as the risk of experiencing a more severe form of NAFLD, including cirrhosis, hepatocellular carcinoma, and death. Advanced fibrosis has been reported in 5-7% of asymptomatic subjects with T2D [39]. The alanine aminotransferase (ALT) level alone is not sufficient to rule out the presence of hepatic steatosis [40]. In a study published in 2019, Gawrieh et al. have evaluated 534 adults with biopsy-proven NAFLD and ALT and aspartate aminotransferase (AST) levels < 40 U/L within 3 months of their liver biopsy. The prevalence of stage F2-F3 nonalcoholic steatohepatitis (NASH) and cirrhosis was 19% and 7%, respectively. Detecting, assessing, and treating NAFLD in DP are thus required.

A meta-analysis of 49 studies including 4720 patients has found that the sensitivity and specificity of US were 85% and 94%, respectively, when using liver biopsy as the gold standard [41]. Different findings have been found in NAFLD: a hyperechoic texture or a bright liver due to a diffuse fatty infiltration and parenchyma heterogeneity, bright hepatic echoes, an increased hepatorenal echogenicity, a vascular blurring of the portal or hepatic vein (Figure 1(e)), and a rapid attenuation of the image within 4-5 cm of depth making deeper structures difficult to appreciate. The liver fills the entire field with no visible edges (considered helpful but not necessary for the diagnosis) [42]. When steatosis affects >30% of the liver, a bright liver echo pattern is present in 89% of cases [43]. In this study, the sensitivity, specificity, and positive and negative predic-

tive values of a bright liver echo pattern for steatosis were 64%, 97%, 96%, and 65%, respectively, and in the subgroup of patients with steatosis of ≥30%, these values were 91%, 93%, 89%, and 94%, respectively.

The subcutaneous tissue thickness (Figure 1(c)), mainly made of fatty tissue, measured as the distance between the skin surface and the liver surface, also called the "skin capsular distance" (SCD), has been shown to be another characteristic sonographic finding that can be easily assessed. It has been shown that the SCD may be used in patients to diagnose NASH. In 101 patients with NASH, Shen et al. have shown that 70% of patients had a SCD > 25 mm. When the SCD was <25 mm, only 20% of patients had NASH [44]. Riley et al. [45] have found in a comparative study that NAFLD patients had a thicker subcutaneous tissue, with a mean thickness of 25.6 ± 5.6 mm. In comparison, non-NAFLD patients had a mean subcutaneous tissue thickness of 19.5 ± 5.2 mm ($p < 0.001$). In addition, NAFLD was unlikely when the subcutaneous tissue thickness was <20 mm.

The US evaluation of the liver can be performed using a low-frequency probe and the general findings of liver US can be assessed with no need for extensive training (Figure 1(d)) [46].

Two studies have specifically focused on the efficiency of pocket-sized US for assessing the liver. In the first study, 100 adults undergoing conventional abdominal US examinations for various indications were screened by POCUS immediately prior to conventional US. POCUS was only used to assess the presence or the absence of excess fat. Other liver disorders were not assessed. The investigators (conventional US: an experienced radiologist and POCUS: a general internist recently trained in the use of POCUS) were blinded to the results of the alternative imaging. Forty patients (40%) showed fatty infiltration of the liver on both conventional US and POCUS, and 49 (49%) were negative on both modalities. A consensus was reached in two out of the 11 remaining subjects whose results were initially discordant. The overall sensitivity and specificity of POCUS compared to conventional US were 91% and 88%, respectively [47]. These data were concordant with the study by Reily et al. showing that after a 20-minute teaching session, physicians are able to diagnose fatty liver infiltration with a positive predictive value of 94% and a negative predictive value of 96% [48]. Despite the fact that liver US is an easy to use and efficient tool allowing assessing the presence of NAFLD, its use is limited in severely obese patients and in patients with steatosis of less than 20-30% [42].

2.2. Lipohypertrophy. Lipohypertrophy (LH) occurs in the subcutaneous tissue as a result of the lipogenic effect of repeated insulin injections and repeated trauma induced by the needle [49, 50]. LH lesions are histologically characterized by decreased vascularity, fibrosis, and both hypertrophic and small neomitotic adipocytes. The risk factors include needle reuse, the absence of site rotation, a low level of education, the number of injections, and diabetes duration. Clinically, LH is characterized by thickened, "rubbery" tissue swelling and may be assessed by inspection and palpation. However, this method is poorly reliable with a high interobserver variation. Most studies suggest that insulin absorption from LH sites may be delayed and erratic [51], and the consequences are potentially dramatic with glycemic variability and an increased risk of severe hypoglycemia [52, 53]. The prevalence of LH varies considerably between the studies from 14.5% to 88%, reflecting diagnosis difficulties [51]. In 2013, Blanco et al. [54] have shown that 40% of patients with LH experienced unexplained hypoglycemia and 49% showed glycemic variability compared to only 5.9% and 6.5%, respectively, in patients without LH. These patients have increased insulin needs leading to an additional cost of €122 million in Spain. In China, the LH-related excess annual insulin consumption cost is estimated at $297 million [55]. Detecting LH is therefore crucial. The use of US could help to improve the diagnosis of LH.

The US findings of LH include the simplest subcutaneous hypertrophy, diffuse hyperechoic subcutaneous dystrophy, nodular hyperechoic dystrophy, focal and diffuse hyperechoic subcutis dystrophy, nodular hypoechoic subcutaneous dystrophy, subcutaneous atrophy, or complex multilayer dystrophy [56].

In an observational retrospective study, Bertuzzi et al. [57] have assessed 20 type 1 diabetes patients with LH by US using a linear probe (6-18 MHz). They have shown that the tissue affected by LH showed fibrotic changes (hyperechogenic) and interstitial edema (hypoechogenic). They have thus advised patients to avoid insulin injections in the LH areas seen on US. After 3 months, the HBA1c level was reduced from $7.87 \pm 0.56\%$ to $7.67 \pm 0.52\%$ ($p = 0.029$). In their study, LH areas showed at least three different aspects on US: an isohyperechogenic aspect with a predominant fibrotic component, an isoechogenic aspect with "large tangle" fibrotic components, and an isohypoechogenic aspect with no fibrotic components. No significant improvements in HbA1c were found in the control matched group in which LH was only clinically assessed through inspection and palpation. Thus, US can help to identify and characterize LH areas and could be useful to improve the glycemic control. A study has compared clinical and US examinations for the diagnosis of LH [58]. In this study, 103 patients, mainly with T2D treated with insulin for more than 2 years, were examined by 2 specialized nurses and then underwent US performed by a research associate trained by a certified radiologist. US identified subjects with LH significantly more frequently than the inspection or palpation (55% versus 72%; $p < 0.0001$). Among the subjects with LH lesions detected by US, 24% had lesions only detected by US. These findings show that US could be a promising tool to be used as an adjunct to palpation, but so far, no study has investigated whether US alone could detect LH independently of palpation.

2.3. Muscle. T2D facilitates the occurrence and progression of chronic complications such as diabetic neuropathy and sarcopenia. Diabetes accelerates the loss of muscle mass and strength over time, particularly in the lower extremities, which are associated with an increased risk of mortality in subjects with T2D [59–61]. DP have an altered body composition and a low musculoskeletal strength with a faster loss of

knee extension strength compared to older NDS [62]. There is an age-related increased fatty infiltration of the midthigh skeletal muscle in men and women as shown by increases in intermuscular fat [63]. This fat infiltration worsens over 5 years in both men and women, regardless of weight changes and changes in subcutaneous adipose tissue in the thighs. Glucose fluctuations are also associated with a low muscle mass [64]. Thus, assessing and preserving the muscle mass is a critical point in these patients.

The quadriceps architecture that reflects the muscle mass (mainly by determining the thickness of the vastus intermedius, rectus, and anterior quadriceps) (Figure 1(f)) may be assessed using a high-frequency linear probe. The probe is positioned at half of the distance between the greater trochanter and the interarticular line of the knee, transversally to the muscle for measuring the thickness and cross-sectional area, and longitudinally for measuring the pennation angle (PA) in patients in prone position. Chiaramonte et al. [65] have shown the accuracy, precision, and repeatability of US in assessing the muscle architecture between physiatrists, radiologists, and general internists, and the quadriceps femoris muscle thickness assessed by US is already used as a parameter for assessing the nutritional risk that is more accurate than serum levels of prealbumin, albumin, or transferrin that may vary with the intravascular volume excess, infection, and inflammation [66].

Only one study [67] has assessed the reliability and applicability of quadriceps muscle architecture measurements in T2D patients. They have used a 10-13 MHz probe to assess the thickness of the rectus femoris (RF), vastus intermedius (VI), anterior quadriceps (sum of RF and VI), and the PA of the RF. T2D patients had neuropathy without osteoarticular injury and were older than 50. The PA of the RF was determined at the intersection between the muscle fascicles of the RF and the internal aponeurosis. Intra- and interrater analyses have shown a high to very high reliability between the three raters except for the PA.

Further studies are needed to precisely determine the role of US in the evaluation of the muscle mass and osteoarticular complications in DP, but it seems promising.

2.4. Gastroparesis. Gastroparesis is characterized by a delayed gastric emptying of solid food in the absence of a mechanical obstruction of the stomach, resulting in the cardinal symptoms of early satiety, postprandial fullness, nausea, vomiting, belching, and bloating [68]. It usually affects DP with other neuropathic diseases, affecting 30 to 50% of DP (T1D or T2D). Gastroparesis should be investigated because it induces a risk of stasis (full stomach) and aspiration upon anesthetic induction. Delayed gastric emptying and the resultant "full stomach" are the most important risk factors for perioperative regurgitation and aspiration, which remain common, disastrous complications associated with high morbidity and mortality in patients undergoing general anesthesia [69]. US examinations performed 2 h after ingesting a clear fluid or 6 h after a light meal using a low-frequency (2-5 MHz) curvilinear array probe from a Philips device (CX50) have shown that almost half of the T2D patients with a median diabetes duration of 6 years had a full stomach when the current preoperative fasting guidelines were followed [70]. Other studies have confirmed that US allows determining the gastric residual volume [71].

2.4.1. Questions about Overdiagnosis. The question of overdiagnosis should be raised. Although the studies remain limited, the first data are quite reassuring. The rate of incidentalomas is lower in symptomatic patients (0.05%) and can reach up to 25% in asymptomatic patients [48].

3. Conclusion

POCUS is a diagnostic aid already used in many fields of internal medicine. Its use in diabetology is promising, but further studies are needed to confirm the data from the studies reported here. It allows improving the determination of the CV profile of DP but also allows monitoring the complications.

References

[1] P. Saeedi, I. Petersohn, P. Salpea et al., "Global and regional diabetes prevalence estimates for 2019 and projections for 2030 and 2045: results from the International Diabetes Federation Diabetes Atlas, 9th edition," *Diabetes Research and Clinical Practice*, vol. 157, p. 107843, 2019.

[2] K. Papatheodorou, M. Banach, E. Bekiari, M. Rizzo, and M. Edmonds, "Complications of diabetes 2017," *Journal Diabetes Research*, vol. 2018, p. 3086167, 2018.

[3] A. P. Murchison, L. Hark, L. T. Pizzi et al., "Non-adherence to eye care in people with diabetes," *BMJ Open Diabetes Research & Care*, vol. 5, no. 1, p. e000333, 2017.

[4] H. Tanaka, N. Ihana-Sugiyama, T. Sugyiama, and M. Ohsugi, "Contribution of diabetes to the incidence and prevalence of comorbid conditions (cancer, periodontal disease, fracture, impaired cognitive function, and depression): a systematic review of epidemiological studies in Japanese populations," *Journal of Epidemiology*, vol. 29, no. 1, pp. 1–10, 2019.

[5] E. Giovannucci, D. M. Harlan, M. C. Harcher et al., "Diabetes and cancer: a consensus report," *Diabetes Care*, vol. 33, no. 7, pp. 1674–1685, 2010.

[6] B. Jeffrey, M. Bagala, A. Creighton et al., "Mobile phone applications and their use in the self-management of type 2 diabetes mellitus: a qualitative study among app users and non-app users," *Diabetology and Metabolic Syndrome*, vol. 11, no. 1, p. 84, 2019.

[7] M. M. Kebede, C. Schuett, and C. R. Pischke, "The role of continuous glucose monitoring, diabetes smartphone applications, and selfcare behavior in glycemic control: results of a multinational online survey," *Journal of Clinical Medicine*, vol. 8, no. 1, p. 109, 2019.

[8] E. G. Umpierrez and D. C. Klonoff, "Diabetes technology update: use of insulin pumps and continuous glucose monitoring in the hospital," *Diabetes Care*, vol. 41, no. 8, pp. 1579–1589, 2018.

[9] M. C. Peterson, J. H. Holbrook, D. von Hales, N. L. Smith, and L. V. Staker, "Contributions of the history, physical examination, and laboratory investigation in making medical diagnoses," *The Western Journal of Medicine*, vol. 156, no. 2, pp. 163–165, 1992.

[10] G. Sandler, "The importance of the history in the medical clinic and the cost of unnecessary tests," *American Heart Journal*, vol. 100, no. 6, pp. 928–931, 1980.

[11] I. Edler and C. H. Hertz, "The use of ultrasonic reflectoscope for the continuous recording of the movements of heart walls," *Clinical Physiology and Functional Imaging*, vol. 24, no. 3, pp. 118–136, 2004.

[12] S. Campbell, "A short history of sonography in obstetrics and gynaecology," *Facts Views Vis Obgyn*, vol. 5, no. 3, pp. 213–229, 2013.

[13] P. L. McCluskey, R. A. Prinz, R. Guico, and H. B. Greenlee, "Use of ultrasound to demonstrate gallstones in symptomatic patients with normal oral cholecystograms," *American Journal of Surgery*, vol. 138, no. 5, pp. 655–657, 1979.

[14] S. M. Mazur and J. Rippey, "Transport and use of point-of-care ultrasound by a disaster medical assistance team," *Prehospital and Disaster Medicine*, vol. 24, no. 2, pp. 140–144, 2009.

[15] J. A. Nations and R. F. Browning, "Battlefield applications for handheld ultrasound," *Ultrasound Quarterly*, vol. 27, no. 3, pp. 171–176, 2011.

[16] J. Boldt, "Clinical review: hemodynamic monitoring in the intensive care unit," *Critical Care*, vol. 6, no. 1, pp. 52–59, 2002.

[17] X. Vandemergel, "Point-of-care-ultrasound for hospitalists and general internists," *Acta Clinica Belgica*, vol. 9, pp. 1–7, 2019.

[18] A. J. Halupa, R. J. Strony, D. H. Bulbin, and C. K. Kraus, "Pseudogout diagnosed by point-of-care ultrasound," *Clinical Practice and Cases in Emergency Medicine*, vol. 3, no. 4, pp. 425–427, 2019.

[19] S. L. Kobal, L. Trento, S. Baharami et al., "Comparison of effectiveness of hand-carried ultrasound to bedside cardiovascular physical examination," *The American Journal of Cardiology*, vol. 96, no. 7, pp. 1002–1006, 2005.

[20] G. Mouratev, D. Howe, R. Hoppmann et al., "Teaching medical students ultrasound to measure liver size: comparison with experienced clinicians using physical examination alone," *Teaching and Learning in Medicine*, vol. 25, no. 1, pp. 84–88, 2013.

[21] N. J. Morrish, S. L. Wang, L. K. Stevens, J. H. Fuller, and H. Keen, "Mortality and causes of death in the WHO multinational study of vascular disease in diabetes," *Diabetologia*, vol. 44, no. S2, pp. S14–S21, 2001.

[22] M. C. Bertoluci and V. Z. Rocha, "Cardiovascular risk assessment in patients with diabetes," *Diabetology & Metabolic Syndrome*, vol. 9, no. 1, p. 25, 2017.

[23] K. Gu, C. C. Cowie, and M. I. Harris, "Mortality in adults with and without diabetes in a national cohort of the U.S. population, 1971–1993," *Diabetes Care*, vol. 21, no. 7, pp. 1138–1145, 1998.

[24] R. K. Simmons, R. L. Coleman, H. C. Price et al., "Performance of the UK prospective diabetes study risk engine and the Framingham risk equations in estimating cardiovascular disease in the EPIC-Norfolk cohort," *Diabetes Care*, vol. 32, no. 4, pp. 708–713, 2009.

[25] J. W. Stephens, G. Ambler, P. Vallance, D. J. Betteridge, S. E. Humphries, and S. J. Hurel, "Cardiovascular risk and diabetes. Are the methods of risk prediction satisfactory?," *European*

Journal of Cardiovascular Prevention and Rehabilitation, vol. 11, no. 6, pp. 521–528, 2004.

[26] G. M. Allan, F. Nouri, C. Korownyk, M. R. Kolber, B. Vandermeer, and J. McCormack, "Agreement among cardiovascular disease risk calculators," *Circulation*, vol. 127, no. 19, pp. 1948–1956, 2013.

[27] The Ascend Study Collaborative Group, "Effects of aspirin for primary prevention in persons with diabetes mellitus," *The New England Journal of Medicine*, vol. 379, no. 16, pp. 1529–1539, 2018.

[28] N. Katakami, T. A. Matsuoka, and L. Shimomura, "Clinical utility of carotid ultrasonography: application for the management of patients with diabetes," *Journal of Diabetes Investigation*, vol. 10, no. 4, pp. 883–898, 2019.

[29] T. H. Park, "Evaluation of carotid plaque using ultrasound imaging," *Journal of Cardiovascular Ultrasound*, vol. 24, no. 2, pp. 91–95, 2016.

[30] J. L. Wofford, F. R. Kahl, G. R. Howard, W. M. Mac Kinney, J. F. Toole, and J. R. Crouse, "Relation of extent of extracranial carotid artery atherosclerosis as measured by B-mode ultrasound to the extent of coronary atherosclerosis," *Arteriosclerosis and Thrombosis: A Journal of Vascular Biology*, vol. 11, no. 6, pp. 1786–1794, 1991.

[31] J. Hulthe, J. Wisktrand, H. Emanuelsson, O. Wiklund, P. J. de Feyter, and I. Wendelhag, "Atherosclerotic changes in the carotid artery bulb as measured by B-mode ultrasound are associated with the extent of coronary atherosclerosis," *Stroke*, vol. 28, no. 6, pp. 1189–1194, 1997.

[32] S. Akazama, M. Tojikumo, Y. Nakano et al., "Usefulness of carotid plaque (sum and maximum of plaque thickness) in combination with intima-media thickness for the detection of coronary artery disease in asymptomatic patients with diabetes," *Journal of Diabetes Investigation*, vol. 7, no. 3, pp. 396–403, 2016.

[33] V. Nambi, L. Chambless, A. R. Folsom et al., "Carotid Intima-Media Thickness and Presence or Absence of Plaque Improves Prediction of Coronary Heart Disease Risk: The ARIC (Atherosclerosis Risk In Communities) Study," *Journal of the American College of Cardiology*, vol. 55, no. 15, pp. 1600–1607, 2010.

[34] S. Novo, P. Carita, A. Lo Voi et al., "Impact of preclinical carotid atherosclerosis on global cardiovascular risk stratification and events in a 10-year follow-up," *Journal of Cardiovascular Medicine*, vol. 20, no. 2, pp. 91–96, 2019.

[35] Y. Irie, N. Katakami, H. Kaneto et al., "Maximum carotid intima-media thickness improves the prediction ability of coronary artery stenosis in type 2 diabetic patients without history of coronary artery disease," *Atherosclerosis*, vol. 221, no. 2, pp. 438–444, 2012.

[36] S. de Vigili de Kreutzenberg, G. P. Fadini, S. Guzzinati et al., "Carotid plaque calcification predicts future cardiovascular events in type 2 diabetes," *Diabetes Care*, vol. 38, no. 10, pp. 1937–1944, 2015.

[37] R. M. Williamson, J. F. Price, S. Glancy, E. Perry, L. D. Nee, and P. C. Hayes, "Prevalence of and risk factors for hepatic steatosis and nonalcoholic fatty liver disease in people with type 2 diabetes: the Edinburgh Type 2 Diabetes Study," *Diabetes Care*, vol. 34, no. 5, pp. 1139–1144, 2011.

[38] G. Targher, L. Bertolini, R. Padovani, S. Rodella, R. Tessari, and L. Zenari, "Prevalence of nonalcoholic fatty liver disease and its association with cardiovascular disease among type 2

diabetic patients," *Diabetes Care*, vol. 30, no. 5, pp. 1212–1218, 2007.

[39] R. M. Williamson, J. F. Price, P. C. Hayes, S. Glancy, B. M. Frier, and G. I. Johnston, "Prevalence and markers of advanced liver disease in type 2 diabetes," *QJM*, vol. 105, no. 5, pp. 425–432, 2012.

[40] S. Gawrieh, L. A. Wilson, O. W. Cummings et al., "Histologic findings of advanced fibrosis and cirrhosis in patients with nonalcoholic fatty liver disease who have normal aminotransferase levels," *The American Journal of Gastroenterology*, vol. 114, no. 10, pp. 1626–1635, 2019.

[41] R. Hernaez, M. Lazo, S. Bonekamp et al., "Diagnostic accuracy and reliability of ultrasonography for the detection of fatty liver: a meta-analysis," *Hepatology*, vol. 54, no. 3, pp. 1082–1090, 2011.

[42] N. Khov, A. Sharma, and T. R. Riley, "Bedside ultrasound in the diagnosis of nonalcoholic fatty liver disease," *World Journal of Gastroenterology*, vol. 20, no. 22, pp. 6821–6825, 2014.

[43] B. Palmienteri, I. de Sio, V. la Mura et al., "The role of bright liver echo pattern on ultrasound B-mode examination in the diagnosis of liver steatosis," *Digestive and Liver Disease*, vol. 38, no. 7, pp. 485–489, 2006.

[44] F. Shen, R. D. Zheng, J. P. Shi et al., "Impact of skin capsular distance on the performance of controlled attenuation parameter in patients with chronic liver disease," *Liver International*, vol. 35, no. 11, pp. 2392–2400, 2015.

[45] T. R. Riley and M. A. Bruno, "Sonographic measurement of the thickness of subcutaneous tissues in nonalcoholic fatty liver disease versus other chronic liver diseases," *Journal of Clinical Ultrasound*, vol. 33, no. 9, pp. 439–441, 2005.

[46] S. Arora, A. C. Cheung, U. Tarique, A. Argawal, M. Firdouse, and J. Ailon, "First-year medical students use of ultrasound or physical examination to diagnose hepatomegaly and ascites: a randomized controlled trial," *Journal of Ultrasound*, vol. 20, no. 3, pp. 199–204, 2017.

[47] D. A. Miles, C. S. Levi, J. Uhanova, S. Cuvelier, K. Hawkins, and G. Y. Minuk, "Pocket-sized versus conventional ultrasound for detecting fatty infiltration of the liver," *Digestive Diseases and Sciences*, vol. 65, no. 1, pp. 82–85, 2020.

[48] T. R. Riley, A. Mendoza, and M. A. Bruno, "Bedside ultrasound can predict nonalcoholic fatty liver disease in the hands of clinicians using a prototype image," *Digestive Diseases and Sciences*, vol. 51, no. 5, pp. 982–985, 2006.

[49] H. Hauner, B. Stockamp, and B. Haastert, "Prevalence of lipohypertrophy in insulin-treated diabetic patients and predisposing factors," *Experimental and Clinical Endocrinology & Diabetes*, vol. 104, no. 2, pp. 106–110, 1996.

[50] T. Richardson and D. Kerr, "Skin-related complications of insulin therapy," *American Journal of Clinical Dermatology*, vol. 4, no. 10, pp. 661–667, 2003.

[51] S. Gentile, G. Guarino, A. Giancaterini, P. Guida, and F. Strollo, "A suitable palpation technique allows to identify skin lipohypertrophic lesions in insulin-treated people with diabetes," *SpringerPlus*, vol. 5, no. 1, pp. 1–7, 2016.

[52] S. Famulla, U. Hovelmann, A. Fischer et al., "Insulin injection into lipohypertrophic tissue: blunted and more variable insulin absorption and action and impaired postprandial glucose control," *Diabetes Care*, vol. 39, no. 9, pp. 1486–1492, 2016.

[53] U. B. Johansson, S. Amsberg, L. Hannerz et al., "Impaired absorption of insulin aspart from lipohypertrophic injection sites," *Diabetes Care*, vol. 28, no. 8, pp. 2025–2027, 2005.

[54] M. Blanco, M. T. Hernandez, K. W. Strauss, and M. Amaya, "Prevalence and risk factors of lipohypertrophy in insulin-injecting patients with diabetes," *Diabetes & Metabolism*, vol. 39, no. 5, pp. 445–453, 2013.

[55] L. Ji, Z. Sun, Q. Li et al., "Lipohypertrophy in China: prevalence, risk factors, insulin consumption and clinical impact," *Diabetes Technology & Therapeutics*, vol. 19, no. 1, pp. 61–67, 2017.

[56] R. Percium, "Ultrasonographic aspect of subcutaneous tissue dystrophies as a result of insulin injections," *Med Ultrasonogr*, vol. 12, pp. 104–109, 2010.

[57] F. Bertuzzi, E. Meneghini, E. Bruschi, L. Luzi, M. Nichelatti, and O. Epis, "Ultrasound characterization of insulin induced lipohypertrophy in type 1 diabetes mellitus," *Journal of Endocrinological Investigation*, vol. 40, no. 10, pp. 1107–1113, 2017.

[58] J. Kapeluto, B. W. Paty, S. D. Chang, and G. S. Meneilly, "Ultrasound detection of insulin-induced lipohypertrophy in type 1 and type 2 diabetes," *Diabetic Medicine*, vol. 35, no. 10, pp. 1383–1390, 2018.

[59] H. Umegaki, "Sarcopenia and diabetes: hyperglycemia is a risk factor for age-associated muscle mass and functional reduction," *Journal of Diabetes Investigation*, vol. 6, no. 6, pp. 623–624, 2015.

[60] N. Guerrero, D. Bunout, S. Hirsch et al., "Premature loss of muscle mass and function in type 2 diabetes," *Diabetes Research and Clinical Practice*, vol. 117, pp. 32–38, 2016.

[61] H. Myake, I. Kanazawa, K. Tanake, and T. Sugimoto, "Low skeletel muscle mass is associated with the risk of all-cause mortality in patients with type 2 diabetes mellitus," *Therapeutic Advances in Endocrinology and Metabolism*, vol. 10, pp. 1–9, 2019.

[62] S. W. Park, B. H. Goodpaster, E. S. Strotmeyer et al., "Decreased muscle strength and quality in older adults with type 2 diabetes: the health, aging, and body composition study," *Diabetes*, vol. 55, no. 6, pp. 1813–1818, 2006.

[63] A. L. Schafer, E. Vittinghoff, T. F. Lang et al., "Fat infiltration of muscle, diabetes, and clinical fracture risk in older adults," *The Journal of Clinical Endocrinology and Metabolism*, vol. 95, no. 11, pp. E368–E372, 2010.

[64] N. Ogama, T. Sakurai, S. Kawashima et al., "Association of glucose fluctuations with sarcopenia in older adults with type 2 diabetes mellitus," *Journal of Clinical Medicine*, vol. 8, no. 3, pp. 319–334, 2019.

[65] R. Chiaramonte, M. Bonfiglio, E. G. Castorina, and S. Antoci, "The primacy of ultrasound in the assessment of muscle architecture: precision, accuracy, reliability of ultrasonography. Physiatrist, radiologist, general internist, and family practitioner's experiences," *Revista da Associação Médica Brasileira*, vol. 65, no. 2, pp. 165–170, 2019.

[66] U. Ozdemir, M. Ozdemir, G. Aygencel, B. Kaya, and M. Turkoglu, "The role of maximum compressed thickness of the quadriceps femoris muscle measured by ultrasonography in assessing nutritional risk in critically-ill patients with different volume statuses," *Revista da Associação Médica Brasileira*, vol. 65, no. 7, pp. 952–958, 2019.

[67] C. R. de Souza Silva, A. dos Santos Costa, T. Rocha, D. A. Martins de Lima, T. do Nascimento, and S. R. A. de Moraes, "Quadriceps muscle architecture ultrasonography of individuals with type 2 diabetes: reliability and applicability," *PLoS One*, vol. 13, no. 10, p. e0205724, 2018.

[68] M. Camilleri, V. Chedid, A. C. Ford et al., "Gastroparesis," *Nature Reviews Disease Primers*, vol. 1, p. 41, 2018.

[69] S. M. Green, P. L. Leroy, M. G. Roback et al., "An international multidisciplinary consensus statement on fasting before procedural sedation in adults and children," *Anaesthesia*, vol. 75, no. 3, pp. 374–385, 2020.

[70] G. Cheisson, S. Jacqueminet, E. Cosson et al., "Perioperative management of adult diabetic patients. Preoperative period," *Anaesthesia Critical Care & Pain Medicine*, vol. 37, pp. S9–19, 2018.

[71] R. Sabry, A. Hasanin, S. Refaat, S. Abdel Raouf, A. S. Abdallah, and N. Helmy, "Evaluation of gastric residual volume in fasting diabetic patients using gastric ultrasound," *Acta Anaesthesiologica Scandinavica*, vol. 63, no. 5, pp. 615–619, 2019.

25

Chronic Diseases Multimorbidity among Adult People Living with HIV at Hawassa University Comprehensive Specialized Hospital, Southern Ethiopia

Endrias Markos Woldesemayat ⓘ

College of Medicine and Health Sciences, School of Public Health, Hawassa University, Ethiopia

Correspondence should be addressed to Endrias Markos Woldesemayat; endromark@yahoo.com

Academic Editor: Tadeusz Robak

Background. Due to the wide implementation of antiretroviral therapy (ART), people living with HIV (PLWHIV) are now living longer. This increased the risk of developing noncommunicable chronic diseases (NCCDs) among them. *Objective.* We aimed to describe prevalence of NCCDs multimorbidity among PLWHIV at Hawassa University Comprehensive Specialized Hospital (HUCSH). *Method.* In April 2016, institution-based cross-sectional study was conducted among PLWHIV, aged ≥ 18 years at the ART unit of HUCSH. A nurse working in the ART unit interviewed patients and reviewed medical records. Data on the NCCDs and its risk factors were obtained. List of diseases considered in this study were arthritis, diabetes mellitus, hypertension, congestive heart failure (CHF), rheumatic heart diseases (RHD), chronic bronchitis, asthma, and cancer. *Results.* More than half of the respondents (196) had at least one of the NCCDs and 34 (8.9%) had multimorbidity. The main system of the body affected were the musculoskeletal system, 146 (38.2%) and respiratory system, 46 (12.0%). There was no significant difference in the prevalence of individual NCCDs by gender. Patients aged above 44 years, patients with ART duration of at least 6 years, and patients with higher CD4 counts had increased odds of having any one of the NCCDs. Multimorbidity patients with a longer ART duration had an increased risk. *Conclusion.* The prevalence of NCCD multimorbidity among PLWHIV was high. Monitoring the occurrence of NCCDs among PLWHIV and noncommunicable disease care is recommended.

1. Introduction

Due to an increased access and utilization of antiretroviral therapy (ART), people living with HIV (PLWHIV) are now living longer [1]. This in turn raised the risk of having noncommunicable chronic diseases (NCCDs) among them. Aging, the HIV itself, and the adverse effect of antiretroviral medications may escalate the risk of having NCCD morbidity [2–5]. Having NCCDs among the PLWHIV may deteriorate the quality of life and prognosis of HIV. Considering these facts, investigating the NCCD comorbidities and multimorbidity among PLWHIV has a public health importance [6, 7].

In 2016, the prevalence of HIV in Ethiopia was 1.1% [8]. In the other hand, in the study setting, a hospital-based study reported the prevalence of diabetes mellitus (DM) and hypertension (HTN) to be 12.2% and 10.5%, respectively [9]. In a retrospective cohort study conducted in South Ethiopia, the prevalence of NCCDs was 29.7% and this was in line with the WHO country profile report of 2014 [10, 11].

In HIV-negative people, the risk of having NCCDs and multimorbidity is higher among the elderly [1, 12, 13]. Diabetes mellitus, cardiovascular diseases like HTN, and chronic obstructive pulmonary diseases (COPDs) are among the most common comorbidities in patients living with HIV [14, 15]. Certain study reported, HIV-positive status is associated with an increased likelihood of having the NCCDs [16]. Increased age, immune suppression or advanced stage of AIDS, coexisting infections (viral and tuberculosis), social deprivation, longer duration with HIV infection, longer survival, and the traditional risk factors of NCCDs are among the factors associated with having NCCDs among HIV patients [17].

Having NCCDs decreases the functional status and quality of life of patients and it increases drug side effects, medical costs, disability, and mortality of patients in HIV-negative people [18–21]. There is an increased risk of NCCDs in PLWHIV [16], and the NCCD comorbidities increase with the HIV severity [4]. NCCD comorbidities would negatively affect the quality of life and the cost of patient care of PLWHIV [22–24]. Due to the combined effect of the HIV and the NCCDs, patients living with HIV may have a complex healthcare needs. An increasing number of comorbid conditions in PLWHIV is directly linked to an increase in the number of total medications [2]. NCCDs are the major causes of death among PLWHIV [17]. In countries like Ethiopia, multimorbidity associated with HIV could affect healthy aging and overwhelm the healthcare systems [25]. Investigating the NCCDs among PLWHIV is thus an important issue [7]. The investigator aimed to describe the prevalence of NCCDs multimorbidity among PLWHIV at Hawassa University Comprehensive Specialized Hospital (HUCSH). This is the first study to estimate the prevalence of NCCDs and multimorbidity among PLWHIV in the study area.

2. Methods

A cross-sectional institutional study was conducted among PLWHIV attending HUCSH. Hawassa town is the capital of both the Sidama Zone and the Southern Nations and Nationalities Peoples Region (SNNPR) in Ethiopia. The town is located at 275 Km to the South of Addis Ababa with a total population of more than 400,000. HUCSH is the largest hospital in southern Ethiopia with more than 300 beds. The hospital was established in 2004; and currently, it provides a comprehensive and specialized health services to peoples of the region and other peoples coming from the neighboring Oromia Region. The ART unit in the hospital started its service in June 2006.

The study was conducted in April 2016. During the study period, over 4,000 PLWHIV were under follow-up in the ART unit with a median duration of 6 years of follow-up. Of this, about 2,000 patients were taking ART. For this cross-sectional study, the study participants were recruited from adult patients (aged at least 18 years) taking ART in the hospital.

A questionnaire format was developed based on the objective of the study. Questions were first developed in English and translated into Amharic and then back translated to English. The investigator provided training to the data collector. Training included explanation of the study objectives and techniques for interviewing. A few days prior to the actual data collection, pretesting was done on 5% of the calculated sample size of PLWHIV. Based on the pretest, necessary amendments were done on the questionnaire. Having NCCDs was measured by an open question. Each study participant was interviewed after consulting the physician and taking his pills. Patient's cards were reviewed to

obtain additional information from the history, physical examination, investigations, and the medications used. Weight and height of the patients were measured. A nurse working at the ART unit collected data. Supervision was done throughout the data collection process, and daily checking of the collected data was done and problems encountered were managed accordingly.

Chronic disease was defined as a nonreversible and non-infectious disease affecting specific body systems which was diagnosed by a physician. Presence of NCCDs was assessed mainly by interview, which was supplemented with the review of medical records. The lists of diseases considered in this study were rheumatoid arthritis, gouty arthritis, diabetes mellitus, HTN, congestive heart failure (CHF), rheumatic heart diseases (RHD), chronic bronchitis, asthma, and cancer in any of the body parts. Rheumatoid arthritis refers to a chronic, autoimmune inflammatory disease of the joint [26]. Gouty arthritis was defined as an inflammatory arthritis caused by the deposition of urate crystals in the joints, which occurs due to chronic hyperuricemia [27]. Physicians diagnosed arthritis based on clinical data (history, physical examination, and investigations) obtained from each patient. Diabetes mellitus was considered if a patient presented with episodes of hyperglycemia and glucose intolerance, as a result of lack of insulin or its defective action [28]. A participant having systolic blood pressure of 140 mmHg and/or diastolic blood pressure of 90 mmHg was considered hypertensive [29]. Asthma was defined as an incurable lung disease that causes breathing difficulties due to narrowing of the tubes that carry air to and from the lungs. Its symptoms is relieved with treatment [30]. Chronic bronchitis was defined as a condition characterized by bronchial hypersecretion, chronic cough, and sputum production [31]. A patient suffering from dyspnea, fatigue, and clinical signs of congestion was diagnosed as a case of congestive heart failure [32]. Rheumatic heart disease was considered if permanent damage to the valves of the heart was developed due to repeated episodes of acute rheumatic fever [33]. Study participants without symptom of the NCCDs described above because of taking medications for the conditions were also considered cases of the specific NCCD. Multimorbidity refers to the presence of at least two of the NCCDs.

Normal body mass index (BMI) considered in this study was 18.5–24.9 kg/m^2. Social support refers to obtaining any kind of regular support from individuals or organizations, which was provided in kind or in the form of money. ART duration was defined as the time period measured since the initiation of the ARV medications up to the date of interview.

The outcome variables considered in this study were having any of the NCCDs and multimorbidity among PLWHIV. Explanatory variables determining having a NCCD or multimorbidity were sociodemographic variables (gender, age, literacy status, monthly household income) and other variables such as smoking, alcohol drinking, khat chewing, high BMI, lack of physical activity, and low consumption of fruits and vegetables. ART duration and the CD4 count level were clinical factors expected to determine the outcome measures.

Assuming a prevalence of multimorbidity of 65% [34], 95% confidence interval (CI), a precession of 5%, and adding 10% for possible nonresponse, the sample size required for this study was 380. We added 10% to what we have calculated. Every 3rd PLWHIV who were on ART during the study period were interviewed until the required sample size was obtained.

The investigator entered and analyzed data using SPSS version 20 statistical packages (SPSS Inc., Chicago, IL, USA). BMI refers to the calculated value of an individual weight in kilogram divided by height in meter square. Age was grouped in to 18–29 years, 30–44 years, and >44 years, considering the availability of values in cells for each age group. Education was categorized into two values, people with no education and literates. People with no education are participants without formal education. Participants with any of the formal schooling were considered as literate. Exercise was defined as performing of at least 30 minutes of physical activity of moderate intensity for at least 4 days per week [12]. Insufficient consumption of fruits and vegetables refers to the consumption of less than 125 ml or 400 grams fruit and vegetable per day [35]. Smoking refers to the use of at least one cigarette per day for more than 6 months. Alcohol drinking was considered if the study participant previously or currently habitually consumed any amount of alcoholic beverage. Khat chewing refers to a habitual chewing of any amount of khat (a psychoactive substance).

Descriptive statistics was used to calculate and present the sociodemographic, behavioral, and clinical characteristics of the study participants. The difference in the prevalence of individual chronic diseases among men and women was evaluated. Logistic regression model was used to determine the association between outcome variables and the expected determinants. Variables with a P value of less than 0.2 in the bivariate analysis were included in the multivariate analysis. Odds ratio and a 95% confidence interval (CI) were used to describe the association between the dependent variables and the independent variables.

3. Results

All of the approached eligible PLWHIV participated in the study. The median (interquartile range (IQR)) age of the study participants was 35 (10) years. Majority of the study participants (235 (61.5%)) were female. Employed, married, and literate PLWHIV were 106 (27.7%), 215 (56.3%), and 339 (88.7%), respectively. The median (IQR) household income was 1,500 (2,000) Eth. Birr. More than three-fourth of the study participants had children and get social support. Details of the sociodemographic characteristics of the study participants are described in Table 1.

Study participants with a BMI score of at least 25 were 117 (30.6%). Majority (361 (94.5%)) of the patients had the habit of exercising. Alcohol drinking, khat chewing, and cigarette smoking were experienced by 185 (48.4%), 137 (35.9%), and 49 (12.8%) patients, respectively. Seven (1.8%) of the study participants responded as current alcohol drinkers. The median (IQR) duration on ART and CD4

counts of the study participants were 74 (57) months and 545.1 (314) cells/μl, respectively (Table 2).

More than half (196 (51.3%)) of the respondents were affected by at least one of the NCCDs. While 34 (8.9%) had multimorbidity by these chronic diseases. Musculoskeletal problems like rheumatoid arthritis and gouty arthritis were reported by 146 (38.2%) of the study participants. Of which, the majority (143 (97.9%)) were affected by rheumatoid arthritis. The second leading system of the body affected was the respiratory system, the diseases being chronic bronchitis and asthma 46 (12.0%). Seventeen patients had cardiovascular problems; of this, HTN was reported by 16 (94.1%) of the patients. Malignant cancers affected 15 (8.2%) patients; of which, 8 (53.3%) were reproductive system cancers (Table 3). There was no significant difference in the prevalence of an individual chronic disease among men and women (Table 4).

In a bivariate analysis, factors like age above 44 years, ART duration, alcohol drinking, khat chewing, and CD4 count above 350 cells per μl showed association with having at least one of the NCCDs. In a multivariate analysis, however, age above 44 years (adjusted odds ratio (AOR) = 2.5, 95% CI 1.3–4.9), ART duration of at least 6 years (AOR = 2.1, 95% CI 1.4–3.2), and CD4 count maintained the significance in predicting having a NCCD. Patients with a CD4 count of 200–350 cells per μl (AOR = 2.7, 95% CI 1.1–6.7) and CD4 count of above 350 cells per μl (AOR = 2.3, 95% CI 1.0–5.3) had an increased risk of having at least one of the NCCDs. Concerning multimorbidity, ART duration of at least six years showed statistically significant association both in a bivariate (AOR = 3.0, 95% CI 1.3–6.5) and in a multivariate analysis (AOR = 2.6, 95% CI 1.2–5.9). Tables 5 and 6 show factors associated with having NCCDs and NCCD multimorbidity.

4. Discussion

In this institutional-based cross-sectional study, high prevalence of NCCDs and high prevalence of multimorbidity among PLWHIV were observed. Arthritis was the predominant disease affected the study participants. There was no significant difference on the prevalence of NCCDs by gender. The risk of having any of the NCCD comorbidity was higher among patients above 44 years of age, patients with ART duration of at least 6 years, and patients with high CD4 count, while being on ART for at least six years was associated with an increased risk of NCCD multimorbidity.

A study in Brent UK reported that 29% of PLWHIV had one or more comorbidity [36]. In a population-based study in Canada, 34.4% of PLWHIV had at least one other physical condition [37]. In Tanzania, the proportion of PLWHIV with one or more NCCDs was 57.8% [38]. The prevalence of comorbidity among PLWHIV was 15.3% in Zimbabwe [39]. The current study finding was comparable to the report from Tanzania [38], but it was higher than the reports from the UK, Canada, and Zimbabwe [36, 37, 39]. The difference could be due to variation in the study design [37]. The current study is a facility-based study carried out on PLWHIV who were on ART at a tertiary health care unit, in which

TABLE 1: Sociodemographic characteristics of people living with HIV at HUCSH, April 2016.

Characteristics	Value	Number	%
Gender	Male	147	38.5
	Female	235	61.5
Age in years	Median (IQR)	35 (10)	
Occupation	Employed	106	27.7
	House wife	96	25.1
	Daily laborer	84	22.0
	Merchant	54	14.2
	No job	14	3.7
	Other	28	7.3
Marital status	Single	41	10.7
	Married	215	56.3
	Divorced	60	15.7
	Widowed	59	15.4
	Missing	7	1.8
Household income in Eth. Birr*	Median (IQR)	1,500 (2,000)	
Educational status	No education	43	11.3
	Literate	339	88.7
Having children	Yes	294	77.0
	No	71	18.6
	Missing	17	4.5
Social support	Yes	305	79.8
	No	74	19.4
	Missing	3	0.8

Household income had 8 missing values; exchange rate during the study period was 1 USD to 21.4 Ethiopian Birr.

TABLE 2: Behavioral and clinical characteristics of people living with HIV at HUCSH, April 2016.

Characteristics	Value	Number	%
BMI	<25	265	69.4
	≥25	117	30.6
Exercise	Yes	361	94.5
	No	21	5.5
Fruits and vegetables consumption	Yes	376	98.4
	No	6	1.6
Alcohol drinking	Yes	185	48.4
	No	197	51.6
Khat chewing	Yes	137	35.9
	No	245	64.1
Cigarette smoking	Yes	49	12.8
	No	333	87.2
Duration of ART in months*	Median (IQR)	74 (57)	
Most recent CD4 count (cells/μl)	Median (IQR)	545.1 (314)	

ART: antiretroviral therapy; BMI: body mass index. Duration of ART in months has 4 missing values, CD4 count had 1 missing value.

TABLE 3: Prevalence of chronic diseases by systems of the body among people living with HIV at HUCSH, April 2016.

Body systems affected	Diseases	Cases (%)
Musculoskeletal system	Rheumatoid arthritis, gout	146 (38.2)
Respiratory system	Chronic bronchitis, asthma	46 (12.0)
Cardiovascular system	HTN, CHF, RHD	17 (4.5)
Any cancer	Cancer	15 (3.9)
Endocrine system	Diabetes mellitus	8 (2.1)
Chronic diseases	Any chronic diseases	196 (51.3)
Multimorbidity		34 (8.9)

HTN: hypertension; CHF: congestive heart failure; RHD: rheumatic heart disease.

interview was used as a primary method of data collection for identifying chronic diseases diagnosed by physicians, which was supplemented with a record review. In population-based studies, usually low prevalence of chronic diseases is reported, because relatively more healthy people are involved in such studies. Moreover, participants in community-based studies may prefer responding to the absence of diseases and diagnosing NCCDs in such studies may not be easy and accurate. The method of diagnosis could be another explanation for the observed differences. In Brent England, they did a retrospective study based on a confirmed evidence by investigations [36]. In retrospective studies, patients who do not complain for the presence of symptoms of a chronic disease may not be investigated and thus they may not be diagnosed. This may lower the prevalence of NCCDs. A similar explanation may apply for the observed difference in the prevalence of NCCDs between the current study and the report from Zimbabwe [39].

The commonly observed individual NCCDs occurring among PLWHIV in Australia, London and Ontario, Canada were mental health problems, followed by cardiovascular diseases [36, 37, 40]. In Zimbabwe, HTN, asthma, type 2 diabetes mellitus, cancer, and congestive cardiac failure were among the leading diseases reported [39]. In the current study, the commonest reported disease was arthritis. This finding is comparable to the report from Tanzania, where arthritis was the leading NCD that affected PLWHIV [38].

The prevalence of multimorbidity in the current study was lower than the reports from Canada (65%) and Australia (54.5%) [34, 40]. The differences could be due to the difference in the prevalence of the risk factors. In Canada, almost two-third of participants were overweight (36%) or obese (29%) [34] and various studies confirmed that there is an increased risk of multimorbidity among people with high BMI [34, 41]. In the current study, only 30.4% of PLWHIV had a BMI score of over 24.9. The mean age of the study participants in the Australia study was 51.8 years [40]. Study participants in the current study were younger than the study participants in these settings. There is an increased risk of multimorbidity among older people [37, 41, 42]. The investigator suggests the importance of controlling the modifiable risk factors and follow-up of PLWHIV with the nonmodifiable risk factors of NCCDs to lower the burden.

Current smoking was reported by 12-23% of men and 1-3% of women in Tanzania and Uganda [43]. Similar measure was 14.7% in Cambodia [44]. Only 0.3% of the current study participants were current tobacco smoker and women smoked less than men. This was as expected and in agreement to the finding in another study [44]. Problem of drinking alcohol was 6-15% in Tanzania and Uganda [43] and 54.7% in Cambodia [44]. Only 1.8% of the study participants in the current study responded as current alcohol drunkers. This finding was lower than the reports in other settings [43, 44]. The low level of current tobacco smoking and alcohol drinking among the study participants in the current study could be related to the change in behavior of the PLWHIV after being diagnosed with the HIV and started the ART.

Gender was one of the risk factors of NCCDs among PLWHIV [17, 39]. Contrary to the reports in these studies, in the current study, there was no association between gender and having of any of the NCCDs or having of multimorbidity. Higher age categories were significantly associated with comorbidity risk in Zimbabwe [39]. In agreement to their finding, in the current study, an increase in age predicted the risk of having an individual chronic disease. However, our study did not show the statistical association between age and multimorbidity. In other settings, increasing age was the risk factor for the presence of multiple health problems [37, 41, 42]. The investigator suggests the importance of early identification and management of chronic diseases among the elderly PLWHIV.

Higher CD4 values increased the risk for multimorbidity [17, 45]. Contrary to this report, no association was observed between CD4 level and multi-morbidity in the current study. However, there was a higher risk of having at least one of the NCCDs among PLWHIV with higher CD4 count. Another study reported that increased immune suppression was among the determinants of NCCDs [17]. Continuous monitoring of PLWHIV for having of NCCDs and delivering appropriate intervention is important to reduce the burden of NCCD comorbidity among PLWHIV. Particular attention should be given to patients with higher CD4 level.

In the current study, PLWHIV with at least 6 years of ART had an increased risk of developing both an individual NCCD and multimorbidity. This is in agreement to a previous report [17]. Longer duration of exposure to ART, especially exposure to protease inhibitors, was reported to increase the risk of NCCDs among PLWHIV [17]. Screening of PLWHIV with longer duration on ART could help in timely identifying the NCCDs. This helps to provide appropriate intervention in order to limit the effect of the diseases.

Obesity was associated with an increased odds of multimorbidity [34] and the prevalence of multimorbidity increased with each progressive BMI category [41]. Higher levels of traditional NCCD risk factors among PLWHIV (which includes higher BMI) were also among the associated risk factors reported for having any one of the NCCDs [17]. In the current study, none of the lifestyle factors showed association with having of any one of the NCCDs or multimorbidity by the NCCDs. This could be due to the limitation in the study design used to measure associations. Analytical

TABLE 4: Difference in prevalence of chronic diseases by gender among people living with HIV at HUCSH, April 2016.

Chronic diseases	Value	Men, n (%)	Women, n (%)	Total	P value
Arthritis	Yes	55(37.4)	91 (38.7)	146 (38.2)	0.8
	No	92 (62.6)	144 (61.3)	236 (61.8)	
Chronic bronchitis	Yes	9 (6.1)	19 (8.1)	28 (7.3)	0.47
	No	138 (93.9)	216 (91.9)	354 (92.7)	
Bronchial asthma	Yes	6 (4.1)	16 (6.8)	22 (5.8)	0.27
	No	141 (95.9)	219 (93.2)	360 (94.2)	
Hypertension	Yes	7 (4.8)	9 (3.8)	16 (4.2)	0.7
	No	140 (95.2)	226 (96.2)	366 (95.8)	
Cancer	Yes	4 (2.7)	11 (4.7)	15 (3.9)	0.3
	No	143 (97.3)	231 (95.3)	374 (96.1)	
Diabetes mellitus	Yes	4 (2.7)	4 (1.7)	8 (2.1)	0.5
	No	143 (97.3)	231 (98.3)	374 (97.9)	
Chronic diseases	Yes	72 (49.0)	124 (52.8)	196 (51.3)	0.5
	No	75 (51.0)	111 (47.2)	186 (48.7)	

n = number of respondents for the category.

TABLE 5: Risk factors of having a chronic disease among people living with HIV at HUCSH, April 2016.

Variables	Value	Chronic diseases		COR (95% CI)	AOR (95% CI)
		Yes	No		
Age in years	18–29	39	54		
	30–44	107	107	1.4 (0.9 – 2.2)	1.3 (0.7 – 2.2)
	≥45	50	25	2.8 (1.5–5.2)	2.6 (1.3–5.0)
ART duration	<6 years	77	110		
	≥6 years	119	76	2.3 (1.5–3.4)	2.0 (1.3–3.2)
Social support*	Yes	150	155		
	No	44	30	1.5 (0.9–2.5)	1.4 (0.8–2.5)
Fruit/vegetable consumption	Yes	195	181		
	No	1	5	0.2 (0.0–1.6)	0.2 (0.0–1.6)
Alcohol drinking	Yes	110	75	1.9 (1.2–2.8)	1.6 (0.9–2.9)
	No	86	111		
Khat chewing	Yes	82	55	1.7 (1.1–2.5)	1.1 (0.6–2.1)
	No	114	131		
BMI	<25	128	137		
	≥25	68	49	1.5 (0.9–2.4)	1.6 (0.9–2.6)
CD4 count (cells/μl)*	<200	10	21		
	200–350	36	33	2.3 (0.9–5.6)	2.7 (1.1–6.8)
	>350	149	132	2.4 (1.1–5.2)	2.3 (1.0–5.2)

COR: crude odds ratio; AOR: adjusted odds ratio; 95% CI: 95% confidence interval: BMI: body mass index. *The variables have missing values.

study design could have been used to investigate such associations.

5. Limitation of the Study

This study has limitations. The dataset used had missing values in some of the measured characteristics. However, the missing values were low (less than 2%). Therefore, missing values are less likely to affect conclusion of the study. The study design used in the current study may be inappropriate for measuring association between exposure factors and the outcome variables. A cohort study or a case control study design could have been used to determine such kind of causal relationships.

TABLE 6: Risk factors of multimorbidity among people living with HIV at HUCSH, April 2016.

Variables	Value	Chronic diseases		COR (95% CI)	AOR (95% CI)
		Yes	No		
Age in years	18–29	4	89		
	30–44	22	192	2.6 (0.9–7.9)	2.8 (0.9–8.7)
	≥45	8	67	2.7 (0.8–9.5)	2.3 (0.6–8.5)
ART duration	<6 years	9	178		
	≥6 years	25	170	3.0 (1.3–6.5)	2.6 (1.1–5.8)
Social support*	Yes	23	282		
	No	10	64	1.9 (0.9–4.2)	2.0 (0.9–4.6)
Alcohol drinking	Yes	20	165	1.6 (0.8–3.2)	1.0 (0.4–2.8)
	No	14	183		
Khat chewing	Yes	16	121	1.7 (0.8–3.4)	1.1 (0.4–3.2)
	No	18	227		
Smoking	Yes	8	41	2.3 (0.9–5.3)	2.4 (0.9–6.5)
	No	26	307		

COR: crude odds ratio; AOR: adjusted odds ratio; 95% CI: 95% confidence interval; BMI: body mass index. *The variable has missing value.

6. Conclusion

In conclusion, high prevalence of NCCDs and multimorbidity was observed among PLWHIV. The main chronic disease that affected the patients was arthritis. There was no significant difference in the occurrence of chronic diseases among men and women. Age, ART duration, and CD4 count were determinant factors of having any one of the NCCDs, while being on ART for at least for six years predicted having multimorbidity. Monitoring the occurrence of NCCDs among PLWHIV with the risk factors and noncommunicable diseases care among PLWHIV is recommended.

Consent

The data collector obtained informed verbal consent from each study participant before commencing data collection. Data were collected and analyzed anonymously.

Authors' Contributions

EMW conceptualized, designed, collected, and analyzed data. EMW also performed literature search and wrote the first draft. The author read and approved the final manuscript.

Acknowledgments

The investigator thanks Hawassa University for funding the research and the data collectors and the study subjects for participating in the study.

References

[1] A. C. Justice, "HIV and aging: time for a new paradigm," Current HIV/AIDS Reports, vol. 7, no. 2, pp. 69–76, 2010.

[2] B. Hasse, B. Ledergerber, H. Furrer et al., "Morbidity and aging in HIV-infected persons: the Swiss HIV cohort study," Clinical Infectious Diseases, vol. 53, no. 11, pp. 1130–1139, 2011.

[3] G. Guaraldi, G. Orlando, S. Zona et al., "Premature age-related comorbidities among HIV-infected persons compared with the general population," Clinical Infectious Diseases, vol. 53, no. 11, pp. 1120–1126, 2011.

[4] J. L. Goulet, S. L. Fultz, D. Rimland et al., "Aging and infectious diseases: do patterns of comorbidity vary by HIV status, age, and HIV severity?," Clinical Infectious Diseases, vol. 45, no. 12, pp. 1593–1601, 2007.

[5] M. Rabkin and S. Nishtar, "Scaling up chronic care systems: leveraging HIV programs to support noncommunicable disease services," JAIDS Journal of Acquired Immune Deficiency Syndromes, vol. 57, pp. S87–S90, 2011.

[6] K. M. V. Narayan, M. K. Ali, C. del Rio, J. P. Koplan, and J. Curran, "Global Noncommunicable Diseases — Lessons from the HIV–AIDS Experience," New England Journal of Medicine, vol. 365, no. 10, pp. 876–878, 2011.

[7] N. S. Levitt, K. Steyn, J. Dave, and D. Bradshaw, "Chronic noncommunicable diseases and HIV-AIDS on a collision course: relevance for health care delivery, particularly in low-resource settings–insights from South Africa," The American Journal of Clinical Nutrition, vol. 94, no. 6, pp. 1690S–1696S, 2011.

[8] EPHI, HIV Related Estimates and Projections for Ethiopia-2017, Ethiopian public health institute, Addis Ababa, 2017.

[9] A. Kassa and E. M. Woldesemayat, "Hypertension and diabetes mellitus among patients at Hawassa University Comprehensive Specialized Hospital, Hawassa, Southern Ethiopia," International Journal of Chronic Diseases, vol. 2019, 8 pages, 2019.

[10] M. Endriyas, E. Emebet, T. Dana et al., "Burden of NCDs in SNNP region, Ethiopia: a retrospective study," *BMC Health Services Research*, vol. 18, no. 1, p. 520, 2018.

[11] WHO, *Noncommunicable diseases country profiles 2014*, WHO, Ethiopia, 2014.

[12] E. M. Woldesemayat, K. Andargachew, T. G. Ayana, and M. H. Dangiso, "Chronic diseases multi-morbidity among adult patients at Hawassa University Comprehensive Specialized Hospital," *BMC public health*, vol. 18, no. 1, p. 352, 2018.

[13] L. R. Hirschhorn, S. F. Kaaya, P. S. Garrity, E. Chopyak, and M. C. S. Fawzi, "Cancer and the 'other' noncommunicable chronic diseases in older people living with HIV/AIDS in resource-limited settings: a challenge to success," *AIDS*, vol. 26, pp. S65–S75, 2012.

[14] The Lancet Diabetes & Endocrinology, "HIV and NCDs: the need to build stronger health systems," *The Lancet Diabetes & Endocrinology*, vol. 4, no. 7, pp. 549-550, 2016.

[15] E. Nou, J. Lo, and S. K. Grinspoon, "Inflammation, immune activation, and cardiovascular disease in HIV," *AIDS*, vol. 30, no. 10, pp. 1495–1509, 2016.

[16] T. Nigatu, "Integration of HIV and noncommunicable diseases in health care delivery in low and middle income countries," *Preventing Chronic Disease*, vol. 9, article E93, 2012.

[17] T. N. Haregu, B. Oldenburg, G. Setswe, J. Elliott, and V. Nanayakkara, "Epidemiology of comorbidity of HIV/AIDS and non-communicable diseases in developing countries: a systematic review," *Journal of Global Health Care Systems*, vol. 2, no. 1, pp. 2159–6743, 2012.

[18] M. Fortin, C. Hudon, J. Haggerty, M. Akker, and J. Almirall, "Prevalence estimates of multimorbidity: a comparative study of two sources," *BMC Health Services Research*, vol. 10, no. 1, p. 111, 2010.

[19] M. L. Salter, B. Lau, V. F. Go, S. H. Mehta, and G. D. Kirk, "HIV infection, immune suppression, and uncontrolled viremia are associated with increased multimorbidity among aging injection drug users," *Clinical Infectious Diseases*, vol. 53, no. 12, pp. 1256–1264, 2011.

[20] I. Schafer, E.-C. von Leitner, G. Schön et al., "Multimorbidity patterns in the elderly: a new approach of disease clustering identifies complex interrelations between chronic conditions," *PLoS One*, vol. 5, no. 12, article e15941, 2010.

[21] H. Van-den-Bussche, D. Koller, T. Kolonko et al., "Which chronic diseases and disease combinations are specific to multimorbidity in the elderly? Results of a claims data based cross-sectional study in Germany," *BMC Public Health*, vol. 11, no. 1, p. 101, 2011.

[22] S. Degroote, D. Vogelaers, and D. M. Vandijck, "What determines health-related quality of life among people living with HIV: an updated review of the literature," *Archives of Public Health*, vol. 72, no. 1, p. 40, 2014.

[23] L. Emuren, S. Welles, and A. A. Evans, "Health-related quality of life among military HIV patients on antiretroviral therapy," *PLoS One*, vol. 12, no. 6, article e0178953, 2017.

[24] C. Stefan, W. Eva, A. Julia, and D. C. Helena, "Comorbidities and costs in HIV patients: a retrospective claims database analysis in Germany," *PLoS One*, vol. 14, no. 11, article e0224279, 2019.

[25] S. G. Deeks, S. R. Lewin, and D. V. Havlir, "The end of AIDS: HIV infection as a chronic disease," *Lancet*, vol. 382, no. 9903, pp. 1525–1533, 2013.

[26] A. Gibofsky, "Overview of epidemiology, pathophysiology, and diagnosis of rheumatoid arthritis," *The American Journal of Managed Care*, vol. 18, 13 Suppl, pp. S295–S302, 2012.

[27] G. Nuki and P. A. Simkin, "A concise history of gout and hyperuricemia and their treatment," *Arthritis Research & Therapy*, vol. 8, Supplement 1, p. S1, 2006.

[28] R. Sicree, J. Shaw, and P. Zimmet, *The Global Burden. Diabetes and Impaired Glucose Tolerance. Prevalence and Projections*, Brussels, International Diabetes Federation, 2006.

[29] "The sixth report of the Joint National Committee on prevention, detection, evaluation, and treatment of high blood pressure," *Archives of Internal Medicine*, vol. 157, no. 21, pp. 2413-2446, 1997.

[30] *Asthma*, WHO, 2019, https://www.who.int/news-room/q-a-detail/asthma.

[31] V. Kim and G. J. Criner, "The chronic bronchitis phenotype in chronic obstructive pulmonary disease: features and implications," *Current Opinion in Pulmonary Medicine*, vol. 21, no. 2, pp. 133–141, 2015.

[32] S. F. Gary, W. H. Tang, and R. A. Walsh, "Pathophysiology of heart failure," *Hurst's the Heart*, R. A. Valentin Fuster and R. A. Harrington, Eds., 719–738, 2011.

[33] J. M. Katzenellenbogen, P. R. Anna, W. Rosemary, and R. C. Jonathan, "Rheumatic heart disease: infectious disease origin, chronic care approach," *BMC Health Services Research*, vol. 17, no. 1, p. 793, 2017.

[34] J. K. David, O. W. Andrew, C. Eric et al., "Multimorbidity Patterns in HIV-Infected Patients," *JAIDS Journal of Acquired Immune Deficiency Syndromes*, vol. 61, no. 5, pp. 600–605, 2012.

[35] M. Fortin, H. Jeannie, A. José, B. Tarek, S. Maxime, and L. Martin, "Lifestyle factors and multimorbidity: a cross sectional study," *BMC Public Health*, vol. 14, no. 1, p. 686, 2014.

[36] L. Ava, A. Piriyankan, L. James, B. Ricky, J. Mohamade, and B. Gary, "The prevalence of comorbidities among people living with HIV in Brent: a diverse London borough," *London Journal of Primary Care*, vol. 6, no. 4, pp. 84–90, 2014.

[37] E. K. Claire, W. Jenna, T. Monica et al., "A cross-sectional, population-based study measuring comorbidity among people living with HIV in Ontario," *BMC Public Health*, vol. 14, no. 1, 2014.

[38] M. GMDM, M. Kazuhiko, U. I. Ehimario et al., "Non-communicable diseases in antiretroviral therapy recipients in Kagera Tanzania: a cross-sectional study," *The Pan African Medical Journal*, vol. 16, no. 84, 2013.

[39] M. M. Itai, M. E. Tonya, and C. Tawanda, "A cross-sectional, facility based study of comorbid non-communicable diseases among adults living with HIV infection in Zimbabwe," *BMC Research Notes*, vol. 9, no. 1, 2016.

[40] A. E. Natalie-Edmiston, B. C. Erin-Passmore, J. S. David, and P. Kathy, "Multimorbidity among people with HIV in regional New South Wales, Australia," *Sexual Health*, vol. 12, no. 5, pp. 425–432, 2015.

[41] C. Michael, "Obesity is a risk factor for co-occuring chronic health problems in patients with HIV," *Nutrition*, 2012.

[42] O. Tolu, Y. Elizabeth, B. Andrew, M. C. G. Nuala, J. W. Robert, and S. L. Naomi, "Patterns of HIV, TB, and non-communicable disease multi-morbidity in peri-urban South Africa- a cross sectional study," *BMC Infectious Diseases*, vol. 15, no. 1, 2015.

[43] B. Kavishe, S. Biraro, K. Baisley et al., "High prevalence of hypertension and of risk factors for non-communicable diseases (NCDs): a population based cross-sectional survey of NCDS and HIV infection in Northwestern Tanzania and Southern Uganda," *BMC Medicine*, vol. 13, no. 1, 2015.

[44] P. Chhoun, C. Ngin, S. Tuot et al., "Non-communicable diseases and related risk behaviors among men and women living with HIV in Cambodia: findings from a cross-sectional study," *International Journal for Equity in Health*, vol. 16, no. 1, p. 125, 2017.

[45] A. Mocroft, P. Reiss, J. Gasiorowski et al., "Serious fatal and nonfatal non-AIDS-defining illnesses in Europe," *Journal of Acquired Immune Deficiency Syndromes*, vol. 55, no. 2, pp. 262–270, 2010.

Permissions

List of Contributors

Nurul Akidah Lukman, Annette Leibing and Lisa Merry
Faculty of Nursing, University of Montreal, Canada

Biruk Legese
Infectious Disease Screening Division, Amhara National Regional State Health Bureau, Bahir Dar Blood Bank Laboratory, Bahir Dar, Ethiopia

Molla Abebe and Alebachew Fasil
Department of Clinical Chemistry, School of Biomedical and Laboratory Sciences, College of Medicine and Health Sciences, University of Gondar, Gondar, Ethiopia

V. T. S. Kaluarachchi, D. U. S. Bulugahapitiya, M. D. Jayasooriya, C. H. De Silva, P. H. Premanayaka and A. Dayananda
Diabetes and Endocrinology Unit, Colombo South Teaching Hospital, Kalubowila, Colombo, Sri Lanka

M. H. Arambewela
Department of Physiology, Faculty of Medical Sciences, University of Sri Jayewardenepura, Diabetes and Endocrinology Unit, Colombo South Teaching Hospital, Kalubowila, Colombo, Sri Lanka

Mistire Teshome Guta, Tiwabwork Tekalign and Nefsu Awoke
School of Nursing, College of Health Science and Medicine, Wolaita Sodo University, Wolaita Sodo, Ethiopia

Robera Olana Fite
HaSET Program/Ethiopian Public Health Institute, Adis Abeba, Ethiopia

Getahun Dendir
School of Anesthesia, College of Health Science and Medicine, Wolaita Sodo University, Wolaita Sodo, Ethiopia

Tsegaye Lolaso Lenjebo
School of Public Health, College of Health Science and Medicine, Wolaita Sodo University, Ethiopia

Esileman Abdela Muche, Mohammed Biset Ayalew and Ousman Abubeker Abdela
Department of Clinical Pharmacy, School of Pharmacy, College of Medicine and Health Sciences, University of Gondar, Gondar, Ethiopia

Li Zheng, Feng Deng, Honglin Wang, Biao Yang, Meng Qu and Peirong Yang
Baoji Center for Disease Control and Prevention, Baoji 721000, China

Sebastián Jaurretche
Biophysics and Human Physiology, School of Medicine Instituto Universitario Italiano de Rosario, Rosario, Santa Fe, Argentina
Los Manantiales, Neurosciences Center, Grupo Gamma Rosario, Rosario, Santa Fe, Argentina

Germán Perez
Faculty of Biochemical and Pharmaceutical Sciences, Nacional University of Rosario, Rosario, Santa Fe, Argentina
Gammalab, Grupo Gamma Rosario, Rosario, Santa Fe, Argentina

Norberto Antongiovanni
Center for Infusion and Study of Lysosomal Diseases, Instituto de Nefrología de Pergamino, Pergamino, Buenos Aires, Argentina

Fernando Perretta
Intensive Care Unit, Hospital Dr. Enrique Erill, Belén de Escobar, Buenos Aires, Argentina

Graciela Venera
Research Department, Instituto Universitario Italiano de Rosario, Rosario, Santa Fe, Argentina

Hasan Ahmad Hasan Albitar
Department of Internal Medicine, Mayo Clinic, Rochester, Minnesota, USA

Narjust Duma and Konstantinos Leventakos
Division of Medical Oncology, Mayo Clinic, Rochester, Minnesota, USA

Alice Gallo De Moraes
Division of Pulmonary and Critical Care, Mayo Clinic, Rochester, Minnesota, USA

Arsene T. Signing, Wiliane J. T. Marbou and Victor Kuete
Department of Biochemistry, University of Dschang, Dschang, Cameroon

Veronique P. Beng
Department of Biochemistry, University of Yaoundé 1, Cameroun, Yaoundé, Cameroon

Rasheed Ofosu-Poku and Michael Owusu-Ansah
Directorate of Family Medicine, Komfo Anokye Teaching Hospital, Kumasi, Ghana

John Antwi
Directorate of Internal Medicine, Komfo Anokye Teaching Hospital, Kumasi, Ghana

Emerson Joachin-Sánchez, Aranza Joffre-Torres, Bertha M. Córdova-Sánchez, Guadalupe Ferrer-Burgos and Angel Herrera-Gomez
Department of Critical Care Medicine, Instituto Nacional de Cancerología, Mexico City, Mexico

Octavio González-Chon
Department of Critical Care Medicine, Medica Sur Clinic & Foundation, Mexico City, Mexico

Silvio A. Ñamendys-Silva
Department of Critical Care Medicine, Instituto Nacional de Cancerología, Mexico City, Mexico
Department of Critical Care Medicine, Medica Sur Clinic & Foundation, Mexico City, Mexico
Department of Critical Care Medicine, Instituto Nacional de Ciencias Médicas y Nutrición Salvador Zubirán, Mexico City, Mexico

Mohd Jokha Yahya, Norshariza binti Nordin, Abdah binti Md Akim and Maryam Jamielah Yusoff
Department of Biomedical Sciences, Faculty of Medicine and Health Sciences, Universiti Putra Malaysia, Malaysia

Patimah binti Ismail
Department of Human Development and Growth, Faculty of Medicine and Health Sciences, Universiti Putra Malaysia, Malaysia

Wan Shaariah binti Md. Yusuf and Noor Lita binti Adam
Department of Medicine (Endocrinology & Nephrology), Hospital Tuanku Ja'afar, Malaysia

Gabriel S. Pena, Hector G. Paez, Trevor K. Johnson, Jessica L. Halle, Joseph P. Carzoli, Nishant P. Visavadiya, Michael C. Zourdos, Michael A. Whitehurst and Andy V. Khamoui
Department of Exercise Science and Health Promotion, Florida Atlantic University, Boca Raton, Florida 33431, USA

Donny Ard
Department of Surgery, Holy Cross Hospital, Silver Spring, MD 20910, USA

Naa-Solo Tettey
Department of Public Health, William Paterson University, Wayne 07470, USA

Shinga Feresu
Department of Public Health, University of Johannesburg, Auckland Park 2006, South Africa

Nafiu Amidu, Lawrence Quaye, Peter Paul Mwinsanga Dapare and Yussif Adams
Department of Biomedical Laboratory Science, University for Development Studies, Tamale, Ghana

William Kwame Boakye Ansah Owiredu
Department of Molecular Medicine, Kwame Nkrumah University of Science and Technology, Kumasi, Ghana

Alison Rouncefield-Swales, Bernie Carter, Lucy Bray and Lucy Blake
Faculty of Health, Social Care & Medicine, Edge Hill University, Ormskirk, UK

Stephen Allen
Liverpool School of Tropical Medicine, Liverpool, UK

Chris Probert
Institute of Translational Medicine, University of Liverpool, Liverpool, UK

Kay Crook
St. Mark's & Northwick Park, London North West University Healthcare NHS Trust, London, UK

Pamela Qualter
Manchester Institute of Education, University of Manchester, Manchester, UK

Richard S. Henry, Paul B. Perrin, Ashlee Sawyer and Mickeal Pugh Jr.
Department of Psychology, Virginia Commonwealth University, Richmond, Virginia, USA

Belachew Kebede
Public Health, John Snow Inc., Ethiopia

Gistane Ayele and Desta Haftu
School of Public Health, Arba Minch University, Ethiopia

Gebrekiros Gebremichael
School of Public Health, Mekelle University, Ethiopia

Carlos M. Galmarini
Topazium Artificial Intelligence, Paseo de la Castellana 40, 28046 Madrid, Spain

Kennedy Dodam Konlan
Department of Social & Behavioural Sciences, School of Public Health, University of Ghana, Legon, Accra, Ghana

Charles Junior Afam-Adjei and Jeremiah Bella-Fiamawle
Department of Medicine, Nursing Directorate, Korle-Bu Teaching Hospital, Accra, Ghana

Christian Afam-Adjei and Jennifer Oware
Department of Nursing, St. Karol School of Nursing, Aplaku-Accra, Ghana

Theresa Akua Appiah
School of Business, Ghana Institute of Management & Public Administration (GIMPA), Accra, Ghana

Kennedy Diema Konlan
Department of Public Health Nursing, School of Nursing and Midwifery, University of Allied Health Sciences, Ho, Ghana

Andargachew Kassa
College of Medicine and Health Sciences, School of Nursing and Midwifery, Hawassa University, Ethiopia

George Owusu
Department of Pharmacology, Faculty of Pharmacy and Pharmaceutical Sciences, College of Health Sciences, Kwame Nkrumah University of Science and Technology (KNUST), Kumasi, Ghana
Department of Pharmacology, School of Medicine and Health Sciences, University for Development Studies, Tamale, Ghana

David D. Obiri, George K. Ainooson, Newman Osafo, Aaron O. Antwi and Charles Ansah
Department of Pharmacology, Faculty of Pharmacy and Pharmaceutical Sciences, College of Health Sciences, Kwame Nkrumah University of Science and Technology (KNUST), Kumasi, Ghana

Babatunde M. Duduyemi
Department of Pathology, School of Medical Sciences, Kwame Nkrumah University of Science and Technology (KNUST), Kumasi, Ghana

Daniel Gululi, Jianping Li and Haohuan Li
Department of Orthopaedics, Renmin Hospital of Wuhan University, Wuhan, 430060 Hubei, China

Guy-Armel Bounda
Department of Clinical Pharmacy, School of Basic Medicine and Clinical Pharmacy, China Pharmaceutical University, 24# Tong Jia Xiang, Nanjing, 210009 Jiangsu, China
Sinomedica Co., Ltd., 677# Nathan Road, Mong Kok, Kowloon, Hong Kong
Gabonese Scientific Research Consortium B.P. 5707, Libreville, Gabon

X. Vandemergel
Department of Endocrinology and Diabetology, EpiCURA, Belgium

Endrias Markos Woldesemayat
College of Medicine and Health Sciences, School of Public and Environmental Health, Hawassa University, Ethiopia

Index

Printed in the USA
CPSIA information can be obtained
at www.ICGtesting.com
JSHW051624061123
51533JS00005B/95